Intestinal Toxicology
Target Organ Toxicology Series

Target Organ Toxicology Series

Editor-in-Chief: Robert L. Dixon

National Institute of Environmental Health Sciences
Research Triangle Park, North Carolina

Target Organ Toxicology Series

Intestinal Toxicology

Editor

Carol M. Schiller, Ph.D., J.D.
Senior Scientist
Laboratory of Pharmacology
National Institute of Environmental Health Sciences
National Institutes of Health
Research Triangle Park, North Carolina

Raven Press ■ New York

Raven Press, 1140 Avenue of the Americas, New York, New York 10036

Made in the United States of America

Library of Congress Cataloging in Publication Data
Main entry under title:

Intestinal toxicology.

(Target organ toxicology series)
Includes bibliographies and index.
1. Intestines—Diseases. 2. Toxicology. 3. Environmentally induced diseases. I.Schiller, Carol M.
II. Series. [DNLM: 1. Intestinal Absorption—drug effects.
2. Intestinal Diseases—chemically induced. 3. Intestines
—drug effects. WI 400 I605]
RC860.I58   1984   616.3′4   84-6959
ISBN 0-89004-841-X

Preface

> *"There was once a town where all life seemed to live in harmony with its surroundings . . .*
> *Then a strange blight crept over the area . . .*
> *Mysterious maladies swept the flocks of chickens; the cattle and sheep sickened and died.*
> *Everywhere was the shadow of death. The farmers spoke of much illness in their families.*
> *In the town, the doctors had become more and more puzzled by new kinds of sickness . . .*
> *In the gutters under the eaves and between the shingles of the roofs, a white granular powder still showed a few patches; some weeks before, it had fallen like snow upon the roofs and the lawns, the fields and streams . . .*
> *This town does not actually exist . . . I know of no community that has experienced all the misfortunes I describe . . ."*

When author Rachel Carson described these events in her book *Silent Spring* in 1962, the story was a myth, a legend. Her critics were quick to seize on this point. Her foresight was rejected by her tunnel-visioned contemporaries. Since World War II, when the widespread use of DDT and other organic insecticides began, there has been a dramatic surge in the development of synthetic organic chemicals. Presently, there are an estimated two million recognized chemical compounds. Chemical sales are now $100 billion per year, with over 30,000 chemical substances in commerical use. To this number, a thousand new ones may be introduced each year.

Even though chemicals play an important role in protecting, prolonging, and enhancing our lives, in the past few years, many have been found to present significant health and environmental dangers. More often than not, these chemicals leak out slowly and insidiously. In some instances, the chemical insult is sudden, direct, concentrated, and awesome. These events symbolize the complex problems inherent in regulating chemical production and usage without compromising the quality of the environment and the health of workers and residents. While current regulatory agencies are examining production and utilization of chemicals, various other institutions in both the private and government sectors are concerned with the evaluation of the health effects of many of these chemicals.

This volume reviews the methods used in the assessment of chemically induced toxicity and focuses on intestinal function and toxicology. This volume represents a scientific landmark since it is an indication of the increasing awareness of the wide variety of chemicals and the level of insult that the intestinal tract is being exposed to, and of the possible intestinal damage that these exposures might cause. The intestinal wall serves both as a barrier to ingested environmental substances and, also, as a modifier of specific compounds. Alterations to these natural defense mechanisms may, in turn, allow for additional harm to other organ systems because of changes in the absorption of natural and foreign substances.

A better understanding of the basic principles of normal intestinal functions should permit greater appreciation for the unique roles of this organ in absorption and metabolism. In addition, this understanding of normal function may lead to better methods for the detection of dysfunction and malabsorption. The possible interactions of ingested substances, both in natural and metabolized forms, are rapidly increasing as are the nature and degree of intentional and unintentional contamination of ingested substances.

The purpose of this volume is to emphasize the importance of the intestines as a target organ and to provide a forum for the exchange of information among basic scientists, toxicologists, and clinicians.

It is hoped that the review of the basic sciences and the methodologies concerning the intestines and the review of the status of intestinal toxicological research will provide the groundwork for future studies in this area of target orgran toxicology. The current volume presents a reexamination of the progress within this growing research area and an elaboration of many important aspects of this new area of toxicology.

Carol M. Schiller

Acknowledgments

The National Institute of Environmental Health Sciences and the Society of Toxicology co-sponsored the symposium on which this book is based. We are indebted to them and to the community of academic, biomedical, and federal scientists for their respective contributions to the initial symposium and to the final monograph.

Foreword

The *Target Organ Toxicology* monographs have evolved from the need for periodic review of the methods used to assess chemically induced toxicity. In each monograph, experts focus on the following areas of a particular organ system: (a) review of the morphology, physiology, biochemistry, cellular biology, and developmental aspects of the system; (b) a description of the means routinely used to assess toxicity; (c) an evaluation of the feasibility of tests used in the assessment of hazards; (d) proposals for applying recent advances in the basic sciences to the development and validation of new test procedures; (e) a description of the incidence of chemically induced human disease; and (f) an assessment of the reliability of laboratory test data extrapolation to humans and of the methods currently used to estimate human risk.

Thus, these monographs should be useful to both students and professionals of toxicology. Each provides a concise description of organ toxicity, including an up-to-date review of the biological processes represented by the target organ, a summary of how chemicals perturb these processes and alter function, and a description of methods by which such toxicity is detected in laboratory animals and humans. Attention is also directed to the identification of probable toxic chemicals and to the establishment of exposure standards that are both economically and scientifically feasible, while adequately protecting human health and the environment.

Robert L. Dixon, Editor-in-Chief

Contents

Contributors

John G. Banwell, M.D.
Division of Gastroenterology
Department of Medicine
Case Western Reserve University
Cleveland, Ohio 44106

Dennis E. Chapman, B.Sc.
Laboratory of Pharmacology
National Institute of Environmental
   Health Sciences
Research Triangle Park,
   North Carolina 27709

**Rajendra S. Chhabra, Ph.D.,
D.V.M.**
Toxicology Research and Testing Program
National Institute of Environmental
   Health Sciences
Research Triangle Park,
   North Carolina 27709

William C. Eastin, Jr., Ph.D.
Toxicology Research and Testing Program
National Institute of Environmental
   Health Sciences
Research Triangle Park,
   North Carolina 27709

William D. Heizer, M.D.
Department of Medicine
School of Medicine
University of North Carolina
Chapel Hill, North Carolina 27514

Susan J. Henning, Ph.D.
Department of Biology
University of Houston
Houston, Texas 77004

Harald P. Hoensch, M.D.
Medizinische Universitatsklinik
Abteilung Allgemeine Invere Medizin
Hufelandstrabe 55
D 4300 Essen 1, Federal Republic of
   Germany

W. C. Hülsmann, Ph.D.
Department of Biochemistry I
Erasmus University Rotterdam
Postbus 1738
3000 DR Rotterdam, The Netherlands

D. D. Joel, Ph.D.
Medical Research Center
Brookhaven National Laboratory
Upton, New York 11973

George A. Kimmich, Ph.D.
Department of Radiation Biology and
   Biophysics
University of Rochester Medical Center
400 Elmwood Avenue
Rochester, New York 14642

A. Kuksis, Ph.D.
Banting and Best Department of Medical
   Research
University of Toronto
112 College Street
Toronto, Ontario M5G 1L6, Canada

James G. Lecce, Ph.D.
Department of Animal Science
North Carolina State University
P.O. Box 5127
Raleigh, North Carolina 27650

M. E. LeFevre, Ph.D.
Medical Research Center
Brookhaven National Laboratory
Upton, New York 11973

Harold P. Schedl, M.D., Ph.D.
Department of Internal Medicine
The University of Iowa
College of Medicine
Iowa City, Iowa 52242

Carol M. Schiller, Ph.D., J.D.
Laboratory of Pharmacology
National Institute of Enviromental Health
  Sciences
Research Triangle Park,
  North Carolina 27709

Michael Schwenk, Ph.D.
Institut für Toxikologie
Universität Tübingen
Wilhemstrabe 56
D-7400 Tübingen,
  Federal Republic of Germany

Chon R. Shoaf, Ph.D.
Laboratory of Pharmacology
National Institute of Environmental
  Health Sciences
Research Triangle Park,
  North Carolina 27709

Ramsey Walden, B.Sc.
Laboratory of Pharmacology
National Institute of Environmental
  Health Sciences
Research Triangle Park,
  North Carolina 27709

Carol T. Walsh, Ph.D.
Department of Pharmacology and
  Experimental Therapeutics
Boston University Medical Center
80 East Concord Street
Boston, Massachusetts 02118

Intestinal Toxicology

Intestinal Toxicology, edited by C. M. Schiller.
Raven Press, New York © 1984.

Introduction: Intestines as a Barrier and as an Absorptive and Metabolic Organ

Carol M. Schiller and Ramsey Walden

Laboratory of Pharmacology, National Institute of Environmental Health Sciences, National Institutes of Health, Research Triangle Park, North Carolina 27709

This volume on intestinal toxicology is concerned with the critical appraisal of experimental methods and data obtained from research past and present and attempts to define those regions of research that should prove to be productive for our future efforts. Within these two broad objectives, the volume focuses on a number of specific areas of intestinal research. These areas of research reflect the increasing awareness and documentation of the multiple roles of the intestines, including the well-recognized and major roles of nutrient absorption and of penetrant barrier. In addition, emphasis is given to the expanding body of knowledge that relates to the intestines as a major metabolic organ involved in the synthesis and degradation of both natural and foreign substances. A further dimension is the inclusion of several discussions aimed directly at the function and dysfunction of the human absorptive processes and the possible effects of environmental toxins on these processes.

The gastrointestinal tract is assumed to be an impenetrable barrier to the uptake of intraluminal substances. Increasing experimental evidence, however, suggests that the mucosal barrier to foreign substances may be incomplete. Some macromolecules are absorbed to a degree and, although not in sufficient amounts to be of nutritional significance, may have an antigenic role or be biologically active within the organism. The development of the gastrointestinal tract during the perinatal and neonatal periods to the level of that of the adult involves a unique continuum of morphological and biochemical maturations. It is this maturation process that culminates in the highly complex organ with its many and complex functions.

A wide range of approaches and methodologies have been employed to evaluate the maturation and functions of the gastrointestinal tract. Because of its unusual morphology, the intestines can be examined *in vivo* and *in vitro* by a variety of techniques, each providing different kinds of relevant information and understanding. Utilization of sacs, loops, rings, and cells have provided ample data to reveal the importance of the gastrointestinal tract as a barrier and absorptive organ and also as a highly active major metabolic tissue. Examination of the development of

1

intestinal enzymes and metabolic pathways reveals an understanding of nutrient active transport and metabolism as well as metabolism of foreign substances. The relatively large mass of this organ provides additional significance to its metabolic roles in the homeostasis of the organism as a whole.

Since ingestion is a major route of exposure to foreign substances, significant research involving the absorption and metabolism of these substances is needed. In addition, the effects of the foreign substances on the normal intestinal functions is an area of research requiring further attention. Currently, more Americans are affected by serious diseases of the gastrointestinal tract than any other system except the cardiovascular system, which provides emphasis for the increasing concern for understanding the possible environmental elements to gastrointestinal disease.

Intestinal Toxicology, edited by C. M. Schiller.
Raven Press, New York © 1984.

Methods for the Analysis of Intestinal Function

Carol T. Walsh

Department of Pharmacology and Experimental Therapeutics, Boston University Medical Center, Boston, Massachusetts 02118

The intestinal tract is an organ of considerable complexity, comprised of numerous tissue types and subserving multiple functions. Analysis of the physiology of this system has therefore involved, and continues to require, the application of research tools from many disciplines within the sciences (63,64). The following chapter analyzes the primary function of the intestinal tract, namely the processing of orally ingested substances. Major emphasis is on determining intestinal structural integrity, absorptive function, and contractile properties responsible for transit of luminal contents.

ASSESSING THE STRUCTURAL INTEGRITY OF THE INTESTINAL TRACT

Examination of intestinal tissue by histologic techniques is useful for the detection of generalized structural alterations (58). Altered organ function may be induced, however, without changes in the microanatomy of the tissue. Lesions may be highly localized and consequently they are missed by selective sampling techniques. A noninvasive approach for monitoring the structural integrity of the mucosal lining of the intestinal tract is based on estimating gastrointestinal bleeding. The procedure entails determining occult blood in the feces by colorimetric or radioisotopic methods. The detection of fecal occult blood, an important clinical diagnostic tool (68), has application to the screening of substances for potential toxic effects on the gut and to the testing of agents with suspected or probable ulcerogenic properties such as nonsteroidal anti-inflammatory agents (44), certain food additives (38), and radiation exposure (40).

A number of procedures are available for assaying fecal occult blood. Colorimetric techniques (1,13,27,30,45) are based on the use of phenolic compounds, such as guaiac or *o*-tolidine, whose oxidation to color-emitting substances by hydrogen peroxide is catalyzed by hemoglobin. These reagents differ in their sensitivity and in their potential toxicity. Certain of these reagents are commercially available in convenient formulation for clinical use, e.g., Hemoccult, in which a slide is impregnated with guaiac. Numerous factors affect this colorimetric assay

(27). A primary variable is the peroxidase activity in the feces that originates from the diet rather than from gastrointestinal bleeding. In addition to interference from dietary factors, the results of this type of assay depend on the extent to which hemoglobin loses peroxidase activity by its metabolism in the gut lumen during transit from the site of bleeding (54). Since bleeding may be intermittent, the results will depend on the fecal sampling technique. Because of these problems, this technique is usually applied semiquantitatively.

A second approach for assessing gastrointestinal bleeding is based on quantitating radioactivity in the feces following labeling of erythrocytes with ^{59}Fe or ^{51}Cr. This procedure, which requires greater experimental intrusion than colorimetric methods, entails intravenous administration of ferrous 59-sulfate for *in vivo* labeling of erythrocytes (32,44) or of erythrocytes prelabeled with ^{51}Cr *in vitro* (39). These techniques, based on the use of radioisotopes, require the experimenter to exercise considerably greater attention to the proper housing of animals, handling of excreta, disposal of carcasses, and to other problems related to contamination and exposure. However, such approaches are more sensitive than colorimetric methods and are not subject to invalid results caused by interference from dietary sources. In addition, metabolism of hemoglobin during its transit through the gut lumen has less of an effect on a radioisotopic assay than on a colorimetric one.

Macroscopic injury to the gastrointestinal wall may also be detected by sacrificing the animal and inspecting the mucosa for lesions (50) or the serosa for perforations or adhesions (6). This technique can be made more sensitive by pretreating test animals with a nonerythrocytic vascular marker followed by its visualization on the mucosal surface or its quantitation in the gut lumen. Examples of such markers include the dye pontamine sky blue 6 BX (7) and ^{51}Cr-labeled albumin.

ANALYZING THE PROLIFERATION OF INTESTINAL MUCOSAL CELLS

A potential effect of toxic substances on the intestine is alteration of the proliferative process that occurs in the intestinal crypts. This effect may be a primary event as occurs with antineoplastic agents that impair cell division. Or, the effect may be a secondary one that occurs in response to changes in one of the many factors regulating intestinal renewal such as hormones, microorganisms, and food intake (37). Alterations in crypt cell division and migration up the villous surface may in some cases be inferred from histologic evaluation of morphology of crypt and villous cells and villous height. More definitive assessment is based on techniques of cell kinetic analysis (8). These procedures are based on pulse exposure of cells to tritiated thymidine, which is incorporated into DNA of crypt cells undergoing DNA replication. Tissue is collected at various times after thymidine exposure and thin sections processed using autoradiography. From these samples it is possible to determine the time for complete migration of newly formed cells from the crypt to the site of extrusion on the villous tip. In addition, by evaluating the fraction of mitoses in the crypt, which are labeled with ^{3}H-thymidine as a function of time, one can estimate the characteristics of the cell cycle, including the duration of the various phases as well as the complete cell cycle time.

As new cells are formed in the intestinal crypts and subsequently migrate up the villus, they differentiate from proliferative, secretory cells into absorptive ones. There are numerous structural and functional indicators of this differentiation process. Several enzymes, whose activities differ markedly in crypt cells and fully differentiated villous cells, have been used as markers to assess the differentiation process. These tools also have application in verifying procedures for separating crypt and villous cells. Examples include thymidine kinase, whose activity is highest in proliferating crypt cells where DNA synthesis is occurring (26), and the oligosaccharidases such as lactase and maltase, whose activities are highest in differentiated villous cells (11). The activities of these enzymes are dependent not only on their rate of formation but also on their rate of degradation. Recent studies have demonstrated, for example, that sucrase activity can be altered by conditions that affect its degradation rate (20). This factor must be taken into account when interpreting studies where activity of a mucosal enzyme is altered.

DETERMINATION OF INTESTINAL ABSORPTION

Study of the absorptive function of the intestinal tract can be carried out with numerous methods. Among the primary considerations in choosing an experimental technique to assess an aspect of the absorption process are the following:

1. The test species to be used, i.e., must the study be conducted in humans with all the accompanying complications or is there an appropriate experimental animal model?
2. The aspect of the absorption process of interest, e.g., is it the overall absorption from the gut lumen to the systemic circulation and tissues, or is it the process of transport across the brush border or basolateral membrane of the intestinal mucosal cell?
3. Which experimental or physiological variables should be controlled, e.g., the presence of anesthetic agents, the electrochemical potential difference across the gut wall, or the pH of the luminal gut contents?

The answers to these questions will determine the particular method that may be chosen from among the *in vivo* and *in vitro* methods available for studying absorptive function (33,41). These methods can be categorized according to (a) the method by which the test substance is administered and (b) the method for assessing the extent and/or rate of absorption.

Methods of Administering Test Substance

Among the various techniques for administering the test substance in an *in vivo* study are the following:

1. Incorporating the test substance into the diet, which is then administered to the subject. This procedure may be specially relevant to the analysis of the absorption of toxic substances that are contaminants of the diet (61).

2. Intubating the test substance into the stomach, a procedure that allows more precise control of the total dose administered. (With both these methods the rate and possibly the extent of absorption of the test substance may be markedly affected by the gastric emptying pattern of the subject.)

3. Directly administering the test substance into the intestinal lumen, which eliminates the influence of gastric emptying. In human studies, substances can be administered through small-bore intubating tubes localized to particular sites by radiographic techniques (16). In animal experimentation, test substances may be perfused through the gut lumen as a single pass, analogous to the perfusion method in man, or recirculated in the perfusate. Such a technique, illustrated in Fig. 1, requires cannulation of the intestine, an external heating device for maintaining the perfusate at body temperature, and a pump for maintaining constant flow (3). An advantage of perfusion procedures, over techniques described below, is that the influence of flow rate on absorption kinetics can be directly determined. Analyses

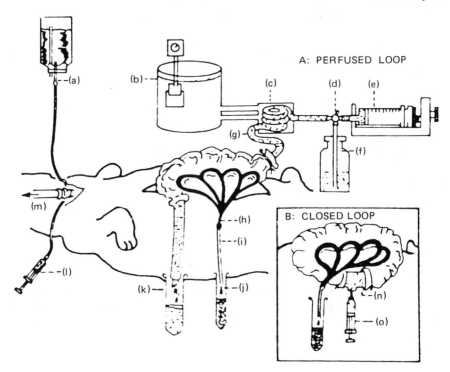

FIG. 1. *In vivo* apparatus for perfusion of the small intestine of the rabbit with complete venous collection. Note the constant temperature water bath (b), the perfusion pump (e), and the infusion of blood (a) to permit complete venous collection (i). Reprinted from W. H. Barr and S. Riegelman (3), with permission.

have indicated that for many substances, such as long-chain fatty acids, bile acids, and cholesterol (56), diffusion through an unstirred water layer overlying the mucosal surface is a rate-limiting step in the overall absorption process (69).

Another method of direct administration in experimental animals consists of placing a test substance into a segment of the intestine that is closed by ligatures both proximally and distally (33,35). The construction of the closed segment and the injection of the test dose do require the use of anesthetic agents. However, the animal, typically small animals such as rats, can be allowed to recover from anesthesia and to become ambulatory for the majority of the absorption period. This procedure has the additional advantage of not requiring perfusion pumps or heating devices.

Substances may also be administered directly into the intestinal lumen following surgical creation of exteriorized fistulas (41). Studies are then carried out in unanesthetized larger animals, typically dogs. This approach, of historical importance, has the disadvantage of requiring considerable surgical manipulation.

Methods for Quantitating Degree of Absorption

Appearance in Systemic Fluids

In addition to the method of administering the test substance, the second critical aspect of a technique is the sampling procedure for quantitating the extent and/or rate of absorption. With *in vivo* methods the least invasive techniques entail the collection of blood, urine, or breath samples for determining the appearance of the absorbed test substance (and its metabolites) in body fluids. Comparing the time course of plasma concentrations or excretory rates in urine or breath after oral administration with results after intravenous administration may permit quantitation of the extent of absorption of the test substance and the rate constant of this process (62). This approach is relatively imprecise and may be confounded by numerous factors such as the "first pass" effect (17), the enterohepatic circulation of the agent, and the status of elimination processes such as hepatic and renal function. Nevertheless, this technique is useful in the diagnosis of malabsorption syndromes associated with gastrointestinal diseases (19). For example, one test of the transport capacity of the small intestine for carbohydrates entails oral administration of the pentose sugar D-xylose followed by its determination in plasma or in urine. Similarly, assessment of intestinal lactase, the disaccharide that cleaves lactose into the absorbable sugars glucose and galactose, involves an oral lactose load followed by determination of blood sugars. A test of fat absorption can include determination of serum carotene. One test of ileal absorptive function entails the oral administration of radiolabeled vitamin B_{12} with determination of its urinary recovery.

Currently receiving clinical attention as an approach for analyzing intestinal function is the sampling of excretory products in breath (21,48). This technique entails analyzing breath for hydrogen, which is generated by the body exclusively by the action of intestinal bacteria on unabsorbed carbohydrates, or for carbon dioxide, which is derived from metabolism of an orally administered isotopically labeled test substance. These tests, which can provide an indication of the rate and extent of absorption of a test substance, can be used to detect biliary, pancreatic, and mucosal cell malfunction as well as bacterial overgrowth in the small intestine (Table 1). For example, the bile salt glycocholic acid is normally absorbed intact from the ileum and reexcreted in the bile. However, in patients with impaired ileal function or with bacterial overgrowth in the small intestine there is increased bacterial deconjugation of glycocholic acid with release of glycine. Glycine is then metabolized to CO_2, primarily by bacterial enzymes. Consequently, the administration of glycocholic acid, labeled in the glycine moiety with ^{14}C, results in an increased excretion of [14]CO_2 in patients with ileal disease or bacterial overgrowth. Generally, clinical validation of CO_2 breath tests has been carried out using ^{14}C radioisotopes. However, use of the stable ^{13}C analogs with quantitation of [13]CO_2 by mass spectroscopy has also been used (52,65), an approach that may be of special importance for diagnosing malabsorption in children (2) and in women of childbearing age.

The technique of administering an oral load and of sampling body fluids not only has clinical diagnostic importance but is a useful approach for determining the overall rate and extent of absorption of environmental contaminants. Such determinations may be important in the theoretical prediction of systemic concentrations of toxic substances following various ingestion rates. Analyses of this sort, referred to by the recently coined term "toxicokinetics," apply mathematical tools extensively used to describe the disposition of pharmacologic agents (42).

A more direct approach for analyzing absorption characteristics than the sampling of systemic or excreted body fluids entails the sampling of portal blood (43) or the collection of the mesenteric blood draining the sites of absorption of the test substance (3) as shown in Fig. 1. Such a procedure requires considerably more complicated surgical techniques than that of sampling systemic blood, urine, or breath. Furthermore, transfusions of blood into the animal may be required. An important advantage of this procedure is the capacity to determine *in vivo* the kinetics of metabolism of a test substance by intestinal tissues. In certain studies, the appearance of the test substance in lymph may be critical, as in the absorption

TABLE 1. *Breath tests in diagnosing gastrointestinal function*

Function	Test dose	Analysis
Lactase activity	^{14}C-Lactose	Exhaled [14]CO_2
Lactase activity	Lactose	Exhaled H_2
Fat absorption	Triglyceride, e.g., glyceryl esters of ^{13}C or ^{14}C triolein	Exhaled [13]CO_2 or [14]CO_2
Fat absorption: Pancreatic lipase activity	^{14}C-triglyceride, ^{14}C free fatty acid	Ratio of exhaled [14]CO_2 from the two sources
Bacterial activity	^{14}C-Xylose	Exhaled [14]CO_2
Bacterial activity	Cholylglycine [14]C	Exhaled [14]CO_2

of fats: Cannulation of the mesenteric lymphatic vessel may be carried out even in a small animal such as the rat (12).

Disappearance from Intestine

Another approach to quantitating absorption entails monitoring the disappearance of a test substance from the intestine after its administration into the lumen. The perfusion method, for example, monitors differences in the amount infused from the amount appearing at a site distal to the area of infusion. Such perfusion techniques have been exceedingly useful in determining the transport of electrolytes and nutrients in man. The determination of the amount unabsorbed in the sample taken at a distal site is made possible by the use of a marker substance that is neither metabolized nor absorbed, commonly polyethylene glycol 4000 (28). This particular marker has the advantages of lack of adsorption to the gut, high water solubility, stability during frozen storage, and ease of determination by radioisotopic or spectrophotometric methods (51). However, one drawback to techniques in which only the luminal contents are sampled is that retention of the test substances in the intestinal mucosa is not quantitated.

In the closed segment procedure, referred to above, the extent of absorption is calculated on the basis of disappearance of the test substance from both the lumen and the intestinal tissue. With this method, at the end of the absorption period the entire segment, both intestinal wall and contents, is assayed quantitatively for the amount of the test substance remaining. A disadvantage to this technique when compared with perfusion methods is that sequential samples cannot be taken from a single animal. However, this method is readily used in small animals and can therefore be relatively economical.

In both the perfusion and the closed segment procedures, equating loss of a test substance with its absorption requires verification that disappearance does not result as a consequence of metabolism in the intestine. If metabolism of the substance does occur, then assay of the intestine alone is inadequate for a description of its absorption kinetics, unless the metabolite is poorly absorbed and can be completely recovered in the intestinal samples.

In Vitro Methods

Numerous advances in the understanding of cellular mechanisms of electrolyte flux and nutrient absorption in the intestine have been made using *in vitro*, as opposed to *in vivo*, techniques. With *in vitro* procedures, physiological variables such as intestinal motility and mesenteric blood flow can be eliminated or controlled. In addition, the experimenter has the option of control over factors such as the composition of the solutions bathing both the mucosal and the systemic side of the intestine and the electrochemical potential difference between the mucosal and serosal sides. *In vitro* techniques include those analogous to *in vivo* methods already discussed. Investigators, for example, have studied the absorption of substances from isolated gut sections with perfusions of the lumen or with perfusions of the vasculature (24).

One *in vitro* method, with no *in vivo* analog, is the everted sac technique (67). This method has been useful in characterizing the energy-dependent, carrier-mediated transport processes. In this procedure, small lengths of the intestine are everted, filled with fluid, and tied at both ends. Absorption is quantitated by monitoring the appearance of a test substance inside the sac in the fluid bathing the serosal surface of the intestine. Therefore, unlike the *in vivo* condition, absorption of a test substance is considered equivalent in this model to its passage not only through the mucosa but also through the submucosa, the external muscle layers, and serosal tissue of the gut wall. Modifications have included cannulation permitting sequential sampling of the serosal fluid and control of the serosal fluid volume (10).

Problems with the everted segment technique include inadequate oxygen diffusion into the tissue and distension and hydration of the gut segment. Consequently, the preparation of the tissue and the experimental incubations must be short in duration. Everted sacs of the duodenum from rats exhibit structural abnormalities after 5-min incubation at 37°C (34). After 1 hr, marked distention of the villus as well as complete loss of the villous architecture occurs. These dramatic structural changes are associated, not surprisingly, with changes in transport kinetics. For example, with this preparation the absorption of large polar molecules such as riboflavin, normally incompletely absorbed from the gut, begins to increase significantly within 30 min (18). One approach to improve tissue viability has been the use of intestinal segments from which the longitudinal and circular muscle layers and serosa have been stripped (70).

Other *in vitro* procedures include rings cut from the whole wall of the intestine (9). This approach is designed to improve oxygenation of the tissue but only permits measurement of the accumulation of test substances by all cell types of the intestinal wall. Several other methods have been developed for quantitating uptake of substances specifically by gut mucosal cells. Methods for recovering mucosal cells such as scraping the inner surface of the gut with a glass slide (14) or vibrating a gut segment everted on a glass spiral (36) have been improved upon to reduce contamination from cells of the lamina propria (57). In addition, isolation of the mucosal brush border membrane recovered as vesicles following differential centrifugation (25,29) has been important to analysis of carbohydrate digestion and absorption (25,29). Baso-lateral membranes of mucosal cells have also been isolated by use of differential and discontinuous sucrose-gradient centrifugation (15).

An additional *in vitro* preparation has been of major significance in the elucidation of mechanisms controlling electrolyte absorption and secretion (46). This procedure, using the Ussing chamber (60), entails *in vitro* short-term exposure of a segment of intestine to defined mucosal and serosal solutions (47). The electrical potential difference across the intestine is measured with a voltmeter and short-circuit current with an external microamp source. Flux of electrolytes is determined by the addition of an isotope to the solution, bathing one surface of the intestinal segment and monitoring its accumulation in the tissue or solution bathing the other surface. More recently, studies have been carried out using microelectrode impalement of individual cells of the intestinal wall to differentiate the active chloride-secreting activity of crypt and villous cells (66). Presumably, this procedure could also be applied to distinguish cellular sites of action of toxic substances.

An *in vitro* preparation with the advantage of more prolonged viability is the organ culture of mucosal biopsies. This technique permits the *in vitro* maintenance of mucosal explants for 24 to 48 hr, depending on the species and region of the intestine biopsied (58). A major advantage of this approach is that the normal anatomical arrangement of the mucosal cells is maintained, and the processes of mucosal cell proliferation and differentiation can be studied. Successful applications of this technique have included analysis of hormonal control of mucosal metabolism, proliferation, and development and analysis of the biochemical basis of diseases such as celiac sprue.

ASSESSMENT OF INTESTINAL MOTILITY

A second major function of the intestinal tract depends on its contractility. Intestinal motility is responsible for appropriate mixing of ingested materials with endogenous secretions required for digestion and for appropriate delivery of substances to the site of absorption or elimination.

One approach to the study of intestinal motility *in vivo* is the use of an intraluminal marker substance whose transit through the gut lumen can be quantitated. Substances used as valid markers should not be absorbed from the intestine, nor adsorbed onto the mucosal surface. In addition, ideal markers do not affect any aspect of intestinal function. Furthermore, since the contractile properties of the intestinal musculature may have different effects on solid as opposed to liquid components of the gut contents, markers should be chosen to correspond to the physical composition of the endogenous substance of greatest interest. This point is specially relevant to the study of gastric emptying (31). Markers used in the tracing of solid substances include, for example, [99m]Technitium incorporated into a chicken liver meal (31). Markers such as this gamma emitter can be readily monitored for stomach content in humans using a gamma camera. Other solid markers, used primarily in analysis of total gastrointestinal transit time in humans, include radiopaque pellets made from polythene impregnated with barium sulfate (5,23).

A technique developed by Summers et al. (55) permits investigation of intestinal transit in animals by administering markers into the duodenum. This procedure allows interpretation of effects on intestinal transit without any influence of gastric emptying. Permanent, indwelling catheters are surgically implanted in the duodenum of rats and exteriorized behind the head. Markers such as ^{51}Cr can be administered directly into the small intestine without the disruptive effect of anesthesia or of oral intubation procedures. In animal studies the content of markers in the intestine can be determined by analyzing sequential gut segments after the animals have been killed.

Other approaches to the *in vivo* analysis of the motor function of the gut (22) include determination of intraluminal pressure changes. These changes can be measured using small balloons or fluid-filled open-tipped tubes connected to external strain gauges, or internal miniaturized strain gauges monitored by telemetry or by means of exteriorized wires (49). Analysis of the function of the intestinal musculature may also entail measurement of its electrical activity, which in a chronic *in vivo* preparation can be carried out with a recording electrode surgically implanted on or in the intestinal wall or intubated into the intestinal lumen using a balloon to ensure its juxtaposition to the mucosal surface (4).

The contractile properties of intestinal smooth muscle can also be assessed using *in vitro* preparations of this organ. Such *in vitro* techniques are valuable in screening potentially toxic substances for effects on intestinal contractility and for elucidating mechanisms of effect on propulsion observed with *in vivo* methodology. Use of *in vitro* techniques to study intestinal motility has certain advantages over *in vivo* procedures. Generally, they are technically simpler to execute. They isolate the tissue from extrinsic neural and hormonal influences. The tissue can be directly exposed to the test substance. These advantages are at the expense of loss of prediction of *in vivo* effects of a test substance (46).

The choice of a particular *in vitro* technique depends on the specific aim of the experimentation. Those techniques that are most commonly used differ in several ways (53). First, the species from which the intestinal segment is taken markedly affect the basal contractile activity. The rabbit jejunum, for example, maintains rhythmic contractions *in vitro* and therefore is especially useful for analysis of substances suspected of having inhibitory effects on intestinal smooth muscle. The guinea pig ileum, in contrast, exhibits little spontaneous activity *in vitro*. This preparation is therefore widely used in the bioassay of agents causing contraction of intestinal smooth muscle. To test for depressant effects, the investigator must induce contraction of this tissue as with electrical stimulation. Second, there are differences in the responses of the smooth muscle, depending on the site within the intestine under investigation. This limits the investigator's ability to generalize from an experiment carried out with a muscle preparation from a single region of the intestine and reinforces the importance of strictly controlling the tissue region studied in a series of experiments.

CONCLUSION

In analyzing intestinal function and its perturbations, as in all experimental undertakings, it is critical that the investigator devote considerable attention to the choice of methodology. It is imperative that the limitations of the procedure be carefully considered, as well as factors such as technical difficulty, cost, reproducibility, and precision. In addition, successful experimental outcome from application of a chosen method necessitates appropriate use of the tools of experimental design and statistical analysis.

ACKNOWLEDGMENT

This chapter was prepared with support in part from the National Institute of Environmental Health Sciences grant ES 02665–01.

REFERENCES

1. Andrews, J. S., and Oliver-Gonzalez, J. (1942): The quantitative determination of blood in human feces. *J. Lab. Clin. Med.*, 27:1212–1217.
2. Barr, R. G., Perman, J. A., Schoeller, D. A., and Watkins, J. D. (1978): Breath tests in pediatric gastrointestinal disorders: new diagnostic opportunities. *Pediatrics*, 62(3):393–401.
3. Barr, W. H., and Riegelman, S. (1970): Intestinal drug absorption and metabolism. I. Comparison of methods and models to study physiologic factors of *in vitro* and *in vivo* intestinal absorption. *J. Pharm. Sci.*, 59:154–163.
4. Bass, P. (1968): *In vivo* electrical activity of the small bowel. In: *Handbook of Physiology, Sect. 6: Alimentary Canal, Vol. IV: Motility*, edited by C. F. Code. pp. 2051–2076. American Physiological Society, Washington, D.C.
5. Branch, W. J., and Cummings, J. H. (1978): Comparison of radio-opaque pellets and chromium sesquioxide as inert markers in studies requiring accurate faecal collections. *Gut*, 19(5):371–376.
6. Brodie, D. A., Cook, P. G., Bauer, B. J., and Dagle, G. E. (1970): Indomethacin-induced intestinal lesions in the rat. *Toxicol. Appl. Pharmacol.*, 17:615–624.
7. Brodie, D. A., Tage, C. L., and Hooke, K. F. (1970): Aspirin:Intestinal damage in rats. *Science*, 170:183–185.
8. Cairnie, A. B., Lamerton, L. F., and Steel, G. G. (1965): Cell proliferation studies in the intestinal epithelium of the rat. I. Determination of the kinetic parameters. *Exp. Cell Res.*, 39:528–538.
9. Crane, R. K., and Mandelstam, P. (1960): The active transport of sugars by various preparations of hamster intestine. *Biochim. Biophys. Acta*, 45:460–476.
10. Crane, R. K., and Wilson, T. H. (1958): *In vitro* method for the study of the rate of intestinal absorption of sugars. *J. Appl. Physiol.*, 12:145–146.
11. Dahlqvist, A., and Nordstrom, C. (1966): The distribution of disaccharidase activities in the villi and crypts of the small intestinal mucosa. *Biochim. Biophys. Acta*, 113:624–626.
12. DeMarco, T. J., and Levine, R. R. (1969): Role of the lymphatics in the intestinal absorption and distribution of drugs. *J. Pharmacol. Exp. Ther.*, 169:142–151.
13. Dent, N. J. (1973): Occult blood detection in feces of various animal species. *Lab. Pract.*, 22:674–676.
14. Dickens, F., and Weil-Malherbe, H. (1941): Metabolism of normal and tumor tissue. 19. The metabolism of intestinal mucous membrane. *Biochem. J.*, 35:7–15.
15. Douglas, A. P., Kerley, R., and Isselbacher, K. J. (1972): Preparation and characterization of the lateral and basal plasma membranes of the rat intestinal epithelial cell. *Biochem. J.*, 128:1329–1338.
16. Fordtran, J. S., Rector, F. C., Jr., Ewton, M. F., Soter, N., and Kinney, J. (1965): Permeability characteristics of the human small intestine. *J. Clin. Invest.*, 44:1935–1944.
17. Gibaldi, M., Boyes, R. N., and Feldman, S. (1971): Influence of first-pass effect on availability of drugs on oral administration. *J. Pharm. Sci.*, 60:1338–1340.
18. Gibaldi, M., and Grundhofer, B. (1972): Drug transport VI: Functional integrity of the rat everted small intestine with respect to passive transfer. *J. Pharm. Sci.*, 61:116–119.
19. Gray, G. (1978): Maldigestion and malabsorption—clinical manifestations and specific diagnosis. In: *Gastrointestinal Disease: Pathophysiology, Diagnosis, Management*, edited by M. H. Sleisenger and J. S. Fordtran, p. 272. W. B. Saunders, Philadelphia.
20. Gray, G. (1981): Carbohydrate absorption and malabsorption. In: *Physiology of the Gastrointestinal Tract*, edited by L. R. Johnson, pp. 1063–1072. Raven Press, New York.
21. Hepner, G. W. (1978): Breath tests in gastroenterology. *Adv. Intern. Med.*, 23:25–45.
22. Hightower, N. C. (1968): Motor action of the small bowel. In: *Handbook of Physiology, Section 6, Alimentary Canal, Vol. IV, Motility*, edited by C. F. Code, pp. 2001–2024. American Physiological Society, Washington, D.C.
23. Hinton, J. M., Lennard-Jones, J. E., and Young, A. C. (1969): A new method for studying gut transit times using radio-opaque markers. *Gut*, 10:842–847.

24. Hohenlietner, F. J., and Senior, J. R. (1969): Metabolism of canine small intestine vascularly perfused *in vitro*. *J. Appl. Physiol.*, 26:119–128.
25. Hopfer, V., Sigrist-Nelson, K., and Murer, H. (1975): Intestinal sugar transport: studies with isolated plasma membranes. *Ann. NY Acad. Sci.*, 264:414–427.
26. Imondi, A. R., Balis, M. E., and Lipkin, M. (1969): Changes in enzyme levels accompanying differentiation of intestinal epithelial cells. *Exp. Cell Res.*, 58:323–330.
27. Irons, G. V., Jr., and Kirsner, J. B. (1965): Routine chemical tests of the stool for occult blood: an evaluation. *Am. J. Med. Sci.*, 249:247–260.
28. Jacobson, E. D., Bondy, D. C., Broitman, S. A., and Fordtran, J. S. (1963): Validity of polyethylene glycol in estimating intestinal water volume. *Gastroenterology*, 44:761–767.
29. Kessler, M., Acuto, O., Storelli, C., Murer, H., Müller, M., and Semenza, G. (1978): A modified procedure for the rapid preparation of efficiently transporting vesicles from small intestinal brush border membranes. *Biochim. Biophys. Acta*, 506:136–154.
30. Kohn, J., and O'Kelly, T. (1955): An ortho-tolidine method for the detection of occult blood in feces. *J. Clin. Pathol.*, 8:249–251.
31. Lavigne, M. E., Wiley, Z. D., Meyer, J. H., Martin, P., and MacGregor, I. L. (1978): Gastric emptying rates of solid food in relation to body size. *Gastroenterology*, 74:1258–1260.
32. Leonards, J. R. (1963): Aspirin and gastrointestinal blood loss. *Gastroenterology*, 44:617–619.
33. Levine, R. R. (1971): Intestinal absorption. In: *Absorption phenomena*, edited by J. L. Rabinowitz and R. M. Myerson, pp. 27–96. Wiley-Interscience, New York.
34. Levine, R. R., McNary, W. F., Kornguth, P. J., and LeBlanc, R. (1970): Histological reevaluation of everted gut technique for studying intestinal absorption. *Eur. J. Pharmacol.*, 9:211–219.
35. Levine, R. R., and Pelikan, E. W. (1961): The influence of experimental procedures and dose on the intestinal absorption of an onium compound, benzomethamine. *J. Pharmacol. Exp. Ther.*, 131:319–327.
36. Levine, P. H., and Weintraub, L. R. (1970): Preparation of suspensions of small bowel mucosal epithelial cells. *J. Lab. Clin. Med.*, 75:1026–1029.
37. Lipkin, M. (1981): Proliferation and differentiation of gastrointestinal cells in normal and disease states. In: *Physiology of the Gastrointestinal Tract, Vol. 1*, edited by L. R. Johnson, pp. 145–168. Raven Press, New York.
38. McGill, H. C., Jr., McMahan, C. A., Wigodsky, H. S., and Spring, H. (1977): Carrageenan in formula and infant baboon development. *Gastroenterology*, 73:512–517.
39. Morris, D. W., Hansell, J. R., Ostrow, J. D., and Lee, C.-S. (1976): Reliability of chemical tests for fecal occult blood in hospitalized patients. *Am. J. Dig. Dis.*, 21:845–852.
40. Nakamura, W., Kankura, T., and Eto, H. (1971): Occult blood appearance in feces and tissue hemorrhages in mice after whole body x-irradiation. *Radiat. Res.*, 48:169–178.
41. Parsons, D. S. (1968): Methods for investigation of intestinal absorption. In: *Handbook of Physiology. Section 6. Alimentary Canal. Volume III. Intestinal absorption*, edited by C. F. Code, pp. 1177–1216. American Physiological Society, Washington, D. C.
42. Pelikan, E. W. (1983): Basic concepts in toxicokinetics. In: *A Guide to General Toxicology*, edited by F. Homburger, J. A. Hayes, and E. W. Pelikan, S. Karger, A. G., Basel, New York.
43. Pelzmann, K. S., and Havemeyer, R. N. (1971): Portal vein blood sampling in intestinal drug absorption studies. *J. Pharm. Sci.*, 60:331.
44. Phillips, B. M. (1973): Aspirin-induced gastrointestinal microbleeding in dogs. *Toxicol. Appl. Pharmacol.*, 24:182–189.
45. Rider, J. A., and Owens, F. J. (1954): Evaluation of an ortho-tolidine test (Fecatest) for determination of occult blood. *JAMA*, 156:31–33.
46. Schultz, S. G., Frizzell, R. A., and Nellans, H. M. (1974): Ion transport by mammalian small intestine. *Ann. Rev. Physiol.*, 36:51–91.
47. Schultz, S. G., and Zalusky, R. (1964): Ion transport in isolated rabbit ileum. I. Short-circuit current and Na fluxes. *J. Gen. Physiol.*, 47:567–584.
48. Schwabe, A. D., and Hepner, G. W. (1979): Breath tests for the detection of fat malabsorption. *Gastroenterology*, 76:216–218.
49. Scott, L. D., and Summers, R. W. (1976): Correlation of contractions and transit in rat small intestine. *Am. J. Physiol.*, 230:132–137.
50. Shriver, D. A., White, C. B., Sandor, A., and Rosenthale, M. E. (1975): A profile of the rat gastrointestinal toxicity of drugs used to treat inflammatory disease. *Toxicol. Appl. Pharmacol.*, 32:73–83.

51. Soergel, K. H. (1968): Inert markers. *Gastroenterology*, 54:449–452.
52. Solomons, N. W., Schoeller, D. A., Wagonfeld, J. B., Ott, D., Rosenberg, I. H., and Klein, P. D. (1977): Application of a stable isotope (^{13}C)-labelled glycocholate breath test to diagnosis of bacterial overgrowth and ileal dysfunction. *J. Lab. Clin. Med.*, 90:431–439.
53. Staff of the Department of Pharmacology, University of Edinburgh (1970): Pharmacological experiments on isolated preparations. E. S. Livingstone, Edinburgh.
54. Stroehlein, J. R., Fairbanks, V. F., McGill, D. B., and Go, V. L. W. (1976): Hemoccult detection of fecal occult blood quantitated by radio-assay. *Am. J. Dig. Dis.*, 21:841–844.
55. Summers, R. W., Kent, T. H., and Osborne, J. W. (1970): Effects of drugs, ileal obstruction and irradiation on rat gastrointestinal propulsion. *Gastroenterology*, 59:731–739.
56. Thomson, A. B. R., and Dietschy, J. M. (1981): Intestinal lipid absorption: major extracellular and intracellular events. In: *Physiology of the Gastrointestinal Tract, Vol. 2*, pp. 1147–1220. Raven Press, New York.
57. Towler, C. M., Pugh-Humphreys, G. P., and Porteous, J. W. (1978): Characterization of columnar absorptive epithelial cells isolated from rat jejunum. *J. Cell. Sci.*, 29:53–75.
58. Trier, J. S. (1971): Diagnostic value of peroral biopsy of the proximal small intestine. *N. Engl. J. Med.*, 285:1470–1473.
59. Trier, J. S. (1976): Organ culture methods in the study of gastrointestinal-mucosal function and development. *N. Engl. J. Med.*, 295:150–155.
60. Ussing, H. H., and Zerahn, K. (1951): Active transport of sodium as the source of electric current in the short-circuited isolated frog skin. *Acta Physiol. Scand.*, 23:110–127.
61. Van Harken, D. R., and Hottendorf, G. H. (1978): Comparative absorption following the administration of a drug to rats by oral gavage and incorporation in the diet. *Toxicol. Appl. Pharmacol.*, 43:407–410.
62. Wagner, J. G. (1975): Fundamentals of clinical pharmacokinetics. p. 173. Drug Intelligence Publications, Inc., Hamilton, IL.
63. Walsh, C. T. (1982): Methods in gastrointestinal toxicology. In: *Principles and Methods of Toxicology*, edited by A. W. Hayes, pp. 475–486. Raven Press, New York.
64. Walsh, C. T., and Levine, R. R. (1979): Methods for the analysis of intestinal function. *Environ. Health Perspec.*, 33:17–23.
65. Watkins, J. B., Schoeller, D. A., Klein, P. D., Ott, D. G., Newcomer, A. D., and Hofmann, A. F. (1977): C-trioctanoin: a nonradioactive breath test to detect fat malabsorption. *J. Lab. Clin. Med.*, 90:422–430.
66. Welsh, M. J., Smith, P. L., Fromm, M., and Frizzell, R. A. (1982): Crypts are the site of intestinal fluid and electrolyte secretion. *Science*, 218:1219–1221.
67. Wilson, T. H., and Wiseman, G. (1954): The use of sacs of everted small intestine for the study of the transference of substances from the mucosal to the serosal surface. *J. Physiol. (Lond.)*, 123:116–125.
68. Winawer, S. J. (1976): Fecal occult blood testing. *Am. J. Dig. Dis.*, 21:885–888.
69. Winne, D. (1977): The influence of unstirred layers on intestinal absorption. In: *Intestinal Permeation. Workshop Conferences, Hoechst. Vol. 4*, edited by M. Kramer and F. Lauterbach, pp. 58–64. International Congress series, No. 391, Exerpta Medica, Amsterdam.
70. Wolfe, D. L., Forland, S. C., and Benet, L. Z. (1973): Drug transfer across intact rat intestinal mucosa following surgical removal of serosa and muscularis externa. *J. Pharm. Sci.*, 62:200–205.

Intestinal Toxicology, edited by C. M. Schiller.
Raven Press, New York © 1984.

Hormonal and Dietary Regulation of Intestinal Enzyme Development

Susan J. Henning

Department of Biology, University of Houston, Houston, Texas 77004

In this chapter the rat is used as a model system for a discussion of the postnatal development of small intestinal function. Factors affecting the developmental process are reviewed in terms of their implication for toxicological studies.

MORPHOLOGICAL DEVELOPMENT

At birth the intestinal mucosa of the rat displays a high level of structural development characterized by villi lined with a single layer of columnar epithelial cells that have well-defined microvilli at their absorptive surfaces (23,58,73). After birth, continuous proliferation of epithelial cells occurs only in the lower regions of the crypts (7,9), and cells migrate from there onto and along the villi, eventually being extruded from the tips into the intestinal lumen. In adult rats and mice the generation time for the crypt cells is 10 to 14 hr (8), and the transit time along the length of the villus is approximately 48 hr (66). The characteristics of proliferation and migration of enterocytes in adult animals are covered in detail by Lipkin (71). Generation and migration of the cells are much slower in neonatal rats than in adults. Despite the fact that neonatal villi are shorter, the transit time is at least 96 hr (50,66). During the third postnatal week there are significant changes in both cell kinetics and morphology leading to more rapid proliferation and longer villi and crypts, which are characteristic of the adult animal (50). As will be explained later, these changes of cell kinetics may at least partly explain some of the changes in mucosal enzymology in the third postnatal week (90,100).

In both neonatal and adult animals, the crypt-villus unit is a classical example of a system wherein proliferation precedes differentiation. The epithelial cells of the villus have many specialized enzymatic functions concerned with the processes of digestion and absorption (26,83). In contrast, the progenitor cells of the crypt have none of these specialized activities but, as would be expected of proliferating tissue, they contain high activities of various enzymes involved in synthesis of DNA (48,52). Many of the specialized functions of the villous cells are associated with the luminal surface, i.e., with the microvilli.

The continuous renewal of the intestinal epithelium adds a degree of complexity to developmental studies with this organ. When dealing with the development of

17

most other organs, one considers the change, with time, of the enzymatic properties of a stable population of cells. For example, in rat liver the same cells that have high activity of adenosine triphosphate (ATP)-citrate lyase and low activity of tryptophan oxygenase at birth have these enzymatic patterns reversed by the time of weaning (31). In contrast, in the intestine there are two ways in which enzyme patterns can be changed: by changes in a given population of enterocytes within their brief life-span and by simple replacement of one type of cell with another type from the proliferating pool. In a later section evidence is presented showing that it is the latter mechanism that is operative in the ontogenic changes that occur during the third week of life.

BIOCHEMICAL DEVELOPMENT

Biochemically, the rat intestine is relatively immature at birth and for the first 2 postnatal weeks; during the third and fourth weeks it undergoes a dramatic array of functional changes.

One of the most striking features of the neonatal rat intestine is its ability to absorb intact macromolecules, including proteins (16,32,82), by the process of pinocytosis (10,54,91). The capacity for pinocytosis appears in the rat intestine by day 19 or 20 of intrauterine life (38,84), remains high during the first 2 weeks of suckling, and then decreases markedly toward the end of the third week (10,54,101). Correspondingly, the proteolytic enzymes from the stomach and the pancreas, which are low during the first 2 weeks of extrauterine life, increase significantly during the weaning period (27,54,90).

The absence of the adult mode of luminal digestion of protein in the neonatal rat and the presence of pinocytic capacity provides an explanation for the absorption of intact immunoglobulins during the suckling period (32,33). On the other hand, since the developmental pattern of pinocytosis correlates with that for certain lysosomal hydrolases (61,101), including cathepsin B (94), it has been suggested (101) that the process of pinocytosis allows intracellular digestion of macromolecules during the period in which the mechanisms for extracellular digestion have not yet matured. This is not consistent with pinocytosis being important for the transfer of passive immunity to the newborn unless immunoglobulins are selectively protected from the action of lysosomal hydrolases. Various models to explain such selectivity have been proposed (6,45,79), and recent evidence (55,80) supports one of these models (45), namely that immunoglobulins are absorbed predominantly in the jejunum where lysosomal activity is low, whereas other proteins are absorbed and digested in the ileum where lysosomal activity is high.

Two points relevant to toxicology are illustrated here. First, for both the adult intestine and the infant intestine one should always remain open to the possibility that different regions may have quite different biochemical characteristics. Second, during the developmental period, proteins (and any ligands that may be bound to them) have direct access to intestinal epithelial cells as a result of pinocytosis.

In terms of digestive capacity, the neonatal rat intestine has hydrolytic activities that are specific for and restricted to the components of maternal milk. This is demonstrated by a consideration of carbohydrate digestion. Milk is relatively low in total carbohydrates, and the carbohydrates present are those not generally found in adult diets. The major carbohydrate in the milk of most placental mammals is lactose (53), and high activities of its disaccharidase, lactase, are found in the intestinal mucosa of the suckling animals (4,17,67). In the rat, lactase is detectable on day 18 of gestation, has maximal activity during the first week after birth, and then begins to decline, reaching adult values by the end of the fourth week (20). Many other species, including the human, have lower lactase activity in the adult than the newborn (17) and, accordingly, show an inability to utilize ingested lactose in the postweaning period (67).

Although lactose is the major carbohydrate received by the suckling mammal, the milks of various species are also known to contain sialic acid. Interestingly, the digestive enzyme for this component, namely neuraminidase, has been found to have an ontogenic profile very similar to that of lactase (19).

Intestinal hydrolases that are involved in digestion of carbohydrate components of solid food are absent or low at birth, then appear and/or increase in activity. Maltase has low activity during the first 2 postnatal weeks then undergoes a 5- to 10-fold increase during the next 2 weeks (88,92). For sucrase, isomaltase, and trehalase, the transition is even more sudden. These enzymes cannot be detected in the intestine during the first and second postnatal week, but their activities appear on approximately day 16 and rise rapidly, reaching adult levels by the end of the fourth week (21,88,92). The activity changes of the disaccharidases are paralleled by changes in the protein bands of microvillous membrane preparations studied by electrophoresis (28,29,95).

These developmental changes in the nature of the disaccharidases activities of the intestine clearly have physiological significance in allowing the young animal to make the dietary change from lactose as the major carbohydrate during suckling, to maltose, isomaltose, and sucrose as the major disaccharides after weaning (41). The temporal relationship between the developmental rise of sucrase activity and the process of weaning can be seen in Fig. 1. The possibility of a causal relationship between these two phenomena is discussed below.

In addition to the disaccharidases, there are various other hydrolytic enzymes of the intestine that show distinct developmental patterns. Many workers have measured the marked increase in duodenal alkaline phosphatase activity that occurs during the third week of life in rats and mice (17). Much of the pioneer work by Moog on the development of intestinal function was accomplished with this enzyme (75,76). The function of alkaline phosphatase in the intestine is not understood, although its distribution along the crypt-villus unit (83) and its localization in the microvilli of enterocytes (11,25,51) are suggestive of some role in digestion or absorption.

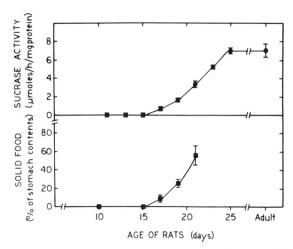

FIG. 1. Top: Activity of jejunal sucrase during postnatal development. **Bottom:** Pattern of weaning in the same animals as indicated by the amount of chow in stomach contents at various ages. Values were obtained by dissecting the chow away from coagulated milk, weighing each component, then expressing the weight of chow as a percent of the weight of milk plus chow. Values are given as mean ± SEM ($N = 5$). Reproduced from Henning (41), with permission.

Role of Diet in the Regulation of Intestinal Development

The possibility of dietary influence over the regulation of intestinal development is an obvious one considering the temporal correlation between the major enzymic changes in the intestine and the onset of weaning (Fig. 1). In terms of nutrition, weaning represents a transition from a high-fat/low-carbohydrate diet to a low-fat/high-carbohydrate diet and from a diet whose sole disaccharide is lactose to one in which the major disaccharides are sucrose and maltose. It is clear, however, that this dietary change cannot be considered the primary cause of the various enzymic and morphologic changes that occur in the intestine during the third postnatal week. We have shown (Fig. 2) that when weaning is prevented, the appearance of sucrase activity in the jejunum is not delayed. Correspondingly, prolonged suckling does not delay the usual decrease in the capacity of the neonatal rat intestine to transport intact antibodies (34), and it delays, but does not prevent, the usual decline of lactase activity (69). Conversely, oral administration of sucrose to 12-day-old rats has no effect on the developmental pattern for sucrase (92). If sucrose is administered by gastrostomy to suckling rats, precocious increase of sucrase is observed; however, since this does not occur if the animals have been previously adrenalectomized, it is probably a stress response rather than a dietary response (68). The same comment applies to the precocious appearance of sucrase, maltase, isomaltase, and alkaline phosphatase following early weaning (30,87). These conclusions are supported by the observations that sucrase develops normally in by-passed intestinal segments (99) and that when intestinal explants from 6-day-old rats are cultured in the presence of various sugars there is no stimulatory effect on sucrase or maltase activity (86).

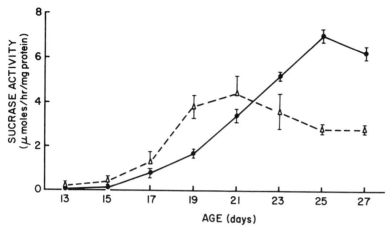

FIG. 2. Effect of weaning-prevention on sucrase development for four control litters (●————●) raised in the regular manner and four experimental litters (Δ-----Δ) raised on a schedule that prevented weaning. One pup from each litter was removed for sucrase assay every second day from days 13 to 27 inclusive. Results are given as mean ± SEM (*N* = 4). Reproduced from Henning and Sims (47), with permission.

Given, then, that the intestinal changes of the third week are initiated by some factor other than the dietary change of weaning (probably glucocorticoids; see below), there still remains the question of whether the dietary change modulates the extent or the timing of the ontogenic events. The case of sucrase development is particularly interesting. Figure 2 shows that although the timing of the appearance of jejunal sucrase is not affected by prevention of weaning, the activity at which the enzyme plateaus (days 25 and 27) is approximately half that seen in control (weaned) animals. A subsequent study (42) demonstrated that the critical difference between milk and chow is the relative proportions of carbohydrate and fat. A diet like chow, which is high-carbohydrate/low-fat, will elicit a high plateau activity of sucrase whereas a diet like milk, which is low-carbohydrate/high-fat, will elicit a low plateau (42). Correspondingly, in intestinal explants from suckling rats that have been treated with dexamethasone to elicit sucrase and maltase, addition of sugars to the culture medium increases the activities of these enzymes (86).

Another characteristic that appears during the fourth postnatal week is the occurrence of a diurnal rhythm of enzyme activity. We have measured jejunal sucrase activity every 3 hr during 24-hr periods (3). At 19 days of age, this enzyme shows arrhythmic variation, whereas on days 22 and 27, a distinct rhythm with a nocturnal peak has developed. The appearance of this rhythm is unrelated to the corticosterone rhythm which appears at this time (1,3), but rather is due to the fact that the onset of feeding becomes coordinated with the onset of darkness around 22 days of age (43).

Here again, in relation to toxicological studies, there are two important points. First, that although diet seems to have little influence on intestinal biochemistry during the suckling phase, from the weanling phase onward, dietary changes may have dramatic effects on the enzymology of this tissue. Second, that at least from day 22 onward, significant diurnal variations may be present, thus making the timing of experiments (with respect to the light cycle) a variable that must be critically controlled.

Role of Hormones in the Regulation of Intestinal Development

Glucocorticoids

The glucocorticoids are attractive candidates for the regulation of intestinal development because circulating concentrations of corticosterone (the principal glucocorticoid in the rat) increase greatly at the beginning of the third postnatal week (40,89). Since the serum-binding protein CBG also increases at this time (40), it was important to determine the developmental pattern for the free hormone, which is believed to be the biologically active component (85,98). Figure 3 shows that plasma concentrations of free corticosterone are low through day 12 and then increase markedly. Analysis of jejunal sucrase and lactase activities in the same animals (Fig. 3) revealed that the rise of free corticosterone begins about 48 hr before the enzymic changes are initiated. This delay is consistent with the fact that glucocorticoid action on the intestinal epithelium is mediated by the crypt cells (see below).

Administration of glucocorticoids to suckling rats during the first 2 postnatal weeks causes precocious increases in the activities of sucrase (21,29,44), maltase (29,77), trehalase (29), amino peptidase (29,76), and alkaline phosphatase (75), as well as precocious disappearance of various lysosomal hydrolases (65), and of the capacities for pinocytosis (12,16,54,78) and for the absorption of intact immunoglobulins (35,54,81). Correspondingly, addition of glucocorticoids to intestinal explants from rats aged 4 to 13 days elicits a precocious appearance of sucrase and a stimulation of maltase activity (21,59,96,97).

Conversely, it has been shown that if rats are subject to neonatal adrenalectomy or hypophysectomy, the usual decrease of pinocytosis (15) and lysosomal hydrolases (64) and the usual increase of alkaline phosphatase (75,104), sucrase (62,64,72,104), and maltase (64,72,104) are delayed, although not prevented. In hypophysecto-mized infant rats, cortisone administration restores sucrase development to normal (105), indicating that, at least for this enzyme, the critical effect of ablation of the anterior pituitary is the removal of adrenocorticotrophic hormone (ACTH) and thus of corticosterone.

In view of the dramatic effects of changes of glucocorticoid status on the intestinal enzymes of infant rats, it is perhaps surprising that the adult intestine seems insensitive to these hormones. In the adult, jejunal sucrase is not decreased by adrenalectomy nor increased by administration of glucocorticoids (18). We found that this adult characteristic of glucocorticoid independence appears on day 17 through 18, i.e., very soon after the sucrase rise begins (47). Similar results were reported for alkaline phosphatase in mouse duodenum (75), for maltase and lactase

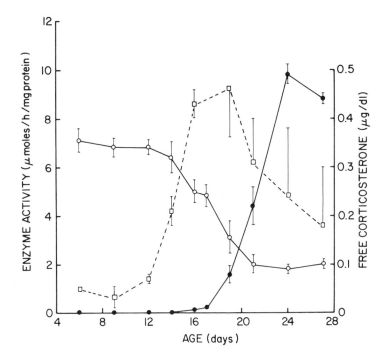

FIG. 3. Developmental patterns for the activities of the enzymes lactase and sucrase in jejunal mucosa as compared with free corticosterone in plasma: (○——○) lactase activity; (●——●) sucrase activity; (□-----□) free corticosterone. Values are given as mean ± SEM ($N = 5$). Absence of error bars indicates that the SEM was smaller than the symbol. Reproduced from Henning (40), with permission.

in rat jejunum (46), and for acid β-galactosidase in rat ileum (46). Thus, with respect to these enzymes, glucocorticoids seem to be required only for the initiation of the developmental changes, not for their maintenance. The possibility that the intestine abruptly loses its sensitivity to certain toxic substances at this time is equally intriguing.

It was pointed out earlier that there are two possible mechanisms by which enzymic changes of the intestinal epithelium could occur: by alteration of the enzyme levels in the differentiated cells that are present on the villi or by replacement of one population of villous cells by another which has altered enzymology. There is now considerable evidence to indicate that it is the latter method that is operative in the various postnatal changes that are observed in the rat intestine. When the distribution of sucrase along the length of the crypt-villus unit after glucocorticoid administration to 9-day-old rats was studied by cryostat sectioning of the intestine (44,49), it was found that 24 hr after administration of the steroid, no sucrase activity was detectable on the villi but a small amount was present at the mouths of the crypt. By day 11 this activity had increased and extended along the lower halves of the villi. The process continued and by day 13 sucrase activity had reached the tips of the villi, and the pattern through the whole depth of the mucosa was similar to that for adult animals (83).

These results indicate that the ability of hydrocortisone to cause precocious appearance of sucrase is mediated via the cells of the crypt. The cells that are on the villi at the time of administration are apparently unaffected by the hormone. The rate at which the enzyme activity appeared at the base of the villi and then spread along the lengths of the villi correlated with reported migratory rates for the epithelial cells (49,66).

Similar results for the pattern of sucrase appearance have been obtained by immunological techniques (22,37). The same series of events apparently occurs when endogenous glucocorticoids participate in the normal appearance of sucrase during the third postnatal week (37). Likewise, during both the normal and the precocious loss of pinocytic capacity from the jejunum, pinocytosis does not decrease in enterocytes already present in the villi, but rather these cells are gradually replaced by new ones from the crypts that do not engage in pinocytosis (12,101).

As detailed above, the involvement of glucocorticoids in intestinal development has been extensively studied. However, the question of whether intestinal maturation is absolutely dependent on glucocorticoids has not been addressed in the literature. As indicated earlier, several studies have shown that enzymic development is delayed but not abolished in adrenalectomized rat pups (15,62,64,75). The problem with these studies is that none of them included either mineralocorticoid replacement or measurement of serum corticosterone following the adrenalectomy. We have recently found that without mineralocorticoid administration following neonatal adrenalectomy, the only pups that survive long enough to study have substantial amounts of corticosterone in the serum. Even with mineralocorticoid replacement, it is essential to measure serum corticosterone in all adrenalectomized pups so as to eliminate those with detectable levels of corticosterone (72). Data from a recent study incorporating these precautions are shown in Fig. 4. It can be seen that

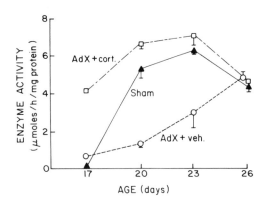

FIG. 4. Effect of adrenalectomy on the development of jejunal sucrase. Enzyme activities are shown for the sham-operated animals (▲——▲), for adrenalectomized animals receiving vehicle injections (○-----○), and for adrenalectomized animals receiving corticosterone injections (□-----□). For the adX + veh. group, only pups having undetectable concentrations of serum corticosterone were included for sucrase assay. Results are given as mean ± SEM. The number of animals represented for each group at each age ranged from 4 to 7. Absence of error bars indicates the SEM was smaller than the symbol. From Martin and Henning *(unpublished data).*

although adrenalectomy greatly suppressed the rate of the sucrase rise, the time of appearance of the enzyme (day 17) was not delayed, and by day 26 the activity of the enzyme in the pups having no detectable serum corticosterone (i.e., the "adX + veh." group) was the same as in the sham-operated controls. Corticosterone replacement therapy in adrenalectomized pups caused a slightly precocious rise of sucrase activity, illustrating the difficulty of achieving physiological concentrations of corticosterone by exogenous administration.

The results of this study (Fig. 4) have led us to the conclusion that the developmental rise of jejunal sucrase activity is not absolutely dependent on corticosterone. It is likely that the timing for the initiation of enzyme development is intrinsically programmed into the intestinal tissue and that the developmental surge of serum corticosterone at the beginning of the third postnatal week only controls the rate of expression of the intestinal program. These conclusions are consistent with the fact that sucrase, maltase, lactase, and acid β-galactosidase develop normally in fetal intestinal tissue that is transplanted into the stable hormonal environment of an adult host (60,74).

In view of the above conclusions, we hypothesized that the physiological significance of glucocorticoids in intestinal development might be that they provide a mechanism for precocious maturation if pups are subjected to loss of their dam prior to the usual time of weaning, i.e., that the stress of forced weaning would cause a sufficient elevation of plasma corticosterone to induce precocious maturation of intestinal enzymes. An early-weaning experiment was conducted to test this hypothesis. In order to be able to assess the contribution of diet composition to any observed enzyme changes, the pups were weaned onto either a regular rat chow or a liquid diet resembling rat milk.

Figure 5 shows the development of jejunal sucrase in early-weaned (EW) pups. On day 17, both EW groups had sucrase activities precociously elevated as compared with those of controls remaining with their mother. On day 21, pups early weaned onto chow again had higher sucrase activities than did control pups, whereas pups early weaned onto the liquid diet had reduced sucrase activities. By day 25, the

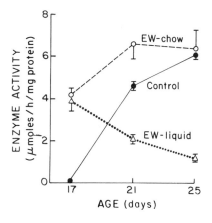

FIG. 5. Effect of early weaning on jejunal sucrase. Enzyme activities are shown from control pups (●——●) as compared with pups weaned at 15 days of age onto either chow (○-----○) or onto a liquid diet (△······△) having a composition similar to rat milk. Values are given as mean ± SEM. For the controls, $N = 4$; EW-liquid, $N = 6$; and EW-chow, $N = 3$. Absence of error bars indicates that the SEM is smaller than the symbol. From Guerin and Henning (*unpublished data*).

controls and the EW-chow pups were not different while activities of the pups remaining on a liquid diet were again substantially lower than those of controls.

It appears that the initial rises in enzyme activities seen in both EW groups (Fig. 5) were a result of stress. The differential activities seen later between the chow-fed and the liquid diet-fed groups are consistent with earlier studies that have shown that by the fourth postnatal week, sucrase activity is proportional to the carbohydrate content of the diet (42,47). Our early-weaning/stress hypothesis is also supported by the data of Boyle and Koldovsky (5), who showed that sucrase activity was precociously elevated in EW pups only if the adrenal glands were present. Taken together, we believe the two studies provide compelling evidence that one of the physiological roles of glucocorticoids is to elicit precocious intestinal maturation in curcumstances where the dam is lost prior to the normal time of weaning.

An important corollary of the above is that any stress may elicit significant changes in intestinal biochemistry during the developmental period. Although the hypothalamus-pituitary-adrenal axis is quiescent from day 3 through day 10 (2,36,70), between days 11 and 18, stress-induced elevation of plasma corticosterone can be expected to cause precocious maturation of intestinal function. The stress effects of drugs, surgery, and sickness during the developmental period have not been systematically studied but would be certainly predicted to cause precocious maturation of the small intestine.

Thyroid Hormones

Thyroxine (T_4) has received considerable attention as a candidate for regulation of intestinal development in the rat because its circulating concentration rises significantly during the second postnatal week (13,24,93,102). Administration of T_4 or triiodothyronine (T_3) has been shown to cause precocious decline of jejunal immunoglobulin transport (56), of jejunal lactase activity (57), and of ileal lysosomal hydrolases (63), as well as precocious increases of jejunal sucrase and maltase (57). Conversely, hypothyroidism delays but does not prevent the usual decline of lysosomal hydrolases (64) and the usual increases of sucrase (39,64,104) and maltase (64,104) activities. The significance of findings such as these must be reexamined in view of the demonstrations that administration of T_4 causes a precocious increase in plasma corticosterone (14) and that hypothyroidism virtually abolishes the developmental rise of corticosterone (14,104). Recent data suggest that, at least for sucrase and maltase development, the effects of thyroid manipulations are secondary to the accompanying changes of serum corticosterone (72,104). Specifically, the suppressive effect of hypothyroidism on the developmental rises of sucrase and maltase can be reversed just as effectively by glucocorticoid administration as by T_4 treatment (72,104). Conversely, when T_4 is administered during the first 2 postnatal weeks there is no stimulation of sucrase and maltase unless serum corticosterone is also allowed to increase (72). The conclusion that T_4 plays no role in the normal development of jejunal sucrase and maltase is supported by the finding that T_4 is unable to elicit increases in the activity of these enzymes in jejunal explants from suckling rats (96).

Thyroxine may play a role in the regulation of enzymes that normally decline during development. For neuraminidase and acid β-galactosidase, administration of T_4 together with a saturating dose of cortisone acetate causes a greater precocious decline of activity than when cortisone acetate is given alone (46). For lactase, the developmental effects of hypophysectomy are fully restored by administration of T_4, but only partially restored by administration of cortisone (103). The involvement of T_4 in the ontogenic decline of these enzymes may reflect the fact that this hormone is a potent stimulator of mitotic activity in the intestinal epithelium (104). There is evidence that, at least for lactase, the declining activity during the third postnatal week is largely due to the decreased life-span of enterocytes that follows the increased rates of proliferation and migration of these cells at this time (100). Thus, if the latter increases are caused by T_4, then this hormone could indirectly contribute to the developmental decline of enzyme activities during the third post-natal week. The finding that T_4 does not cause a decline of lactase activity in intestinal explants (96) could be because some other factors, such as nutrients, limit the rate of proliferation of enterocytes in culture.

SUMMARY

Manipulations of diet, glucocorticoids, and T_4 have substantial, although different, effects on the ontogeny of intestinal enzymes. Thus, each of these factors must be considered as critical variables in toxicological studies of the developing intestine. For instance, any substance that delays weaning will thereby alter the plateau levels of enzymic activities in the fourth postnatal week. It would be important to recognize that the observed changes in enzyme activities were not direct effects of the toxic substance administered, but rather were secondary to the effect on weaning. Likewise, any substance that alters plasma concentrations of corticosterone or T_4 during the critical period of development will indirectly cause dramatic changes in the timing of enzymic maturation of the small intestine.

ACKNOWLEDGMENTS

This work was supported by grant number RO1-HD-14094 from the National Institutes of Health.

REFERENCES

1. Allen, C., and Kendall, J. N. (1967): Maturation of the circadian rhythm of plasma corticosterone in the rat. *Endocrinology*, 80:926–930.
2. Bartova, A. (1968): Functioning of the hypothalamo-pituitary-adrenal system during postnatal development in rats. *Gen. Comp. Endocrinol.*, 10:235–239.
3. Beam, H. E., and Henning, S. J. (1978): Development of the circadian rhythm of jejunal sucrase activity in the weanling rat. *Am. J. Physiol.*, 235:E437–E442.
4. Blaxter, K. L. (1961): Lactation and the growth of the young. In: *Milk: The Mammary and Its Secretion, Vol. 11*, edited by S. K. Kon and A. T. Cowie, pp. 305–361. Academic Press, New York.
5. Boyle, J. T., and Koldovsky, O. (1980): Critical role of adrenal glands in precocious increase in

jejunal sucrase activity following premature weaning in rats: Negligible effect of food intake. *J. Nutr.*, 110:169–177.

6. Brambell, D. W. R. (1966): The transmission of immunity from mother to young and the catabolism of immunoglobulins. *Lancet*, ii:1087–1093.

7. Burholt, D. R., Schultze, B., and Maurer, W. (1976): Mode of growth of the jejunal crypt cells of the rat: an autoradiographic study using double labelling with ^{3}H- and ^{14}C-thymidine in lower and upper parts of crypts. *Cell Tiss. Kinet.*, 9:107–117.

8. Cairnie, A. B., Lamerton, L. F., and Steel, G. G. (1965): Cell proliferation studies of the intestinal epithelium of the rat. I. Determination of kinetic parameters. *Exp. Cell Res.*, 39:528–538.

9. Cheng, H., and Leblond, C. P. (1974): Origin, differentiation and renewal of the four main epithelial cell types in the mouse small intestine. I. Columnar cell. *Am. J. Anat.*, 141:461–480.

10. Clark, S. L. (1959): The ingestion of proteins and colloidal materials by columnar absorptive cells of the small intestine in suckling rats and mice. *J. Biophys. Biochem. Cytol.*, 5:41–50.

11. Clark, S. L. (1961): The localization of alkaline phosphatase in tissues of mice using the electron microscope. *Am. J. Anat.*, 109:57–83.

12. Clark, S. L. (1971): The effects of cortisol and BUDR on cellular differentiation in the small intestine of suckling rats. *Am. J. Anat.*, 132:319–338.

13. Clos, J., Crepel, J., Legrand, C., Legrand, J., Rabie, A., and Vigoroux, E. (1974): Thyroid physiology during the postnatal period in the rat: a study of the development of thyroid function and of the morphogenetic effects of thyroxine with special reference to cellular maturation. *Gen. Comp. Endocrinol.*, 23:178–192.

14. D'Agostino, J. B., and Henning, S. J. (1982): Role of thyroxine in coordinate control of corticosterone and CBG in postnatal development. *Am. J. Physiol.*, 242:E33–E39.

15. Daniels, V.G., Hardy, R. N., and Malinowska, K. W. (1973): The effect of adrenalectomy or pharmacological inhibition of adrenocortical function on macromolecule uptake by the newborn rat intestine. *J. Physiol.*, 229:697–707.

16. Daniels, V. G., Hardy, R. N., Malinowska, K. W., and Nathanielsz, P. W. (1973): The influence of exogenous steroids on macromolecule uptake by the small intestine of the newborn rat. *J. Physiol.*, 229:681–695.

17. Deren, J. J. (1968): Development of intestinal structure and function. In: *Handbook of Physiology, Section 6, Alimentary Canal, Vol. III, Intestinal Absorption*, edited by C. F. Code, pp. 1099–1123. American Physiological Society, Washington, D.C.

18. Deren, J. J., Broitman, S. A., and Zamcheck, N. (1967): Effect of diet upon intestinal disaccharidases and disaccharide absorption. *J. Clin. Invest.*, 46:186–195.

19. Dickson, J. J., and Messer, M. (1978): Intestinal neuraminidase activity of suckling rats and other mammals: relationship to the sialic acid content of milk. *Biochem. J.*, 170:407–413.

20. Doell, R. G., and Kretchmer, N. (1962): Studies of the small intestine during development. I. Distribution and activity of β-galactosidase. *Biochim. Biophys. Acta*, 62:353–362.

21. Doell, R. G., and Kretchmer, N. (1964): Intestinal invertase: precocious development of activity after injection of hydrocortisone. *Science*, 143:42–44.

22. Doell, R. G., Rosen, G., and Kretchmer, N. (1965): Immunological studies of intestinal disaccharidases during normal and precocious development. *Proc. Natl. Acad. Sci. USA*, 54:1268–1273.

23. Dunn, J. S. (1967): The fine structure of the absorptive epithelial cells of the developing small intestine of the rat. *J. Anat.*, 101:57–68.

24. Dussault, J. H., and Labrie, F. (1975): Development of the hypothalamic-pituitary-thyroid axis in the neonatal rat. *Endocrinology*, 97:1321–1324.

25. Etzler, M. E., Birkenmeier, E. H., and Moog, F. (1969): Localization of alkaline phosphatase isozymes in mouse duodenum by immunofluorescence microscopy. *Histochemie*, 20:99–104.

26. Fortin-Magana, R., Hurwitz, R., Herbst, J. J., and Kretchmer, N. (1970): Intestinal enzymes: indicators of proliferation and differentiation in the jejunum. *Science*, 167:1627–1628.

27. Furihata, C., Kawachi, T., and Sugimura, T. (1972): Premature induction of pepsinogen in developing rat gastric mucosa by hormones. *Biochem. Biophys. Res. Commun.*, 47:705–711.

28. Galand, G., and Forstner, G. G. (1974): Soluble neutral and acid maltases in the suckling-rat intestine. *Biochem. J.*, 144:281–292.

29. Galand, G., and Forstner, G. G. (1974): Isolation of microvillus plasma membranes from suckling rat intestine. The influence of premature induction of digestive enzymes by injection of cortisol acetate. *Biochem. J.*, 144:293–302.

30. Goldstein, R., Klein, T., Freier, S., and Menczel, J. (1971): Alkaline phosphatase and disaccharidase activities in the rat intestine from birth to weaning. I. Effect of diet on enzyme development. *Am. J. Clin. Nutr.*, 24:1224–1231.
31. Greengard, O. (1970): The developmental formation of enzymes in rat liver. In: *Biochemical Actions of Hormones, Vol. 1*, edited by G. Litwack, pp. 53–87. Academic Press, New York.
32. Halliday, R. (1955): The absorption of antibodies from immune sera by the gut of the young rat. *Proc. Roy. Soc. (Lond.)*, B143:408–413.
33. Halliday, R. (1955): Prenatal and postnatal transmission of passive immunity to young rats. *Proc. Roy. Soc. (Lond.)*, B144:427–430.
34. Halliday, R. (1956): The termination of the capacity of young rats to absorb antibody from the milk. *Proc. Roy. Soc. (Lond.)*, B145:179–185.
35. Halliday, R. (1959): The effect of steroid hormones on the absorption of antibody by the young rat. *J. Endocrinol.*, 18:56–66.
36. Haltmeyer, G. C., Denenberg, V. H., Thatcher, J., and Zarrow, M. X. (1966): Response of the adrenal cortex of the neonatal rat after subjection to stress. *Nature*, 212:1371–1373.
37. Hauri, H.-P., Quaroni, A., and Isselbacher, K. J. (1980): Monoclonal antibodies to sucrase/isomaltase: Probes for the study of postnatal development and biogenesis of the intestinal microvillus membrane. *Proc. Natl. Acad. Sci. USA*, 77:6629–6633.
38. Hayward, A. F. (1967): Changes in the fine structure of developing intestinal epithelium associated with pinocytosis. *J. Anat.*, 102:57–70.
39. Henning, S. J. (1978): Permissive role of thyroxine in the ontogeny of jejunal sucrase. *Endocrinology*, 102:9–15.
40. Henning, S. J. (1978): Plasma concentrations of total and free corticosterone during development in the rat. *Am. J. Physiol.*, 235:E451–E456.
41. Henning, S. J. (1979): Biochemistry of intestinal development. *Environ. Health Perspect.*, 33:9–16.
42. Henning, S. J., and Guerin, D. M. (1981): Role of diet in the determination of jejunal sucrase activity in the weanling rat. *Pediatr. Res.*, 15:1068–1072.
43. Henning, S. J., and Guerin, D. M. (1983): Role of nocturnal feeding in the development of the diurnal rhythm of jejunal sucrase activity. *Proc. Soc. Exp. Biol. Med.*, 172:232–238.
44. Henning, S. J., Helman, T. A., and Kretchmer, N. (1975): Studies on normal and precocious appearance of jejunal sucrase in suckling rats. *Biol. Neonate*, 26:249–262.
45. Henning, S. J., and Kretchmer, N. (1973): Development of intestinal function in mammals. *Enzyme*, 15:3–23.
46. Henning, S. J., and Leeper, L. L. (1982): Coordinate loss of glucocorticoid responsiveness by intestinal enzymes during postnatal development. *Am. J. Physiol.*, 242:G89–G94.
47. Henning, S. J., and Sims, J. M. (1979): Delineation of the glucocorticoid-sensitive period of intestinal development in the rat. *Endocrinology*, 104:1158–1163.
48. Herbst, J. J., Fortin-Magana, R., and Sunshine, P. (1970): Relationship of pyrimidine biosynthetic enzymes to cellular proliferation in rat intestine during development. *Gastroenterology*, 59:240–246.
49. Herbst, J. J., and Koldovsky, O. (1972): Cell migration and cortisone induction of sucrase activity in jejunum and ileum. *Biochem. J.*, 126:471–476.
50. Herbst, J. J., and Sunshine, P. (1969): Postnatal development of the small intestine of the rat. *Pediatr. Res.*, 3:27–33.
51. Hugon, J. S., and Borgers, M. (1969): Ultrastructural differentiation and enzymatic localization of phosphatases in the developing duodenal epithelium of the mouse. I. The foetal mouse. *Histochemie*, 19:13–30.
52. Imondi, A. R., Balis, M. E., and Lipkin, M. (1969): Changes in enzyme levels accompanying differentiation of intestinal epithelial cells. *Exp. Cell Res.*, 58:323–330.
53. Jenness, R., Regehr, E. A., and Sloan, R. E. (1964): Comparative biochemical study of milks. II. Dialysable carbohydrates. *Comp. Biochem. Physiol.*, 13:339–352.
54. Jones, R. E. (1972): Intestinal absorption and gastrointestinal digestion of protein in the young rat during the normal and cortisone-induced closure period. *Biochim. Biophys. Acta*, 274:412–419.
55. Jones, R. E. (1978): Degradation of radioactivity labelled protein in the small intestine of the suckling rat. *Biol. Neonate*, 34:286–294.
56. Jones, R. E. (1982): Effects of thyroxine on the transmission of immunoglobulin across the small intestine of young rats. *Biol. Neonate*, 41:246–251.

57. Jumawan, J., and Koldovsky, O. (1978): Comparison of the effect of various doses of thyroxine on jejunal disaccharidases in intact and adrenalectomized rats during the first 3 weeks of life. *Enzyme*, 23:206–209.
58. Kammeraad, A. (1942): The development of the gastrointestinal tract of the rat. I. Histogenesis of the epithelium of the stomach, small intestine and pancreas. *J. Morphol.*, 20:323–349.
59. Kedinger, M., Simon, P. M., Raul, F., Grenier, J. F., and Haffen, K. (1980): The effect of dexamethasone on the development of rat intestinal brush border enzymes in organ culture. *Develop. Biol.*, 74:9–21.
60. Kendall, K., Jumawan, J., Koldovsky, O., and Krulich, L. (1977): Effect of the host hormonal status on development of sucrase and acid β-galactosidase in isografts of rat small intestine. *J. Endocrinol.*, 74:145–146.
61. Koldovsky, O., and Herbst, J. J. (1971): N-acetyl-β-glucosaminidase in small intestine and its changes during postnatal development of the rat. *Biol. Neonate*, 17:1–9.
62. Koldovsky, O., Jirsova, V., and Heringova, A. (1965): Effect of aldosterone and corticosterone on β-galactosidase and invertase activity in the small intestine of rats. *Nature*, 206:300–301.
63. Koldovsky, O., Jumawan, J., and Palmieri, M. (1974): Thyroxine-evoked precocious decrease of acid hydrolases in the ileum of suckling rats. *Proc. Soc. Exp. Biol. Med.*, 146:661–664.
64. Koldovsky, O., Jumawan, J., and Palmieri, M. (1975): Effect of thyroidectomy on the activity of α-glucosidases and acid hydrolases in the small intestine of rats during weaning. *J. Endocr.*, 66:31–36.
65. Koldovsky, O., and Palmieri, M. (1971): Cortisone-evoked decrease in acid β-galactosidase, β-glucuronidase, N-acetyl-β-glucosamidase and arylsulphatase in the ileum of suckling rats. *Biochem. J.*, 125:697–701.
66. Koldovsky, O., Sunshine, P., and Kretchmer, N. (1966): Cellular migration of intestinal epithelia in suckling and weaned rats. *Nature*, 212:1389–1390.
67. Kretchmer, N. (1971): Lactose and lactase—a historical perspective. *Gastroenterology*, 61:805–813.
68. Lebenthal, E., Sunshine, P., and Kretchmer, N. (1972): Effect of carbohydrate and corticosteroids on activity of α-glucosidases in intestine of infant rat. *J. Clin. Invest.*, 51:1244–1250.
69. Lebenthal, E., Sunshine, P., and Kretchmer, N. (1973): Effect of prolonged nursing on the activity of intestinal lactase in rats. *Gastroenterology*, 64:1136–1141.
70. Levine, S., and Treiman, L. J. (1969): Role of hormones in programming the central nervous system. In: *Ciba Foundation Symposium on Foetal Autonomy*, edited by G. E. W., Wolstenholme and M. O'Connor, pp. 271–281. Churchill, London.
71. Lipkin, M. (1973): Proliferation and differentiation of gastrointestinal cells. *Physiol. Rev.*, 53:891–915.
72. Martin, G. R., and Henning, S. J. (1982): Relative importance of corticosterone and thyroxine in the postnatal development of sucrase and maltase in rat small intestine. *Endocrinology*, 111:912–918.
73. Mathan, M., Moxey, P. C., and Trier, J. S. (1976): Morphogenesis of fetal rat duodenal villi. *Am. J. Anat.*, 146:73–92.
74. Montgomery, R. K., Sybicki, M. A., and Grand, R. J. (1981): Autonomous biochemical and morphological differentiation in fetal rat intestine transplanted at 17 and 20 days of gestation. *Develop. Biol.*, 87:76–84.
75. Moog, F. (1953): The functional differentiation of the small intestine. III. Influence of the pituitary-adrenal system on the differentiation of phosphatases in the duodenum of the suckling mouse. *J. Exp. Zool.*, 124:329–346.
76. Moog, F. (1971): Corticoids and the enzymic maturation of the intestinal surface: alkaline phosphatase, leucyl naphthylamidase and sucrase. In: *Hormones in Development*, edited by M. Hamburgh and E. J. W. Barrington, pp. 143–160. Meridith, New York.
77. Moog, F., Denes, A. E., and Powell, P. M. (1973): Disaccharidases in the small intestine of the mouse: normal development and influence of cortisone, actinomycin D, and cycloheximide. *Develop. Biol.*, 35:143–159.
78. Moog, F., and Yeh, K. Y. (1979): Pinocytosis persists in the ileum of hypophysectomized rats unless closure is induced by thyroxine or cortisone. *Develop. Biol.*, 69:159–169.
79. Morris, I. G. (1968): γ-globulin absorption in the newborn. In: *Handbook of Physiology, Section 6, Alimentary Canal, Vol. III, Intestinal Absorption*, edited by C. F. Code, pp. 1491–1512. American Physiological Society, Washington, D.C.

80. Morris, B., and Morris, R. (1977): The digestion and transmission of labelled immunoglobulin G by enterocytes of the proximal and distal regions of the small intestine of young rats. *J. Physiol.*, 273:427–442.
81. Morris, B., and Morris, R. (1980): The effect of exogenous steroids and steroid inhibitors in IgG transmission in young rats. *Biol. Neonate*, 38:169–178.
82. Mosinger, B., Placer, Z., and Koldovsky, O. (1959): Passage of insulin through the wall of the gastrointestinal tract of the infant rat. *Nature*, 184:1245–1246.
83. Nordstrom, C., Dahlqvist, A., and Josefsson, L. (1968): Quantitative determination of enzymes in different parts of the villi and crypts of rat small intestine. Comparison of alkaline phosphatase, disaccharidases and dipeptidases. *J. Histochem. Cytochem.*, 15:713–721.
84. Orlic, D., and Lev, R. (1973): Fetal rat intestinal absorption of horseradish peroxidase from swallowed amniotic fluid. *J. Cell Biol.*, 56:106–119.
85. Rao, M. L., Rao, G. S., Eckel, J., and Breur, H. (1977): Factors involved in the uptake of corticosterone by rat liver cells. *Biochim. Biophys. Acta*, 500:322–332.
86. Raul, F., Kedinger, M., Simon, P. M., Grenier, J. F., and Haffen, K. (1981): Comparative in vivo and in vitro effect of mono- and disaccharides on intestinal brush border enzyme activities in suckling rats. *Biol. Neonate*, 39:200–207.
87. Raul, F., Simon, P. M., Kedinger, M., Grenier, J. F., and Haffen, K. (1978): Sucrase and lactase synthesis in suckling rat intestine in response to substrate administration. *Biol. Neonate*, 33:100–105.
88. Reddy, B. S., and Wostmann, B. S. (1966): Intestinal disaccharidase activities in the growing germfree and conventional rat. *Arch. Biochem. Biophys.*, 113:609–616.
89. Redman, R. S., and Sreebny, L. M. (1976): Changes in patterns of feeding activity, parotid secretory enzymes and plasma corticosterone in developing rats. *J. Nutr.*, 106:1295–1306.
90. Robberecht, P., Deschodt-Lanckman, M., Camus, J., Bruylands, J., and Christophe, J. (1971): Rat pancreatic hydrolases from birth to weaning. *Am. J. Physiol.*, 221:376–381.
91. Rodewald, R. (1970): Selective antibody transport in proximal small intestine of neonatal rat. *J. Cell Biol.*, 45:635–640.
92. Rubino, A., Zimbalatti, F., and Auricchio, S. (1964): Intestinal disaccharidase activities in adult and suckling rats. *Biochim. Biophys. Acta*, 92:305–311.
93. Samel, M. (1968): Thyroid function during postnatal development in the rat. *Gen. Comp. Endocrinol.*, 10:229–234.
94. Seetharam, B., Yeh, K. Y., and Alpers, D. H. (1980): Turnover of intestinal brush-border proteins during postnatal development in the rat. *Am. J. Physiol.*, 239:G524–G531.
95. Simon, P. M., Kedinger, M., Raul, F., Grenier, J. F., and Haffen, K. (1979): Developmental pattern of rat intestinal brush-border enzymic proteins along the villus-crypt axis. *Biochem. J.*, 178:407–413.
96. Simon, P. M., Kedinger, M., Raul, F., Grenier, J. F., and Haffen, K. (1982): Organ culture of suckling rat intestine: Comparative study of various hormones on brush border enzymes. *In Vitro*, 18:339–346.
97. Simon-Assmann, P. M., Kedinger, M., Grenier, J. F., and Haffen, K. (1982): Control of brush border enzymes by dexamethasone in the fetal rat intestine cultured in vitro. *J. Pediatr. Gastro. Nutr.*, 1:257–265.
98. Slaunwhite, W. R., Lockie, G. N., Back, N., and Sandberg, A. A. (1962): Inactivity in vivo of transcortin bound cortisol. *Science*, 125:1062–1063.
99. Tsuboi, K. K., Kwong, L. K., Ford, W. D. A., Colby, T., and Sunshine, P. (1981): Delayed ontogenic development in the bypassed ileum of the infant rat. *Gastroenterology*, 80:1550–1556.
100. Tsuboi, K. K., Kwong, L. K., Neu, J., and Sunshine, P. (1981): A proposed mechanism of normal intestinal lactase decline in the postweaned mammal. *Biochem. Biophys. Res. Commun.*, 101:645–652.
101. Williams, R. M., and Beck, F. (1969): A histochemical study of gut maturation. *J. Anat.*, 105:487–501.
102. Wysocki, S. J., and Segal, W. (1972): Influence of thyroid hormones on enzyme activities of myelinating rat central-nervous tissue. *Eur. J. Biochem.*, 28:183–189.
103. Yeh, K. Y., and Moog, F. (1974): Intestinal lactase activity in the suckling rat: Influence of hypophysectomy and thyroidectomy. *Science*, 182:77–79.

104. Yeh, K. Y., and Moog, F. (1977): Influence of the thyroid and adrenal glands on the growth of the intestine of the suckling rat, and on the development of intestinal alkaline phosphatase and disaccharidase activities. *J. Exp. Zool.*, 200:337–348.
105. Yeh, K. Y., and Moog, F. (1978): Hormonal influences on the growth and enzymic differentiation of the small intestine of the hypophysectomized rat. *Growth*, 42:495–504.

Intestinal Toxicology, edited by C. M. Schiller.
Raven Press, New York © 1984.

Absorption of Macromolecules by Mammalian Intestinal Epithelium

James G. Lecce

*Department of Animal Science, North Carolina State University,
Raleigh, North Carolina 27650*

NEONATES

Fetal development in most mammals takes place in a protective uterine environment. Birth thrusts the fetus out of an area of protection into one of hostility. After being born, the neonate is greeted by a myriad of challenges, including a need for an external source of nutrients and protection from potential microbial pathogens. Nature, in the guise of a mammary gland, supplies the neonate with both nutrients (milk) and passive immunity (immunoglobulins in colostrum and milk). Passive immunity can be both local (immunoglobulin bathing the gut lumen) and humoral (immunoglobulin absorbed from the gut into the blood) (7,23,36). This chapter focuses on how neonates acquire passive immunity postnatally and speculates on possible pathologic consequences of the absorption of macromolecules both in the neonate and in the adult, which has a remnant of the neonatal system.

How Do Neonatal Mammals Acquire Passive Humoral Immunity Postnatally?

There are two major avenues available for the absorption of macromolecules, such as immunoglobulin G (IgG), by the neonatal intestine. One is receptor-mediated endocytosis and the other is nonreceptor-mediated endocytosis (14).

Receptor-Mediated Endocytosis

Coated pits and vesicles are involved in receptor-mediated endocytosis (14,44). Clathrin, with a molecular weight 180,000, is the major structural protein of coated pits and vesicles (44,48). Clathrin defines the cytoplasmic side of endocytotic organelles by enclosing them in a lattice of pentamers and hexamers. Finally, a polyhedral vesicle is produced. This polygone resembles a soccer ball and appears in transmission electronmicrographs like a vesicle surrounded by knobby projections.

In receptor-mediated endocytosis, it is conjectured that specific protein receptors are randomly dispersed in the lipid bilayer of the plasmalemma (43). Clathrin floats freely beneath this bilayer (Fig. 1A). To initiate internalization, the macromolecule

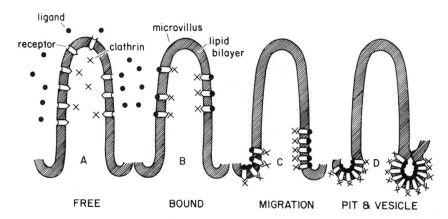

FIG. 1. Microvilli of enterocytes depicting selective internalization of macromolecules in clathrin-coated pits. **A:** Receptor randomly dispersed in lipid bilayer of microvillus, clathrin floats freely beneath the bilayer, and the ligand (IgG) is in the gut lumen. **B:** Ligand binds to luminal side of receptor, which in turn promotes binding of clathrin to the other end. **C:** Ligand-receptor-clathrin complexes migrate down and cluster at the base of the microvillus. **D:** Clustering at the base induces invagination of plasmalemma, forming a coated pit that pinches off into a coated vesicle (43).

or the ligand binds to its receptor. This in turn promotes the binding of clathrin to the other end of the receptor (Fig. 1B). Next, ligand-receptor-clathrin complexes cluster at the base of the microvillus (Fig. 1C), causing the plasmalemma to invaginate or pit (Fig. 1D). The coated pit pinches off forming a coated submicroscopic vesicle that then traverses the cell and fuses with the basal lateral membrane (Fig. 2). Finally, the microvesicle undergoes reverse pinocytosis (exocytosis). This results in the discharge of the ligand into extracellular space (60,61).

Nonreceptor-Mediated Endocytosis

In the case of nonreceptor-mediated endocytosis, the macromolecules are trapped within a submicroscopic apical tubular system which is contiguous with the plasmalemma (Fig. 2) (60,61). The trapped macromolecule flows down the tubule, eventually reaching a blind end in the apical cytoplasm. The blind end pinches off and forms a microvesicle (phagosome) that fuses with other microvesicles, producing a macrovesicle that is visible by light microscopy. These macrovesicles join lysosomes, becoming phagolysosomes. Intracellular digestion is the most probable fate of macromolecules internalized by this nonselective route.

Another mechanism (not involved in acquiring passive immunity) exists for transporting macromolecules across the intestinal epithelium. In this route, M cells absorb macromolecules (soluble antigens, bacteria, viruses, etc.) through endocytosis (9,46,47,64). M cells are specialized cells sandwiched between enterocytes overlying Peyer's patches. These cells may be responsible for initiating a local immune response by transferring antigens from the gut lumen to the lymphoid

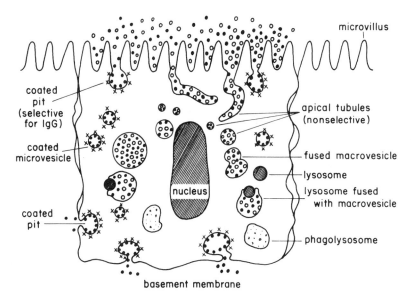

FIG. 2. Enterocyte depicting selective transport (IgG) in coated pits and vesicles. Nonselective internalization and digestion [IgG (●) and albumin (○)] in noncoated apical tubules, macrovesicles, phagosomes, and phagolysosomes (60,61).

tissue in the Peyer's patches. Whether M cells absorb macromolecules by receptor- or nonreceptor-mediated endocytosis is not yet known.

When Do Neonatal Mammals Acquire Passive Humoral Immunity?

Neonatal mammals can be divided into three groups based on when they acquire passive humoral immunity (7,23). Group I mammals acquire passive immunity exclusively postpartum; some examples are pigs, horses, ruminants. Group II mammals acquire passive immunity both pre- and postpartum; examples are mice, rats, hamsters, dogs, cats. Group III mammals acquire passive immunity exclusively prepartum and include humans, other primates, guinea pigs.

Group I: Exclusively Postnatally

Neonates in this category nonselectively absorb macromolecules for a short period postpartum.

Enterocytes on the intestinal epithelium of neonates in Group I nonselectively transport macromolecules from the lumen of the gut into the blood for about 2 days postpartum (1,7,8,23,26,30). However, enterocytes continue to internalize (but do not transport) macromolecules nonselectively for a much longer period. Because of the dichotomy between internalization and transport, the absorption of macromolecules is divided into two phases: (a) uptake or internalization within the enterocyte and (b) transport through the enterocyte. The period after which enterocytes can no longer internalize macromolecules is called "closure" (8,26,27,31).

In the neonatal pig, dietary regimens influence both cessation of transport and closure (21,22,26,27,31,32). For example, piglets denied food from birth transport macromolecules from the gut into the blood for as long as they live (about 3.5 days). Whereas, nursing pigs eating about 300 ml of colostrum or milk cease transporting within 24 hr postpartum (32). It appears as though eating stimulates the release of a humoral signal (hormone) which turns off transport. The reason for suspecting a humoral signal stems from the observation that an intestinal segment isolated surgically at birth from the digestive pathway (Theary-Vealy loops) ceases transporting macromolecules at the same time as the gut remaining in the digestive pathway (21). Although transport is qualitatively nonselective, the process is energy-dependent (24) and preferential; i.e., more immunoglobulin is transported than albumin when ligated segments of neonatal gut are injected with a solution containing both albumin and IgG. Also, the upper half of the small intestine transports more efficiently than the lower half. And, enterocytes in the lower half have more lysosomal-like proteolytic activity (22).

As mentioned above, by the time the pig has nursed for 2 days, the intestine can no longer transport macromolecules; however, the lower half of the small intestine can still internalize them. As the pig ages, more and more of the small intestine (proceeding toward the ileum) ceases internalizing macromolecules. Finally, by 2 to 3 weeks of age all enterocytes, throughout the length of the small intestine, are closed and the pig can not internalize macromolecules (26). As with transport, dietary regimens affect the time of closure. And, the signal for closure again seems to be humoral, since an intestinal segment surgically removed from the digestive pathway, as above, closes at the same time as its counterpart in the digestive pathway (20). Position of the gut in the digestive pathway does not affect closure since ileal sections surgically relocated, shortly after the pig is born, to the upper jejunum do not precociously close but close at the normal time (21).

Histological studies show that enterocytes capable of transporting macromolecules have a submicroscopic noncoated interconnecting tubule system that traverses the enterocytes from plasmalemma to the basal lateral membrane (Fig. 3) (18). These kinds of enterocytes are found mainly in the upper third of the small intestines of newborn pigs. In the lower third of the small intestines of the newborn pigs, enterocytes mainly internalize macromolecules for digestion (Fig. 4). These enterocytes have a few apical tubules and many small vacuoles which appear to fuse, eventually producing a large macroscopic vacuole. Enterocytes in the mid small intestines of newborn pigs contain numerous apical tubules and vacuoles, indicating that they are both internalizing and transporting macromolecules (Fig. 5).

Thus, the neonatal pig has enterocytes that transport macromolecules (mainly upper small intestines), enterocytes that internalize and digest macromolecules (mainly lower small intestines), and enterocytes that do both (mainly mid small intestines). At about 2 days of age, neonatal pigs cease transporting macromolecules from the gut lumen to the blood. At this time, they cease internalizing macromol-

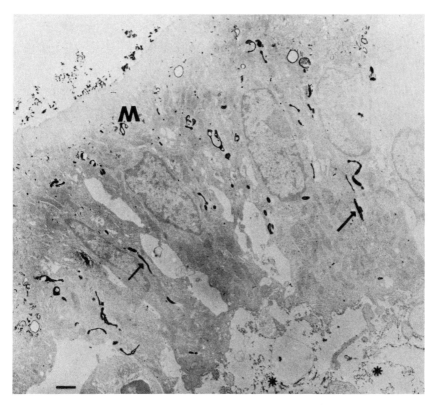

FIG. 3. Transmission electron micrograph of horseradish peroxidase-immunoglobulin G complex (HRP-IgG) in enterocytes of proximal small intestine of a newborn pig. Numerous tubules filled with HRP-IgG are present in the enterocytes *(arrows)*. HRP-IgG is also present in the lamina propria (*). Bar 1 μm (18). Microvilli (M).

ecules in enterocytes in the upper half of the small intestines. They continue to internalize nonselectively macromolecules in the ileal area for 2 more weeks. Both time of cessation of transport and closure are influenced by a humoral signal induced by eating. The separation of transport from digestion would be of value to a neonate requiring intact protein for transport (IgG) and digested protein for amino acid building blocks.

The pig is the most extensively studied neonate in Group I; however, other neonates in this group are also known to nonselectively transport macromolecules. But, in one member of the group (calves), diet does not seem to influence the cessation of transport of macromolecules.

Group II: Prenatal and Postnatal

Neonates in this category selectively absorb macromolecules for an extended period of time, e.g., rats for 21 days, mice for 17 days, and hamsters for 7 days postpartum (7,25,27).

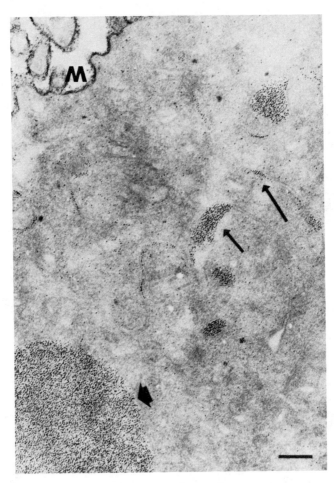

FIG. 4. Transmission electron micrograph of ferritin in the luminal portion of an enterocyte in distal small intestine of a newborn pig. Microvilli (M) at top left. Tubules *(arrows)* and a large vacuole *(arrowhead)* filled with the marker are present. Bar 2 μm (18).

Rats and mice have been extensively studied regarding this phenomenon, and as in the pig, absorption can be divided into a transport phase and an internalization phase. But unlike the pig, the transport in rats and mice occurs exclusively in the upper third of the small intestines and is selective for IgG (25,37,50). The lower third of the small intestine nonselectively internalizes macromolecules and the mid third does both.

Clathrin-like coated pits, coated vesicles, and Fc-receptors for IgG have been associated with an apical tubular system in enterocytes located in the upper part of the small intestines but not with the apical tubular system in the enterocytes in

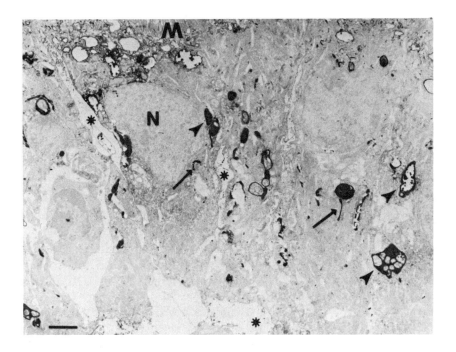

FIG. 5. Transmission electron micrograph of horseradish peroxidase-immunoglobulin complex (HRP-IgG) in enterocytes of mid small intestine of a newborn pig. Microvilli (M) at top center. Tubules *(arrows)* as well as vacuoles *(arrowheads)* are present near the nucleus (N) of one enterocyte. HRP-IgG can also be seen in lateral spaces (*) and lamina propria (*). Bar 1 μm (18).

the ileal area (35,50,60–62). Thus, it seems that IgG is routed through the enterocyte of the upper gut in coated submicroscopic vesicles (60,61) and tubules to the basal lateral membrane, a process not too different from the pig except that the neonatal rat's enterocytes absorb selectively via clathrin-coated organelles.

Enterocytes in the lower part of the small intestine internalize macromolecules nonselectively in uncoated submicroscopic vesicles that fuse with others. Eventually, as with the ileal area in the pig, these fusing vesicles produce a macroscopic vesicle that appears to join the supranuclear vacuole (60). Thus, the internalization of macromolecules in the ileal area leads to the digestion or storage of the macromolecules rather than transport. Again, compartmentation is an elegant way to reconcile the neonate's distinct needs for intact immunoglobulin for transport into the blood and digested proteins for building blocks. Cessation of transport and closure occur at the same time, which is coincident with weaning. These phenomena may be under adrenal hormone control in that glucocorticoids (at unphysiologically high levels) can precociously initiate closure provided the neonate's adrenals have reached the proper maturational state (15,38,39).

Group III: Exclusively Prenatally

Neonates in this category lack the capacity to transport macromolecules post-natally in an appreciable amount (7).

Even though neonates in this group do not transport macromolecules in appreciable amounts, perhaps they can internalize and digest macromolecules for a short period. This notion is supported by evidence from research using guinea pigs. Guinea pigs can nonselectively internalize macromolecules for about 2 days post-natally (27,51). Pinocytotic macrovesicles are present in enterocytes during the internalization phase and probably contribute to the digestion of soluble protein in this early neonatal period (27). Thus, enterocytes in the neonatal guinea pig have internalizing and digesting organelles that are similar to those seen in the neonates in categories I and II.

There are reports of small amounts of antibody transported by the nursing human infant's gut (17,45). Interestingly, the human infant's gut during fetal development undergoes maturational changes analogous to those seen postnatally in pigs and rats (2,34,40–42). These structural changes are apical tubules that appear in enterocytes throughout the entire length of the small intestine at the time villi are formed, around 10 weeks of gestation. (This same kind of structure is seen in the suckling rat and newborn pig as noted above.) Apical tubules and lysosomal elements are more numerous in the lower third of the intestine (again, like the suckling rat and pig). By 22 weeks gestation, apical tubules disappear, and enterocytes in the upper area of the small intestine resemble adult-type enterocytes (a pattern seen in a 2- to 8-day-old pig). At term, or shortly thereafter, the infant's gut is replete with adult-type enterocytes. Although fetal enterocytes in the human seem capable of internalizing macromolecules, there is some doubt regarding the capacity of these enterocytes to transport macromolecules through the cell in an appreciable amount (42).

ADULTS

Normal

Formerly, the mature gut was thought to be relatively impermeable to the absorption of macromolecules. More recently, investigators using a highly sensitive enzymatic macromolecular marker (horseradish peroxidase) have found evidence for transport of this macromolecule through adult rat and rabbit enterocytes (10,16,54,59). Horseradish peroxidase injected into ligated segments of adult jejunum was visualized histochemically within enterocytes in an apical tubular system. Further, this marker was transmitted into the extracellular space of the lamina propria. Others, using horseradish peroxidase and lactoperoxidase, have detected an apical tubular system in enterocytes that are on villi in organ-cultured adult human small intestine (4–6). The feeling is that adult enterocytes internalize macromolecules in a manner analogous to that described for the neonatal rat except that the apical tubular system is less well developed in the adult (10,54,59).

Thus, there is evidence that low levels of macromolecules (antigens) can breach the adult mucosal barrier. They can be absorbed nonselectively by enterocytes via an apical tubular system (which may be a vestige of the neonatal system) or they can be absorbed by M cells.

Abnormal

In the normal adult, low-level absorption of macromolecules does not seem to be a threat to health (53,55). However, disease could result if increased quantities of antigens or toxic substances were absorbed. For example, in adults with gastric and pancreatic insufficiency, macromolecules are less efficiently digested. Thus, higher concentration of macromolecules would be presented to the enterocytes. Therefore, more macromolecules would likely be absorbed (19,52,53,55,58). Also, an increase in absorption would occur if intracellular digestion was decreased because of faulty lysosomes. Mucosa that no longer functions as a viable structure (radiation damage) could serve as a source of the passively transmitted macromolecules. Increased absorption of macromolecules could result from an immune deficiency. In this case, secretory antibodies capable of reacting with antigens and thereby blocking their absorption would be lacking (12,13,56,57). It has been reported that certain diseases—e.g., celiac disease, allergic gastroenteropathies, inflammatory bowel disease, viral and bacterial enteritis, parasitic infestations of the gut, and radiation enteritis—may be associated with increased absorption and transport of macromolecules (3,53,55).

CONCLUSION

Neonatal mammals have a mechanism for absorbing macromolecules. The normal function of the mechanism is to absorb physiologically useful macromolecules such as immunoglobulins. However, if the neonate is ill-managed and placed in an environment replete with toxic macromolecules, then the potential exists for absorbing these toxins. In the neonatal period when the pig and mouse have an immature intestinal epithelium, they are more susceptible to enteric pathogens like *Escherichia coli* and rotavirus, and they can internalize toxins like endotoxins from gram-negative rods (11,28,29,33,49,63). As the intestine matures and can no longer absorb macromolecules, these animals become less susceptible to these enteropathogens.

A remnant of the neonatal system for absorbing macromolecules exists in the adult. Thus, adults can absorb macromolecules at a low level. In the normal adult, the absorption of insignificant quantities of macromolecules produces no ill effects. However, if alteration in the intraluminal digestive process occurs or if the mucosal barrier becomes defective, then increased quantities of antigenic or toxic substances could gain entrance to the body, resulting in local intestinal or systemic disorders.

REFERENCES

1. Balconi, I. R., and Lecce, J. G. (1966): Intestinal absorption of homologous lactic dehydrogenase isoenzyme by the neonatal pig. *J. Nutr.*, 88:233–238.

2. Bierring, F., Andersen, H., Egeberg, J., Bro-Rasmussen, F., and Matthiessen, M. (1964): On the nature of the meconium corpuscles in human foetal intestinal epithelium. I. Electron microscopic studies. *Acta Pathol. Microbiol. Scand.*, 61:365–376.

3. Bloch, K. J., Bloch, D. B., Stearns, M., and Walker, W. A. (1979): Intestinal uptake of macromolecules. VI. Uptake of protein antigen *in vivo* in normal rats and rats infected with *Nippostrongylus brasiliensis* or subjected to mild systemic anaphylaxis. *Gastroenterology*, 77:1039–1044.

4. Blok, J., Mulder-Stapel, A. A., Ginsel, L. A., and Daems, W. Th. (1981a): The effect of chloroquine on lysosomal function and cell-coat glycoprotein transport in the absorptive cells of cultured human small-intestinal tissue. *Cell Tissue Res.*, 218:227–251.

5. Blok, J., Mulder-Stapel, A. A., Ginsel, L. A., and Daems, W. Th. (1981b): Endocytosis in absorptive cells of cultured human small-intestinal tissue: horseradish peroxidase, lactoperoxidase and ferritin as markers. *Cell Tissue Res.*, 216:1–13.

6. Blok, J., Scheven, B. A. A., Mulder-Stapel, A. A., Ginsel, L. A., and Daems, W. Th. (1982): Endocytosis in absorptive cells of cultured human small-intestinal tissue: Effect of cytochalasin B and D. *Cell Tissue Res.*, 222:113–126.

7. Brambell, F. W. R. (1958): The passive immunity of the young mammal. *Biol. Rev.*, 33:488–531.

8. Broughton, C. W., and Lecce, J. G. (1970): Electron-microscopic studies of the jejunal epithelium from neonatal pigs fed different diets. *J. Nutr.*, 100:445–449.

9. Bukinskaya, A. G. (1982): Penetration of viral genetic material into host cell. *Adv. Virus Res.*, 27:141–199.

10. Cornell, R., Walker, W. A., and Isselbacher, K. J. (1971): Small intestinal absorption of horseradish peroxidase: A cytochemical study. *Lab. Invest.*, 25:42–48.

11. Crawford, P. C., and Lecce, J. G. (1979): Internalization of endotoxin (LPS) by enterocytes of neonatal pigs inoculated with *Escherichia coli.* (abstract) *Proc. 79th Annual Meeting A. Soc. Microbiol.*, p. 24.

12. Cunningham-Rundles, C., Brandeis, W. E., Good, R. A., and Day, N. K. (1978): Milk precipitins, circulating immune complexes and IgA deficiency. *Proc. Natl. Acad. Sci. USA*, 75:3387–3389.

13. Cunningham-Rundles, C., Brandeis, W. E., Good, R. A., and Day, N. K. (1979): Bovine antigens and the formation of circulating immune complexes in selective immunoglobulin A deficiency. *J. Clin. Invest.*, 64:272–279.

14. Goldstein, J. L., Anderson, R. G. W., and Brown, M. S. (1979): Coated pits, coated vesicles, and receptor-mediated endocytosis. *Nature.* 279:679–685.

15. Halliday, R. (1959): The effect of steroid hormones on the absorption of antibodies by the young rat. *J. Endocr.*, 18:56–66.

16. Heyman, M., Ducroc, R., Desjeux, J. -F., and Morgat, J. L. (1982): Horseradish peroxidase transport across adult rabbit jejunum in vitro. *Am. J. Physiol.*, 242:G558–G564.

17. Iyengar, L., and Selvaraj, R. J. (1972): Intestinal absorption of immunoglobulins by newborn infants. *Arch. Dis. Child.*, 47:411–414.

18. King, M. W., and Lecce, J. G. (1983): Transport of macromolecules through enterocytes of the neonatal piglet intestine. *(in press).*

19. Kraft, S. C., Rothberg, R. M., Knauer, C. M., Svoboda, A. C., Monroe, L. S., and Farr, R. S. (1967): Gastric acid output and circulating antibovine serum albumin in adults. *Clin. Exp. Immunol.*, 2:321–330.

20. Leary, H. L., and Lecce, J. G. (1976): Uptake of macromolecules by enterocytes on transposed and isolated piglet small intestine. *J. Nutr.*, 106:419–427.

21. Leary, H. L., and Lecce, J. G. (1978): The effect of feeding on the cessation of transport and macromolecules by enterocytes of neonatal piglet intestine. *Biol. Neonat.*, 34:174–178.

22. Leary, H. L., and Lecce, J. G. (1979): The preferential transport of immunoglobulin G by the small intestine of the neonatal pig. *J. Nutr.*, 109:458–466.

23. Lecce, J. G. (1966): Absorption of macromolecules by neonatal intestine. *Biol. Neonat.*, 9:50–61.

24. Lecce, J. G. (1966): In vitro absorption of γ-globulin by neonatal intestinal epithelium of the pig. *J. Physiol.*, 184:594–604.

25. Lecce, J. G. (1972): Selective absorption of macromolecules into intestinal epithelium and blood by neonatal mice. *J. Nutr.*, 102:69–76.

26. Lecce, J. G. (1973): Effect of dietary regimen on cessation of uptake of macromolecules by piglets intestinal epithelium (closure) and transport to the blood. *J. Nutr.*, 103:751–756.

27. Lecce, J. G., and Broughton, C. W. (1973): Cessation of uptake of macromolecules by neonatal guinea pig, hamster and rabbit intestinal epithelium (closure). *J. Nutr.*, 103:744–750.
28. Lecce, J. G., and King, M. W. (1978): Role of rotavirus(reo-like) in weanling diarrhea of pigs. *J. Clin. Microbiol.*, 8:454–458.
29. Lecce, J. G., King, M. W., and Mock, R. (1976): Reovirus-like agent associated with fatal diarrhea in neonatal pigs. *Infect. Immunol.*, 14:816–825.
30. Lecce, J. G., Matrone, G., and Morgan, D. O. (1961): Porcine Neonatal Nutrition: The absorption of unsaltered non-porcine proteins and polyvinylpyrrolidone from the gut of piglets and the subsequent effect of the maturation of the serum protein profile. *J. Nutr.*, 73:158–166.
31. Lecce, J. G., and Morgan, D. O. (1962): The effect of dietary regimen on the cessation of absorption of large molecules (closure) in the neonatal piglet and lamb. *J. Nutr.*, 78:263–268.
32. Lecce, J. G., Morgan, D. O., and Matrone, G. (1964): Effect of feeding colostral and milk components on the cessation of intestinal absorption of large molecules (closure) in neonatal pigs. *J. Nutr.*, 84:43–48.
33. Lecce, J. G., and Reep, B. R. (1962): *Escherichia coli* associated with colostrum-free neonatal pigs raised in isolation. *J. Exp. Med.*, 115:491–501.
34. Lev, R., Siegel, H. I., and Bartman, J. (1972): Histochemical studies of developing human fetal small intestine. *Histochemie*, 29:103–119.
35. Mackenzie, N. M., Morris, B., and Morris, R. (1983): Protein binding to brush borders of enterocytes from the jejunum of the neonatal rat. *Biochim. Biophys. Acta*, 755:204–209.
36. McNabb, P. C., and Tomasi, T. B. (1981): Host defense mechanisms at mucosal surfaces. *Annu. Rev. Microbiol.*, 35:477–496.
37. Morris, B., and Morris, R. (1974): The absorption of ^{125}I-labelled immunoglobulin G by different regions of the gut in young rats. *J. Physiol.*, 241:761–770.
38. Morris, B., and Morris, R. (1976): The effect of corticosterone and cortisone on the transmission of IgG and the uptake of polyvinyl pyrrolidone by the small intestine in young rats. *J. Physiol.*, 255:619–634.
39. Morris, B., Morris, R., and Kenyon, C. J. (1981): Effect of adrenalectomy on the transmission of IgG in young rats. *Biol. Neonat.*, 39:239–245.
40. Moxey, P. C. (1978): Specialized cell types in the human fetal small intestine. *Anat. Rec.*, 191:269–286.
41. Moxey, P. C., and Trier, J. S. (1975): Structural features of the mucosa of human fetal intestine. *Gastroenterology*, 68:102 (Abstract).
42. Moxey, P. C., and Trier, J. S. (1979): Development of villus absorptive cells in the human fetal small intestine: A morphological and morphometric study. *Anat. Rec.*, 195:463–482.
43. Ockleford, C. D., and Munn, E. A. (1980): Dynamic aspects of coated vesicle function. In: *Coated Vesicles*, edited by C. D. Ockleford and A. Whyte, pp. 265. Cambridge University Press, Cambridge, United Kingdom.
44. Ockleford, C. D., and Whyte, A., editors (1980): *Coated Vesicles*. Cambridge University Press, Cambridge, United Kingdom.
45. Ogra, S. S., Weintraub, D. and Ogra, P. L. (1977): Immunologic aspects of human colostrum and milk. III. Fate and absorption of cellular and soluble components in the gastrointestinal tract of the newborn. *J. Immunol.*, 119:245–248.
46. Owen, R. L. (1977): Sequential uptake of horseradish peroxidase by lymphoid follicle epithelium of Peyer's patches in the normal unobstructed mouse intestine: An ultrastructure study. *Gastroenterology*, 72:440–451.
47. Owen, R. L., and Jones, A. L. (1974): Epithelial cell specialization within human Peyer's patches: An ultrastructural study of intestinal lymphoid follicles. *Gastroenterology*, 66:189–203.
48. Pearse, B. M. F. (1978): On the structural and functional components of coated vesicles. *J. Mol. Biol.*, 126:803–812.
49. Riepenhoff-Talty, M., Lee, P. -C., Carmody, P. J., Barrett, H. J., and Ogra, P. L. (1982): Age-dependent rotavirus-enterocyte interactions. *Proc. Soc. Exp. Biol. Med.*, 170:146–154.
50. Rodewald, R. (1970): Selective antibody transport in the proximal small intestine of the neonatal rat. *J. Cell Biol.*, 45:635–640.
51. Rundell, J. O., and Lecce, J. G. (1978): Relationship of incorporation of radioprecursors into protein and phospholipids of the plasmalemma of guinea pig (neonate) intestinal epithelium and the cessation of uptake of macromolecules (closure). *Biol. Neonat.*, 34:278–285.

52. Saffran, M., Franco-Saenz, R., Kong, A., Papahadjopoulos, D., and Szoka, F. (1979): A model for the study of the oral administration of peptide hormones. *Can. J. Biochem.*, 57:548–553.
53. Udall, J. N., and Walker, W. A. (1982): The physiologic and pathologic basis for the transport of macromolecules across the intestinal tract. *J. Pediatr. Gastroenterol. Nutr.*, 1:295–301.
54. Walker, W. A., Cornell, R., Davenport, L. M., and Isselbacher, K. J. (1972): Macromolecular absorption: Mechanism of horseradish peroxidase uptake and transport in adult and neonatal rat intestine. *J. Cell Biol.*, 54:195–205.
55. Walker, W. A., and Isselbacher, K. J. (1974): Uptake and transport of macromolecules by the intestine. Possible role in clinical disorders. *Gastroenterology*, 67:531–549.
56. Walker, W. A., and Isselbacher, K. J. (1977): Intestinal antibodies. *N. Engl. J. Med.*, 297:767–773.
57. Walker, W. A., Isselbacher, K. J., and Bloch, K. J. (1972): Intestinal uptake of macromolecules: Effect of oral immunization. *Science*, 177:608–610.
58. Walker, W. A., Wu, M., Isselbacher, K. J., and Bloch, K. J. (1975): Intestinal uptake of macromolecules. IV. The effect of pancreatic duct ligation on the breakdown of antigen and antigen-antibody complexes on the intestinal surface. *Gastroenterology*, 69:1223–1229.
59. Warshaw, A. L., Walker, W. A., and Isselbacher, K. J. (1974): Protein uptake by the intestine: Evidence for absorption of intact macromolecules. *Gastroenterology*, 66:987–992.
60. Wild, A. E. (1975): Role of the cell surface in selection during transport of proteins from mother to foetus and newly born. *Philos. Trans. R. Soc. Lond. B.*, 271:395–410.
61. Wild, A. E. (1980): Coated vesicles: A morphologically distinct subclass of endocytic vesicles. In: *Coated Vesicles*, edited by C. D. Ockleford and A. Whyte, p. 14. Cambridge University Press, Cambridge, United Kingdom.
62. Wild, A. E. (1981): Distribution of FC receptors on isolated gut enterocytes of the suckling rat. *J. Reprod. Immunol.*, 3:283–296.
63. Wolf, J. L., Cukor, G., Blacklow, N. R., Dambrauskas, R., and Trier, J. S. (1981): Susceptibility of mice to rotavirus infection: Effects of age and administration to corticosteroids. *Infect. Immun.*, 33:565–574.
64. Wolf, J. L., Rubin, D. H., Finberg, R., Kauffman, R. S., Sharpe, A. H., Trier, J. S., and Fields, B. N. (1981): Intestinal M cells: A pathway for entry of reovirus into the host. *Science*, 212:471–472.

Intestinal Toxicology, edited by C. M. Schiller.
Raven Press, New York © 1984.

Peyer's Patch Epithelium: An Imperfect Barrier[1]

M. E. LeFevre and D. D. Joel

Medical Research Center, Brookhaven National Laboratory, Upton, New York 11973

In carrying out its digestive and absorptive functions, the gastrointestinal mucosa encounters not only degradable foodstuffs but also nondegradable macromolecules and particles. The latter classes of substances may be ingested with food and drink, or they may be inhaled and subsequently cleared from the lungs and swallowed. Until recently, the penetration of such nonnutrient material through the mucosal surface of the gut was considered to be of little importance except for the special case of the penetration of pathogenic microorganisms. This situation is now changing. Developments in the field of intestinal immunity together with emerging problems in environmental contamination have led to new questions on the uptake of antigenic and toxic particulate material from the gut. The wide attention given recently to the question of asbestos penetration through the gastrointestinal mucosa is a pertinent example (8,12,14,16,20,24,45).

Immunological and toxicological studies involving the gut tend to focus on different sites of absorption. In toxicological studies, absorption of test substances is usually assumed to take place through all (or at least a large part) of the mucosal epithelium that lines the small intestine. Recent immunological work, however, has focused on absorption through the small fraction of the mucosa that overlies the gut-associated lymphoid tissue (GALT). In the 1970s several groups of immunologically oriented investigators (4,5,23,25,26,39) noted that the GALT epithelium was penetrated by various colloids and protein antigens, findings that corroborated earlier, little-known observations of Kagan (27) and Kumagai (31). In this review, an attempt is made to merge the disparate immunological and toxicological viewpoints; and it is suggested that the quantitatively small portion of the gut mucosa associated with the GALT may contribute disproportionately to the uptake of toxic macromolecules and particulate matter as well as protein antigens.

GUT-ASSOCIATED LYMPHOID TISSUE

The GALT are discrete masses of lymphoid cells located in the wall of the gastrointestinal tract. They differ from diffusely scattered lymphoid cells, present

---

[1]The research described in this chapter involved animals maintained in animal care facilities fully accredited by the American Association for Accreditation of Laboratory Animal Care.

throughout the tract, in their intricate arrangement. This discussion is limited to a type of GALT found in the mammalian small intestine, the Peyer's patches, seen as small protrusions on the antimesenteric border.

Peyer's patches consist of clusters of lymphoid follicles, each of which normally contains a germinal center, surrounding zones of small lymphocytes, and a subepithelial "dome" (Fig.1) (17,63). The germinal center is situated toward the base of the follicle; its prominent features are dividing cells and large macrophages. The dividing cells are B lymphocytes, as are the cells making up the cuff surrounding the germinal center (2). The lateral and interfollicular zones are populated by T lymphocytes, and the dome by macrophages, plasma cells, and both T and B lymphocytes. In histological preparations of the gut wall, an obliquely sectioned Peyer's patch often appears to have no connection with the mucosal epithelium. Illustrations of such sections are found in many texts and atlases (9,18,32,46), and they may lead to the erroneous impression that Peyer's patches are buried deep in the gut wall and are not associated with the epithelial layer. A central, vertically oriented section through the center of a follicle, however, will show that the lymphoid cell mass extends to the epithelial layer. The "Peyer's patch epithelium" is a single cell layer that faces the intestinal lumen and acts as a barrier between gut contents and the cells of the patch.

Peyer's patches from species as divergent as man and mouse are similar, differing primarily in the number of follicles clustered together. In large animals Peyer's patches can reach considerable size, e.g., 6 ft in the distal ileum of the pig (56). The Peyer's patch epithelium, however, comprises only a small percentage of the total surface area of the small intestine. The appearance of the patch epithelium differs from that of nearby villi, often seeming flattened and disorganized. Goblet

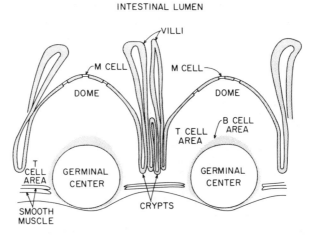

FIG. 1. Diagrammatic representation of a Peyer's patch consisting of two follicles. M cells are enlarged for emphasis. Villi adjacent to follicles tend to be club-shaped. Smooth-muscle layers become attenuated and may disappear entirely beneath follicles. See text for additional details.

cells are reduced in number (3,17), and the epithelium may become infiltrated with lymphocytes (1,44).

Functionally the Peyer's patches are secondary lymphoid organs that are involved in initiating immune responses to certain types of orally ingested antigens (13). They are a source of immunoglobulin A (IgA) precursor cells, which enter the circulation, undergo maturation and division in mesenteric lymph nodes and other tissues, and eventually home to the lamina propria of the gastrointestinal tract (15,19,28,38,48). The production of IgA precursor cells in Peyer's patches is stimulated by the intake and transport of antigenic material from the gut lumen and its delivery to cells within the patch (39). Specialized epithelial cells, discussed in the next section, are believed to be involved in this intake and transfer. The process of bringing in the antigenic material through the epithelium has been called the "sampling" of intestinal contents; it is functionally important in that it provides for controlled contact between antigens in the gut lumen and immunologically responsive cells (4,13,28,39). The passage of toxic substances through the mucosa may be an inadvertent by-product of the sampling process; however, the macro-phages of the dome probably phagocytize and inactivate many kinds of noxious materials. In overall function, the Peyer's patches appear to constitute a system for processing intestinal antigens with little risk to the rest of the body.

M CELLS

Because of their importance in facilitating the penetration of antigenic macro-molecules, the specialized epithelial cells of Peyer's patches are of particular interest. These cells were first described by Bockman and Cooper (5,6,) and were termed the "follicle-associated epithelial (FAE) cells." They were later called "M cells" by Owen and collaborators (41). Owen and Neminac (42) have presented a cogent argument for the adoption of the term M cell, with the reservation of FAE to denote the entire Peyer's patch epithelium (of which M cells are only one component).

M cells are characterized by irregular microvilli or microfolds, numerous vesi-cles, and close association with intraepithelial lymphocytes (Fig. 2). They are true epithelial cells, ultimately derived from proliferating crypt cells (52,53). Whether or not fully differentiated enterocytes become M cells is currently being questioned (10).

Like other epithelial cells, M cells are connected to adjacent cells by tight junctions and desmosomes. They are not susceptible to microbial penetration in general (42), but have recently been shown to endocytose noninvasive *Vibrio cholerae* in the rabbit (43). Owen (39) described their involvement in the passage of horseradish peroxidase (HRP) into Peyer's patches. He reported that HRP was found in vesicles in M cells but not in nearby columnar cells of mouse Peyer's patches 5 min after HRP introduction into the lumen. After 1 hr HRP was detected in intercellular spaces adjacent to M cells as well as within M cell-enfolded lymphocytes. HRP penetration was further characterized by von Rosen et al. (62);

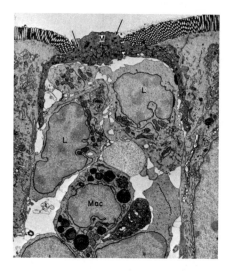

FIG. 2. Electron micrograph of murine Peyer's patch epithelium showing an M cell (M) stretched over a group of lymphoid cells (L) and a macrophage (Mac). Apical surface of the M cell lacks microvilli. *Arrows* mark vesicles containing exogenously administered horseradish peroxidase. (Courtesy of Dr. R. L. Owen, ref. 40.)

the transport of cholera toxin (51) and reovirus (66) through the cytoplasm of M cells has also been shown. In man M cells have been demonstrated in the appendix (7) and in Peyer's patches (41).

PEYER'S PATCH UPTAKE OF PARTICULATE MATTER

The evidence that the Peyer's patch epithelium permits the entry of some macromolecules via the M-cell pathway is overwhelming, although it remains to be determined whether or not M cells take up all classes of ambient macromolecules from the intestinal lumen. In addition, the Peyer's patch epithelium permits penetration of certain types of inert particles. We have demonstrated the accumulation of colloidal carbon and polymeric microspheres (latex particles) in Peyer's patches of mice that ingested the particles (25,26,35–37).

CARBON

Our experiments with carbon particles involved exposure of young adult mice to carbon with subsequent histological demonstration of the particles in tissues (25,26). The carbon particles (Guenther Wagner, Pelikan-Werke, Hanover, West Germany) had a nominal size of 20 to 50 nm (manufacturer's information), but many were present as aggregates. The actual range of particle size was very great.

An important aspect of carbon-particle uptake into Peyer's patches was its cumulative nature. Because of this, chronic experiments in which mice were given carbon suspensions as drinking water were more informative than short-term experiments in which mice were gavaged once or twice with particles. Carbon, which was detected with difficulty at 2 days, was found with ease at 2 months. As illustrated in Fig. 3, carbon deposits were grossly visible in Peyer's patches at this time. The photomicrograph shows a single Peyer's patch follicle containing a mass of finely divided carbon in the subepithelial region. Dense aggregates are scattered

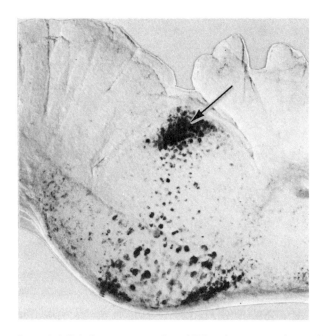

FIG. 3. Peyer's patch follicle from a mouse given 1.5% carbon suspension as drinking water for 2 months. Black carbon particles are abundant in the dome *(arrow)* and at the base of the follicle. Particle aggregates are scattered throughout the follicle, becoming larger and denser toward the base. The barely visible follicle epithelium and the absorptive villi on either side of the follicle contain little or no carbon. Unstained preparation. × 60.

throughout the follicle; most of these are individual carbon-laden macrophages. The germinal center is not visible in this unstained preparation, but two large carbon accumulations demarcate its basal borders.

In the intestines of mice that ingested carbon-containing water for 2 months, particle accumulations such as those illustrated in Fig. 3 were specifically localized in Peyer's patches. They were not visible in the absorptive villi except occasionally in the lamina propria of villi immediately adjacent to Peyer's patches. Even after 6 months of carbon ingestion, mice rarely exhibited carbon particles in the lamina propria of absorptive villi. At this time, however, small black foci barely visible to the naked eye were randomly distributed along the entire length of the small intestine. These were more numerous (150–200 per intestine) than Peyer's patches (10–15 per intestine). Microscopic examination revealed that the small foci were single lymphoid follicles containing carbon and having an epithelium similar to that of Peyer's patches (Fig.4). The presence of these individual follicles, also noted in other species by other investigators (21,29,41), indicates that the capability for particle uptake in the gut is widespread and would be difficult to eliminate. Although it is feasible to remove Peyer's patches surgically, it is not feasible to remove the isolated follicles without extirpation of the entire small intestine.

It required approximately 6 months for murine Peyer's patches to become maximally loaded with carbon particles (25). Additional accumulation was not apparent

fibers in 63% of livers from Duluth residents. Patel-Mandlik et al. (45) found chrysotile fibers in the kidney, liver, and spleen of a neonatal baboon that ingested asbestos in milk for 9 days. Earlier in the decade several investigators reported evidence of intestinal penetration by asbestos fibers in rodents (47,64). More recently Sebastien et al. (49) recovered asbestos fibers in thoracic duct lymph of asbestos-fed rats.

In view of the evidence for asbestos absorption described above, it was surprising to find a lack of asbestos accumulation in the Peyer's patches of mice that chronically drank water suspensions containing 1 mg/ml chrysotile asbestos (Joel and LeFevre, *unpublished data*). The suspensions were prepared as described by Pontrefact and Cunningham (47) and were ingested for 3 months. In addition, the life-span of mice that ingested like suspensions from the time of weaning was not significantly reduced (Joel, *unpublished data*). The median life-span of asbestos-ingesting mice was 19 months; that of controls was 20.5 months ($p > 0.2$, 100 asbestos-fed mice versus 100 controls). Furthermore, certain other chronically fed particles e.g., quartz and carmine, did not accumulate in Peyer's patches in appreciable amounts. Since the histological work utilized light microscopy only, it cannot be said that asbestos, quartz, and carmine were totally absent from Peyer's patches. Nevertheless, in parallel experiments an abundance of carbon and latex aggregates in Peyer's patches contrasted with an absence of aggregates of the other particles and suggested that the uptake process was selective.

FACTORS AFFECTING PARTICLE ENTRY

Since there are marked differences in the readiness with which different types of particles of comparable size accumulate in Peyer's patches, questions arise as to what physicochemical properties of particles influence their uptake. It is possible that the penetration of the Peyer's patch mucosa by particles involves a phagocytic event, either by macrophages or by M or other epithelial cells. Thus, it would be worthwhile to approach the problem by attempting to correlate factors known to influence phagocytosis with the extent of particle uptake into Peyer's patches. Hydrophobicity is one such factor. It has been shown that several types of cells selectively phagocytize particles having a surface more hydrophobic than the cell surface (30,54,57,65). Although no systematic study of particle penetration through the Peyer's patch mucosa versus particle hydrophobicity has been conducted, it is worth noting that particles (carbon and latex) that readily accumulated in Peyer's patches in our experiments were more hydrophobic than particles (asbestos, quartz, and carmine) that did not, as judged by the wettability of dry samples.

Charge is another surface property of potential importance in phagocytic events (54). Both hydrophobicity and charge may be transiently or permanently altered by the adsorption of ambient molecules onto particle surfaces, Since the alimentary tract represents an ever-changing milieu with wide swings in pH and an extraordinary assortment of surface-active molecules, determination of particle surface properties *in situ* in the gut will not be accomplished easily.

FATE OF PARTICLES AFTER PENETRATION INTO
PEYER'S PATCHES

It is pertinent to consider briefly the fate of particles stored in Peyer's patches, remembering, as discussed above, that profound differences in the uptake of various particles may exist.

Our studies with carbon and latex showed that absorbed particles reached all portions of the Peyer's patch follicle, including the germinal center. Macrophages were thought to be instrumental in the transport of particles from the dome to distant regions of the patch (22,25,34). Both carbon latex particles also appeared in mesenteric lymph nodes. In the experiments of Joel et al. (25), carbon-containing macrophages were seen throughout mesenteric lymph nodes in mice 2 months after the initiation of carbon ingestion. These macrophages were adjacent to the subcapsular sinus, in and around germinal centers, on the borders of postcapillary venules, and near the cortico-medullary junction.

Since Volkheimer and collaborators (58–61) have reported finding particles in circulating blood within minutes of their ingestion, it is of interest to examine the possibility that particles entering Peyer's patches pass rapidly into the bloodstream, either by direct entry into portal blood or via lymphatics. Our findings in mice provide little evidence for significant transport of particles from Peyer's patches to the bloodstream. Carbon was not detected in livers, spleen, or lungs of animals exposed to carbon for 2 months (25). Had it reached the bloodstream in appreciable amounts, it would have accumulated in these reticuloendothelial organs. Only after 6 months of carbon ingestion were small amounts seen in liver and lungs. In another series of experiments, 5.7- and 15-μm microspheres were not found in blood or reticuloendothelial organs of mice 20, 60, or 240 min after ingestion of 2×10^8 particles (35). A few hundred 5.7-μm particles were recovered from extra-intestinal tissues (primarily lungs and mesenteric nodes) after ingestion of 4.5×10^8 particles per day for 60 days.

SUMMARY

Findings from this laboratory show the uptake of some but not all types of indigestible particles into murine Peyer's patches and their subsequent transport to mesenteric lymph nodes. Few particles seem to penetrate beyond the mesenteric nodes. The Peyer's patch epithelium is clearly a less effective barrier than the rest of the intestinal epithelium and, for this reason, merits special attention in toxicological studies. Such attention is perhaps most urgent in studies involving intestinal exposure to macromolecules and particulate materials, but, since much remains to be learned about the unique properties of this epithelium, it is also needed in studies utilizing small molecules, heavy metals, and lipid-soluble substances. Attention to the GALT by toxicologists may bring about new insights into the means by which diverse substances penetrate the intestinal barrier and produce injury, whether that injury be localized to the small intestine or expressed throughout the body.

ACKNOWLEDGMENTS

The research described in this report was supported by the U.S. Department of Energy under contract DE-ACO2–76CH-00016 and the U.S. Environmental Protection Agency under contract 79-D-X-05333 and research grant R810140–01.

REFERENCES

1. Abe, K., and Ito, T. (1977): A qualitative and quantitative morphologic study of Peyer's patches of the mouse. *Arch. Histol. Jpn.*, 40:407–420.
2. Abe, K., and Ito, T. (1978): Qualitative and quantitative morphologic study of Peyer's patches of the mouse after neonatal thymectomy and hydrocortisone injection. *Am. J. Anat.*, 151:227–238.
3. Bhalla, D. K., and Owen, R. L. (1982): Cell renewal and migration in lymphoid follicles of Peyer's patches and cecum—an autoradiographic study in mice. *Gastroenterology*, 82:232–242.
4. Bockman, D. E. (1980): Range of function of gut-associated lymphoepithelial tissue. In: *Aspects of Developmental and Comparative Immunology, Vol. 1*, edited by J. B. Solomon, pp. 273–277. Pergamon Press, Oxford.
5. Bockman, D. E., and Cooper, M. D. (1971): Fine structural analysis of pinocytosis in lymphoid follicle-associated epithelium of chick bursa and rabbit appendix. *Fed. Proc.*, 30:511 (abstract).
6. Bockman, D. E., and Cooper, M. D. (1973): Pinocytosis by epithelium associated with lymphoid follicles in the bursa of Fabricius, appendix, and Peyer's patches. *Am. J. Anat.*, 136:455–478.
7. Bockman, D. E., and Cooper, M. D. (1975): Early lymphoepithelial relationships in the human appendix. *Gastroenterology*, 68:1160–1168.
8. Bolton, R. E., Davis, J. M. G., and Lamb, D. (1982): The pathological effects of prolonged asbestos ingestion in rats. *Environ. Res.*, 29:134–150.
9. Borysenko, M., Borysenko, J., Beringer, T., and Gustafson, A. (1979): *Functional Histology*, p. 100. Little, Brown and Co., Boston.
10. Bye, W. A., Allan, C. H., Madara, J. L., and Trier, J. S. (1983): Mature and immature M cells—morphology and distribution. *Gastroenterology*, 84:1118 (abstract).
11. Carter, P. B., and Collins, F. M. (1974): The route of enteric infection in normal mice. *J. Exp. Med.*, 139:1189–1203.
12. Carter, R. E., and Taylor, W. F. (1980): Identification of a particular amphibole asbestos fiber in tissues of persons exposed to a high oral intake of the mineral. *Environ. Res.*, 21:85–93.
13. Cebra, J. J., Kamat, R., Gearhart, P., Robertson, S. M., and Tseung, J. (1977): The secretory IGA system of the gut. In: *Immunology of the Gut*, Ciba Foundation Symposium, pp. 1–29. Elsevier, Amsterdam.
14. Cook, P. M., and Olson, G. F. (1979): Ingested mineral fibers: Elimination in human urine. *Science*, 204:195–198.
15. Craig, S. W., and Cebra, J. J. (1971): Peyer's patches: An enriched source of precursors for IgA-producing immunocytes in the rabbit. *J. Exp. Med.*, 134:188–200.
16. Craighead, J. E., and Mossman, B. Y. (1982): The pathogenesis of asbestos-associated diseases. *N. Engl. J. Med.*, 306:1446–1455.
17. Faulk, W. P., McCormick, J. N., Goodman, J. R., Yoffey, J. M., and Fudenberg, H. H. (1971): Peyer's patches: Morphologic studies. *Cell Immunol.*, 1:500–520.
18. Freeman, W. H., and Bracegirdle, B. (1976): *An Advanced Atlas of Histology*, p. 72. Heinemann Educational Books, London.
19. Guy-Grand, D. C., Griscelli, C., and Vassali, P. (1974): The gut-associated lymphoid system. Nature and properties of the large dividing cells. *Eur. J. Immunol.*, 4:435–443.
20. Hallenbeck, W. H., Markey, D. R., and Dolan, D. G. (1981): Analyses of tissue, blood, and urine samples from a baboon gavaged with chrysotile and crocidolite asbestos. *Environ. Res.*, 25:349–360.
21. Hamilton, S. R., Keren, D. F., Yardley, J. F., and Brown, G. (1981): No impairment of local intestinal immune response to keyhole limpet haemocyanin in the absence of Peyer's patches. *Immunology*, 42:431–435.
22. Hammer, R., Joel, D. D., and LeFevre, M. E. (1983): Ultrastructure of Peyer's patch macrophages. *Exp. Cell Biol.*, 51:61–69.
23. Hess, M. W., Cottier, H., Sordat, B., Joel, D. D., and Chanana, A. D. (1973): The intestinal

barrier to bacterial invasion. In: *Nonspecific Factors Influencing Host Resistance. A Reexamination*, edited by W. Braun and J. Unger, pp. 447–451. Karger, Basel.

24. Hilding, A. C., Hilding, D. A., Larson, D. M., and Aufderheide, A. C. (1981): Biological effects of ingested amosite asbestos, taconite tailings, diatomaceous earth and Lake Superior water in rats. *Arch. Environ. Health*, 36:298–303.

25. Joel, D. D., Laissue, J. A., and LeFevre, M. E. (1978): Distribution and fate of ingested carbon particles in mice. *J. Reticuloendothel. Soc.*, 24:477–487.

26. Joel, D. D., Sordat, B., Hess, M. W., and Cottier, H. (1970): Uptake and retention of particles from the intestine by Peyer's patches in mice. *Experientia*, 26:694 (abstract).

27. Kagan, M. (1931): Zur Kenntnis der Farbstoffresorption durch die Darmschleimhaut. *Z. Zellforsch.*, 14:544–558.

28. Kagnoff, M. F. (1977): Functional characteristics of Peyer's patch lymphoid cells. IV. *J. Immunol.*, 118:992–997.

29. Keren, D. F., Holt, P. S., Collins, H. H., Gemski, P., and Formal, S. B. (1978): The role of Peyer's patches in the local immune response of rabbit ileum to live bacteria. *J. Immunol.*, 120:1892–1896.

30. Kihlstrom, E. (1980): Interaction between Salmonella bacteria and mammalian nonprofessional phagocytes. *Am. J. Clin. Nutr.*, 33:2491–2501.

31. Kumagai, K. (1922): Uber den Resorptions vergang der corpuscularen Bestandteile im Darm. *Kekkaku-Zassi*, 4:429–431.

32. Leeson, T. S., and Leeson, C. R. (1979): *A Brief Atlas of Histology*, p. 125. W. B. Saunders, Philadelphia.

33. LeFevre, M. E., and Joel, D. D. (1977): Intestinal absorption of particulate matter: Minireview. *Life Sci.*, 21:1403–1408.

34. LeFevre, M. E., Hammer, R., and Joel, D. D. (1979): Macrophages of the mammalian small intestine: A review. *J. Reticuloendothel. Soc.*, 26:553–573.

35. LeFevre, M. E., Hancock, D. C., and Joel, D. D. (1980): The intestinal barrier to large particulates in mice. *J. Toxicol. Environ. Health*, 6:691–704.

36. LeFevre, M. E., Olivo, R., Vanderhoff, J. W., and Joel, D. D. (1978): Accumulation of latex in Peyer's patches and its subsequent appearance in villi and mesenteric lymph nodes. *Proc. Soc. Exp. Biol. Med.*, 159:298–302.

37. LeFevre, M. E., Vanderhoff, J. W., Laissue J. A., and Joel, D. D. (1978): Accumulation of 2-μm latex particles in mouse Peyer's patches during chronic latex feeding. *Experientia*, 34:120–122.

38. Mueller-Schoop, J., and Good, R. A. (1975): Functional studies of Peyer's patches: Evidence for their participation in intestinal immune responses. *J. Immunol.*, 114:1757–1760

39. Owen, R. L. (1977): Sequential uptake of horseradish peroxidase of lymphoid follicle epithelium of Peyer's patches in the normal unobstructed mouse intestine. *Gastroenterology*, 72:440–451.

40. Owen, R. L. (1982): Macrophage function in Peyer's patch epithelium. *Adv. Exp. Med. Biol.*, 149:507–513.

41. Owen, R. L., and Jones, A. L. (1974): Epithelial cell specialization within human Peyer's patches: An ultrastructural study of intestinal lymphoid follicles. *Gastroenterology*, 66:189–203.

42. Owen, R. L., and Nemanic, P. (1978): Antigen processing structures of the mammalian intestinal tract: An SEM study of lymphoepithelial organs. *SEM*, II:367–378.

43. Owen, R. L., Pierce, N. F., and Cray, W. C., Jr. (1983): Autoradiographic analysis of M cell uptake and transport of cholera vibrios into follicles of rabbit Peyer's patches. *Gastroenterology*, 84:1269 (abstract).

44. Parrott, D. M. V. (1976): The gut as a lymphoid organ. *Clin. Gastroenterol.*, 5:211–228.

45. Patel-Mandlik, K. J., Hellenbeck, W. H., and Millette, J. R. (1979): Asbestos fibers. 1. A modified preparation of tissue samples for analysis by electron microscopy. 2. Presence of fibers in tissues of baboon fed chrysotile asbestos. *J. Environ. Pathol. Toxicol.*, 2:1385–1395.

46. Piliero, S. J., Jacobs, M. S., and Wischnitzer, S. (1965): Atlas of Histology, p. 133. J. B. Lippincott, Montreal.

47. Pontrefact R. D., and Cunningham, H. M. (1973): Penetration of asbestos through the digestive tract of rats. *Nature*, 243:352–353.

48. Rudzik, O., Perey, D. Y., and Bienenstock, J. (1975): Differential IgA repopulation after transfer of autologous and rabbit Peyer's patch cells. *J. Immunol.*, 114:40–44.

49. Sebastien, P., Morse, R., and Bignon, J. (1980): Recovery of ingested asbestos fibers from the gastrointestinal lymph of rats. *Environ. Res.*, 22:201–216.

50. Selikoff, I. J. (1974): Epidemiology of gastrointestinal cancer. *Environ. Health Perspect.*, 9:229–305.
51. Shakhlamov, V. A., Gaidar, Y. A., and Baranov, V. N. (1980): Electron-cytochemical investigation of cholera toxin absorption by epithelium by Peyer's patches in guinea pigs. *Bull. Exp. Biol. Med.*, 90:1159–1161.
52. Smith, M. W., and Peacock, M. A. (1980): "M" cell distribution in follicle-associated epithelium of mouse Peyer's patch. *Am. J. Anat.*, 159:167–175.
53. Smith, M. W., Jarvis, L. G., and King, I. S. (1980): Cell proliferation in follicle-associated epithelium of mouse Peyer's patch. *Am. J. Anat.*, 159:157–166.
54. Stendahl, O. I., Dahlgren, C., Edebo, M., and Ohman, L. (1981): Recognition mechanisms in mammalian phagocytosis. In: *Endocytosis and Exocytosis in Host Defense*, edited by L. B. Edebo, L. Enerback and O. I. Stendahl, pp. 12–27. Karger, Basel.
55. Stuart, B. O. (1976): Deposition and clearance of inhaled particles. *Environ. Health Perspect.*, 9:299–305.
56. Thompson, H. G. (1938): The lymphoid tissue of the alimentary canal. *Brit. J. Med.*, 1:7–11.
57. Van Oss, C. J. (1978): Phagocytosis as a surface phenomenon. *Annu. Rev. Microbiol.*, 32:19–39.
58. Volkheimer, G. (1974): Passage of particles through the wall of the gastrointestinal tract. *Environ. Health Perspect.*, 9:215–225.
59. Volkheimer, G. (1975): Hematogenous dissemination of ingested polyvinyl chloride particles. *Ann. NY Acad. Sci.*, 246:164–171.
60. Volkheimer, G. (1977): Persorption of particles: Physiology and pharmacology. *Adv. Pharmacol. Chemother.*, 14:163–187.
61. Volkheimer, G., and Schulz, F. H. (1968): The phenomenon of persorption. *Digestion*, 1:213–218.
62. von Rosen, L., Podjaski, B., Bettman, I., and Otto, H. F. (1981): Observations on the ultrastructure and function of the so-called "microfold" or "membranous" cells (M cells) by means of peroxidase as a tracer. *Virchows Arch. (Pathol. Anat.)*, 390:289–312.
63. Waksman, B. H., Ozer, H., and Blythman, H. E. (1973): Appendix and gamma M antibody formation. VI. *Lab. Invest.*, 28:614–626.
64. Westlake G. E. (1974): Asbestos fibers in the colonic wall. *Environ. Health Perspect.*, 9:227.
65. Wilkinson, P. C. (1976): Recognition and response in mononuclear and granular phagocytes. *Clin. Exp. Imm.*, 25:355–366.
66. Wolf, J. L., Rubin, D. H., Finberg, R., Kauffman, R. S., Sharpe, A. H., Trier, J. S., and Fields, B. N. (1981): Intestinal M cells: A pathway for entry of reovirus into the host. *Science*, 212:471–472.

Intestinal Toxicology, edited by C. M. Schiller.
Raven Press, New York © 1984.

Energy Metabolism in Small Intestine

W. C. Hülsmann

Department of Biochemistry I, Medical Faculty, Erasmus University Rotterdam,
3000 DR Rotterdam, The Netherlands

The main objective of this chapter is a discussion on the supply of substrates for the synthesis of adenosine triphosphate (ATP) in small intestinal epithelium. The mechanism of transport of glucose, amino acids, ketone bodies, and long-chain fatty acids into small intestinal epithelium is briefly mentioned. The uptake through the brush border is distinguished from basolateral transport. Literature data for glucose, ketone bodies, fatty acids, glutamine and lactate as major respiratory substrates then follow. Fatty acids as endogenous substrates in isolated epithelial cells are likely to be generated continuously as they are the major source of (cyanide-insensitive) peroxisomal β-oxidation. Moreover, glycerol is continuously produced as a result of endogenous lipolysis. The possible fatty acid-dependent induction of peroxisomal biogenesis might ultimately depend on thyroid (and perhaps also on glucocorticoid) hormones. The short-term regulation of the substrate supply to small intestinal epithelium probably involves the effects of insulin and glucagon on adipose tissue, muscle, and liver, but not on small intestinal epithelium itself.

PENETRATION OF GLUCOSE, AMINO ACIDS, AND MONOCARBOXYLATES INTO SMALL INTESTINAL RESORPTIVE CELLS

As will be seen below, the major energy sources for small intestinal epithelium are glucose, amino acids, fatty acids, ketone bodies, and, perhaps, lactate. During food absorption the first three substrates may enter the cells via the brush border, at least in the upper part of the villi where contact with the succus entericus is intimate. In the lower part of the villi, and in the crypts, the substrates enter the cells mainly through the basolateral cell membrane, both in the fed and fasted state.

UPTAKE THROUGH THE BRUSH BORDER

Miller and Crane (35) succeeded in isolating intestinal mucosal brush borders as an intact subcellular organelle in 1960. It was not only able to digest di- and oligosaccharides, but also to absorb hexoses in an active manner, in which Na^+ cotransport played a role (34). Crane presented a mechanism of cotransport of Na^+ and sugar through the brush border (5). Later it was found that this concept could be extended to cotransport of Na^+ and amino acids (43). With brush border membrane vesicles, Hopfer et al. (12) clearly demonstrated the cotransport in these closed vesicles indeed. The fatty acid transport through the brush border is probably not an active process. After a fatty meal, immediately beyond the terminal web long-chain fatty acids are removed mainly by activation to their coenzyme A derivatives, followed by monoacyl glycerol esterification. As higher concentrations of nonesterified long-chain fatty acids (NEFA) are membrane-toxic, it may be expected that NEFA removal, as in other cell types, is extremely efficient, so that fatty acid resorption occurs along a downhill gradient, created by ATP dependent reesterification in the endoplasmic reticulum. A role of Ca^{2+} in fatty acid transport is presently under investigation in our laboratory Ca^{2+} has been shown to promote luminal fatty acid absorption (42).

TRANSPORT AT THE BASOLATERAL MEMBRANE

Studies with isolated epithelial cells (2,24) and vesicles of basolateral membranes (37) indicated that sugar transport at the basolateral membrane follows a different mechanism than that of brush border transport in that it is energy- and Na^+-independent. Serosal carriers allow the transfer of very hydrophilic molecules, such as sugars and certain amino acids, to pass the hydrophobic membrane barrier. They complement the Na^+-dependent brush border systems for the components to reach the circulatory system. They also provide means of supplying the epithelial cells with metabolizable fuel molecules from the bloodstream during fasting. Also, other substrates for intestinal energy metabolism enter the basolateral membranes in a carrier-mediated fashion. Lactate and pyruvate can be oxidized by small intestinal epithelial cells. When we observed that fatty acids, which may be preferentially oxidized by small intestine (13), inhibit the oxidation of pyruvate in isolated epithelial cells and that pyruvate was not excessively converted to lactate under these conditions, we concluded that pyruvate transport through the cellular membrane was rate-limiting (29,30). Pyruvate transport was characterized by saturation kinetics, competitive inhibition by short-chain fatty acids and counteranion transport. On the basis of these results a carrier-mediated monocarboxylate anion transport mechanism was proposed (30). Such a system probably also exists in heart (49,36), brain (39), and adipose tissue (19). The intestinal monocarboxylate carrier is likely to be present in the basolateral portion of the plasma membrane (cf. ref. 26). Much more could be said about the transport of substrate ions through the cellular membranes of intestinal epithelial cells, but the main emphasis of the present chapter is on the generation of ATP; therefore, ion transport will not be discussed further.

SUBSTRATES FOR ATP SYNTHESIS

Glucose had long been believed a preferred substrate for energy metabolism in small intestine, as *in vitro* preparations such as everted sacs and mucosal scrapings had been shown to produce large amounts of lactate from added glucose. It is clear now that this was probably due to insufficient oxygenation or tissue damage, as small intestine vascularly perfused with glucose and sufficient O_2 displays a normal Pasteur effect and low rates of lactate production (27). These aerobic *in vitro* perfusions, in which fluorocarbons or erythrocytes were used to increase O_2 availability, led to similar energy charges as *in situ* (27). About 84% of the adenine nucleotides was in the form of ATP, 14% as adenosine diphosphate (ADP), and 2% as adenosine monophosphate (AMP), while creatine phosphate had an even higher concentration than ATP. Indeed, *in vivo*, even during glucose transport, also lactate production is slow (25), which points to a high energy charge. Also, enterocytes containing 2 mM ATP, 0.5 mM ADP, negligible AMP, and 1.6 mM creatine phosphate were isolated from everted rat small intestine (14). The energy charge

$$\left(\frac{\text{ATP} + \text{ADP}/2}{\text{ATP} + \text{ADP} + \text{AMP}} \right)$$

of about 0.9 predicts that glycolysis may be limited by the phosphofructokinase reaction in these isolated cells. The experiment also showed that the creatine kinase reaction is intrinsic to the villous cells and not just due to the presence of this enzyme in the muscular part of the intestinal wall. As for the regulation of the rate of glycolysis, not only the phosphofructokinase reaction deserves consideration but also the other two irreversible glycolytic steps: hexokinase and pyruvate kinase. The latter appears to be of the M_2 type and is relatively active (45). The former, however, has a relatively low maximal activity and therefore might limit glycolysis under certain conditions. Two isoenzymes of hexokinase, I and II, appear to be present (44). In guinea pig particulate hexokinase was found to reside in the mitochondrial fraction (44,33). In rat we reported that brush border also contains hexokinase activity (46), but we have subsequently found that this was wrong (14,21) and was based on the presence of mitochondrial outer membranes in the brush border preparation (14,21) and on a histochemical artifact caused by the adsorption of lipophilic formazan formed in a coupled hexokinase and glucose-6-phosphate dehydrogenase assay to structures of the brush border. Hence, also in the rat the bulk of the hexokinase activity is present in the mitochondrial outer membrane. Its activity is of the same order of magnitude as the rate of hypoxia-stimulated glycolysis (14). The mitochondrial hexokinase activity may be 50% inhibited when 2.5 mM ATP in the assay is replaced by 1.5 mM ATP and 1 mM ADP (14). Perhaps then when phosphofructokinase is stimulated by lowering of the energy charge, hexokinase could not cope with this accelerated rate, if hexokinase were not localized on the mitochondrial outer membrane. The energy charge in the epimitochondrial space may well be higher than in the cytosol under aerobic conditions (14). Not only ADP, but also glucose-6-phosphate strongly inhibits rat small intestinal mitochondrial hexokinase (14). This product, in contrast to ADP, might have a physiological role in controlling the rate of hexokinase reaction. Under normal feeding conditions, in the absence of anaerobiosis, ATP levels may not be expected to be low. Even during fructose feeding ATP levels are relatively little affected, thanks to the buffering effect of the creatine kinase activity in rat small intestinal epithelium (28). During sugar absorption, however, glucose-6-phosphate levels might be expected to rise, especially since glucose-6-phosphatase, a gluco-neogenic key enzyme, in small intestinal epithelium is virtually absent. If then, in the vicinity of the upper part of the resorptive cell, mitochondria would produce abundant glucose-6-phosphate (if product inhibitions were to be absent), the se-questration of P_i might result in an inability of the mitochondria to regenerate ATP. However, the energy crisis can be avoided with a number of emergency measures now available, e.g., the presence of creatine kinase and the product inhibition of the hexokinase reaction by both glucose-6-phosphate and ADP.

KETONE BODIES, FATTY ACIDS, LACTATE, AND GLUTAMINE

Not only glucose was rapidly removed from vascularly perfused rat small intes-tine, but also β-hydroxybutyrate, octanoate, and palmitate (13). Assuming complete combustion of the carboxylic acids mentioned, a similar maximal ATP yield for these substrates could be calculated (13). When glucose and fatty acids were perfused together, there was still much glucose utilized; however, this was not combusted, but almost completely converted to lactate. In addition, ketone bodies may also be oxidized in preference to glucose (13). The enzymes required for the conversion of β-hydroxybutyrate to acetyl-coenzyme A, as well as the ability of small intestinal epithelial mitochondria to oxidize β-hydroxybutyrate and acetoac-etate, have been shown by us as well (17,23). Octanoate, β-hydroxybutyrate, and to a lesser extent acetate were found to inhibit the rate of formation of $^{14}CO_2$ from [1-^{14}C]pyruvate simultaneously added to isolated small intestinal epithelial cells (29). During that study evidence showed that the presence of octanoate instead of glucose in isolated cells or in whole intestine caused a decrease of pyruvate dehydrogenase activity (29), so that the preferential oxidation of some carboxylic acids may in part be explained by a decrease of pyruvate dehydrogenase activity in small intestinal epithelium. As may be expected from the raised plasma levels of ketone bodies in the fasted state, ketone bodies may indeed be an important *in vivo* substrate for intestinal epithelium (11,51). Also, lactate may be used as a substrate for oxidative metabolism, as may be expected from the abundant presence of lactate dehydrogenase and pyruvate oxidation. Windmueller and Spaeth (51) reported that when blood lactate levels in rat exceed 1.2 to 1.6 mM, lactate may be utilized. Also, in man lactate may be expected to be an important substrate under certain conditions. In type I gluconeogenesis, glucose levels in blood are often very low, while lactate levels are high. In fact, in this disease in which gluconeogenesis and glycogenolysis are hampered because of glucose-6-phosphatase deficiency in liver, ketosis is absent (because excess fatty acids are trapped as triglyceride, resulting in liver steatosis), and lactate is the only important substrate during fasting. In this disease signs of malabsorption are generally absent, indicating an intact energy metabolism in the gastrointestinal tract.

Windmueller and Spaeth (51) made the important discovery that glutamine is an additionally important substrate for intestinal energy metabolism. They arrived at the conclusion that in the postabsorptive state, in order of importance, glutamine, β-hydroxybutyrate, acetoacetate, glucose, lactate, and free fatty acids are respiratory substrates. The low contribution of the free fatty acids (3.4%) to total CO_2 production has been described by Windmueller and Spaeth (51) as the relative impermeability of the cells to fatty acids as compared with the smaller water-soluble ketone bodies. They may have underestimated fatty acid oxidation as their overall respiratory quotient amounts to 0.85, while the sum of the other substrates amounts to a respiratory quotient close to unity. Labeled long-chain fatty acids indeed do not easily equilibrate between the vascular compartment and the tissue cells. The use of high fatty acid/albumin ratios promotes extraction and oxidation (13,16). Figure 1 shows that increasing the molar ratio of oleate to albumin from 3 to 6 does not alter the rate of fatty acid oxidation by the *in vitro* perfused rat heart, but more than doubles fatty acid oxidation by *in vitro* perfused small intestine. It suggests that serum components are more abundantly present in the lymphatics in intestine than in heart. Abundant transudation of high molecular

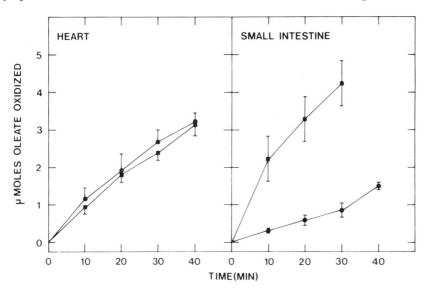

FIG. 1. Comparison of oleate oxidation in heart (37 °C) and small intestine (31 °C). Heart: ●———●, oleate/albumin molar ratio = 3 (*N* = 3); ■———■, oleate/albumin molar ratio = 6 (N = 4). Small intestine: ●———●, oleate/albumin molar ratio = 3 (*N* = 5); ■———■, oleate/albumin ratio = 6 (N = 6). The ordinate shows μmoles oleate oxidized per gram of heart ($^{wt}/_{vol}$) or 60 cm of small intestine. The albumin concentration present in all experiments was 3.4% ($^{wt}/_{vol}$). N, number of experiments. Reprinted from Hülsmann et al. (16), with permission.

complexes from blood to small intestinal lymph is well known. That long-chain fatty acids can be oxidized in small intestine has been observed by a number of workers. Alteveer et al. (1) showed this for dog. Gangl and Ockner (8) infused fatty acids by the intravenous and/or luminal route in rats and found that vascularly applied fatty acids were not incorporated into triacylglycerol, but were oxidized. Hanson and Parsons (11) perfused rat jejunum vascularly with glucose and studied the effect of ketone body addition. They observed ketone body consumption, both in fed and fasted states, and a percentage increase of glucose that was converted to lactate. When ketone bodies were replaced by oleate, lactate production increased, although only significantly in the fasted state. Hanson and Parsons (10) showed earlier that glutamine was an important substrate in both fed and fasted rat jejunum, and they concluded that in the fasted state ketone bodies, fatty acids, and glutamine were preferred substrates of small intestinal energy metabolism (11). In the fed state dietary glutamine, glutamate, and aspartate have a much more important contribution to energy metabolism than does glucose (52). With brush border cells isolated from rat or chick jejunum, Watford et al. (48) and Porteous (41) observed stimulation of respiration by glucose, glutamate, and glutamine. Watford et al. (48) also noted stimulation of rat cell respiration by ketone bodies. Porteous (41) did not see stimulation of chick cell respiration by ketone bodies, but noted that endogenous respiration in the chick cell preparation was higher than in rat cells (41). This endogenous respiration may be due to the utilization of endogenous substrates. Porteous observed considerable formation of glutamine, proline, serine, and alanine during substrate-free incubation of chick cells (41). The extra- and/or intracellular proteolysis is probably accompanied by lipolysis, as fatty acids are present. Therefore, the absence of an effect of added fatty acids, as observed by some investigators, is probably due to the presence of endogenous fatty acids already. This is discussed below. In summing up, it appears that glucose, glutamine, ketone bodies, and fatty acids are important substrates for energy metabolism in small intestinal epithelium.

FATTY ACIDS AS ENDOGENOUS SUBSTRATES

During polarographic measurements of oxygen uptake in isolated epithelial cells, we repeatedly observed that 1 to 10 mM cyanide only partially inhibited respiration. Similar results were obtained during O_2 consumption measurements in vascularly perfused rat small intestine, in which 2 mM cyanide or azide hardly depressed the rate of respiration (40). Later we became aware that this was indicative of the important contribution of (cyanide- or azide-insensitive) peroxisomal fatty acid oxidation to overall oxygen uptake in small intestine. Peroxisomes are present in small intestine (38), and they may shorten (very) long-chain fatty acids in a cyanide-insensitive manner (31,32). The acyl-coenzyme A (CoA) dehydrogenase is an acyl-CoA oxidase, a flavoprotein using O_2 as the electron acceptor with H_2O_2 as the reaction product. The peroxisomal β-oxidation system of rat liver is induced by fat feeding, fasting, or by the administration of clofibrate or other drugs (cf. 3). The mechanism of the adaptation is unknown. Bremer and Norum (3) considered the possibility that fat feeding, fasting, and clofibrate all raised acyl-CoA levels in tissues, which might trigger peroxisomal induction. Other possibilities are increased levels of corticosteroids during stress and fat feeding (15) and particularly increased free thyroid hormone levels, as long-chain fatty acids by binding to albumin may displace protein-bound thyroxin, allowing the formation of more triiodothyronine. This link was considered after the recent observation of Fringes and Reith (7) that hyperthyroidism induces biogenesis of peroxisomes. Some literature data indeed suggest that clofibrate may act via thyroid hormone (cf. 7).

Another indication that fatty acids are formed from endogenous glycerol esters is our observation that glycerol is released from isolated small intestine during vascular perfusion (20). A moderate stimulation of glycerol release was observed after the addition of dibutyryl cyclic AMP and a phosphodiesterase inhibitor, whereas chloroquine and phenothiazines were found to inhibit (20). As the mesenterium may contain adipose tissue (9), the cyclic AMP-sensitive stimulation of endogenous lipolysis might be related to adipocytes and not to enterocytes. Hence, we repeated the demonstration of glycerol release from endogenous sources with isolated small intestinal villous cells. It can be seen from Table 1 that cells isolated from fed rats release glycerol and that some inhibition is obtained by 0.4 mM

TABLE 1. *Lipolysis in isolated small intestinal villous cells*

Additions	N	% Glycerol release	p
None	8	100	—
Dibutyryl cyclic AMP (0.1 mM)	8	113 ± 4	<0.05
Chloroquine (0.4 mM)	8	69 ± 10	<0.005

Villous cells were isolated from everted small intestine of fed Wistar rats (240 ± 20 g) by the vibration method of Harrison and Webster (21). After collection of the cells by centrifugation at 270 × *g* for 3 min, the cells were resuspended in 0.3 M mannitol, containing 0.02 M Tris-HCl (pH 7.4) with the help of a plastic pipette and recentrifuged. This washing procedure was repeated and the cells from 60 cm of small intestine suspended in 24 ml of a modified Tyrode solution containing 141 mM NaCl, 1.06 mM MgCl$_2$, 0.435 mM NaH$_2$PO$_4$, 20.2 mM NaHCO$_3$, 1.35 mM CaCl$_2$, 4.7 mM KCl, and 3% (wt/vol) albumin, defatted according to Chen (4). Plastic materials were used throughout. Two ml of the cell suspension were incubated for 15 or 30 min at 37°C under 95% O$_2$ + 5% CO$_2$ under shaking. The reactions were stopped by the addition of 0.2 ml 30% (wt/vol) perchloric acid followed by neutralization with potassium hydroxide and determination of glycerol fluorimetrically in a glycerol kinase-dependent coupled enzyme system (50). When dibutyryl cyclic AMP was added, it was accompanied by the addition of the phosphodiesterase inhibitor 3-isobutyl-1-methylxanthine (25 μM). In each experiment the glycerol release in the absence of additions was set at 100% (averaging to 18 ± 2 nmoles/min/incubation).
N, number of experiments; *p*, statistical significance.

chloroquine. As the latter is an amphiphilic agent that also inhibits lipolysis in other organs (18,20), it indicates that endogenous lipolysis in enterocytes exists and that the process is chloroquine-sensitive. Only a weak stimulation by dibutyryl cyclic AMP was obtained so that the existence of a hormone-sensitive lipase in enterocytes, like the one that was described by Huttunen and Steinberg for adipocytes (22), is not likely. The necessity of endogenous lipolysis may be appreciated when it is considered that cytoplasmic lipid droplets accumulate under certain conditions, particularly after feeding of $C_{22:1}$ fatty acids (47), as present in erucic acid-rich rapeseed oil or certain marine oils.

In conclusion, it may be stated that enterocytes generate from endogenous sources long-chain fatty acids, which undergo reesterification and β-oxidation, partly in mitochondria and partly in peroxisomes, especially when these microbodies are induced by dietary or other regimens. The presence of endogenous and exogenous intracellular and extracellular fatty acids makes it clear that the oxidation of added fatty acids is sometimes hard to demonstrate. From the literature, however, it appears that preferential fatty acid oxidation exists in small intestinal epithelium.

HORMONAL REGULATION OF SUBSTRATE SUPPLY TO SMALL INTESTINE

Insulin, glucagon, and catecholamines are the most important hormones that regulate the supply of glucose, fatty acids, and ketone bodies to most tissues. In the isolated perfused rat small intestine, we did not find a clear-cut effect on the extraction or metabolism of glucose (13). Nor did we find an acute effect of insulin or glucagon on the cyclic AMP level in isolated enterocytes (6), and the effect of epinephrine was very modest. Therefore we tend to conclude that the direct effect of these hormones on small intestinal epithelium is modest or negligible, although in the streptozotocin-diabetic rat, the vascularly perfused small intestine shows diminished glucose utilization (11). This, however, is probably due to the glucose-sparing action of fatty acids and ketone bodies upon intestinal energy metabolism (13,29), as is suggested by the observation (11) that in diabetes the rate of lactate formation is not decreased.

Discussion of chronic effects of hormones, such as thyroid hormones and glucocorticoids, is not in the scope of this chapter and is dealt with in chapter by S. J. Henning, *this volume.*

ACKNOWLEDGMENTS

The author wishes to acknowledge discussions with Drs. H. R. de Jonge, J. M. J. Lamers, and J. W. Porteous and to thank Miss Cecile Hanson for preparing the manuscript.

REFERENCES

1. Alteveer, R. J., Goldfarb, R. D., Lau, J., Port, M., and Spitzer, J. J. (1973): Effects of acute severe hemorrhage on metabolism of the dog intestine. *Am. J. Physiol.*, 224:197–201.

2. Bihler, I., and Cybulsky, R. (1973): Sugar transport at the basal and lateral aspect of the small intestinal cell. *Biochim. Biophys. Acta*, 298:429–437.
3. Bremer, J., and Norum, K. R. (1982): Metabolism of very long chain monounsaturated fatty acids (22-1) and the adaptation to their presence in the diet. *J. Lipid Res.*, 23:243–256.
4. Chen, R. F. (1967): Removal of fatty acids from serum albumin by charcoal treatment. *J. Biol. Chem.*, 242:173–181.
5. Crane, R. K. (1962): Hypothesis of mechanism of intestinal active transport of sugars. *Fed. Proc.*, 21:891–895.
6. De Jonge, H. R., and Hülsmann, W. C. (1974): Adenylate cyclase activities and adenosine 3′,5′-cyclic monophosphate concentrations in villus and crypt cells of rat small intestinal epithelium. Response to cholera toxin, prostaglandin E_1 and hormones. *Biochem. Soc. Trans.*, 2:416–419.
7. Fringes, B., and Reith, A. (1982): Time course of peroxisome biogenesis during adaptation to mild hyperthyroidism in rat liver. *Lab. Invest.*, 47:19–26.
8. Gangl, A., and Ockner, R. K. (1975): Intestinal metabolism of plasma free fatty acids. Intracellular compartmentation and mechanisms of control. *J. Clin. Invest.*, 55:803–813.
9. Göransson, G., and Olivecrona, T. (1964): The metabolism of fatty acids in the rat. I. Palmitic acid. *Acta Physiol. Scand.*, 62:224–239.
10. Hanson, P. J., and Parsons, D. S. (1977): Metabolism and transport of glutamine and glucagon in vascularly perfused rat small intestine. *Biochem. J.*, 166:509–519.
11. Hanson, P. J., and Parsons, D. S. (1978): Factors affecting the utilization of ketone bodies and other substrates by rat jejunum: effects of fasting and diabetes. *J. Physiol.*, 278:55–67.
12. Hopfer, U., Nelson, K., Perrotto, J., and Isselbacher, K. J. (1973): Glucose transport in isolated brush border membrane from rat small intestine. *J. Biol. Chem.*, 248:25–32.
13. Hülsmann, W. C. (1971): Preferential oxidation of fatty acids by rat small intestine. *FEBS Lett.*, 17:35–38.
14. Hülsmann, W. C. (1977): Energy metabolism in different preparations of rat small intestinal epithelium. In: *Intestinal Permeation. Proceedings of the Fourth Workshop Conference Hoechst*, edited by M. Kramer and F. Lauterbach, pp. 229–239. Excerpta Medica Intern. Congress Series 391, Excerpta Medica, Amsterdam.
15. Hülsmann, W. C. (1978): Abnormal stress reactions after feeding diets rich in (very) long chain fatty acids: high levels of corticosterone and testosterone. *Mol. Cell. Endocrinol.*, 12:1–8.
16. Hülsmann, W. C., Breeman, W. A. P., Stam, H., and Kort, W. J. (1981): Comparative study of chylomicron and fatty acid utilization in small intestine and heart. *Biochim. Biophys. Acta*, 663:373–379.
17. Hülsmann, W. C., Iemhoff, W. G. J., and Van den Berg, J. W. O., and De Pijper, A. M. (1970): Unequal rates of development of mitochondrial enzymes in rat small intestinal epithelium. *Biochim. Biophys. Acta*, 215:553–555.
18. Hülsmann, W. C., and Stam, H. (1978): Intracellular origin of hormone-sensitive lipolysis in the rat. *Biochem. Biophys. Res. Commun.*, 82:53–59.
19. Hülsmann, W. C., and Stam, H. (1979): Lipolysis in heart and adipose tissue; effects of inhibition of glycogenolysis and uncoupling of oxidative phosphorylation. *Biochem. Biophys. Res. Commun.*, 88:867–872.
20. Hülsmann, W. C., Stam, H., and Geelhoed-Mieras, M. M. (1979): Hormone-sensitivity of lipolysis in various rat tissues; effects of chloroquine, phenothiazines, quinidine and lidocaine. In: *Obesity—Cellular and Molecular Aspects*, edited by G. Ailhaud. INSERM, 87:179–192.
21. Hülsmann, W. C., Van den Berg, J. W. O., and De Jonge, H. R. (1974): Isolation of intestinal mucosa cells. In: *Methods in Enzymology*, Vol. 32B, edited by S. Fleischer and L. Packer, pp. 665–673, Academic Press, New York.
22. Huttunen, J. K., and Steinberg, D. (1971): Activation and phosphorylation of purified adipose tissue hormone-sensitive lipase by cyclic AMP-dependent protein kinase. *Biochim. Biophys. Acta.*, 239:411–427.
23. Iemhoff, W. G. J., and Hülsmann, W. C. (1971): Development of mitochondrial enzyme activities in rat-small-intestinal epithelium. *Eur. J. Biochem.*, 23:429–434.
24. Kimmich, G. A., and Randles, J. (1975): A Na^+-independent phloretin-sensitive monosaccharide transport system in isolated intestinal epithelial cells. *J. Mebr. Biol.*, 23:57–76.
25. Kiyasu, J. Y., Katz, J., and Chaikoff, I. L. (1956): Nature of ^{14}C compounds recovered in portal plasma after enteral administration of ^{14}C glucose. *Biochim. Biophys. Acta*, 21:286–290.
26. Lamers, J. M. J. (1977): A monocarboxylate anion carrier in rat small intestinal epithelium. In:

Intestinal Permeation. Proceedings of the Fourth Workshop Conference Hoechst, edited by M. Kramer and F. Lauterbach, pp. 164–172. Excerpta Medica Intern. Congress Series 391, Excerpta Medica, Amsterdam.

27. Lamers, J. M. J., and Hülsmann, W. C. (1972): Pasteur effect in the *in vitro* vascularly perfused rat small intestine. *Biochim. Biophys. Acta*, 275:491–495.

28. Lamers, J. M. J., and Hülsmann, W. C. (1973): The effect of fructose on the stores of energy-rich phosphate in rat jejunum in vivo. *Biochim. Biophys. Acta*, 313:1–8.

29. Lamers, J. M. J., and Hülsmann, W. C. (1974): The effects of fatty acids on oxidative decarboxylation of pyruvate in rat small intestine. *Biochim. Biophys. Acta*, 343:215–225.

30. Lamers, J. M. J., and Hülsmann, W. C. (1975): Inhibition of pyruvate transport by fatty acids in isolated cells from rat small intestine. *Biochim. Biophys. Acta*, 394:31–45.

31. Lazarow, P. B. (1978): Rat liver peroxisomes catalyze the β-oxidation of fatty acids. *J. Biol. Chem.*, 253:1522–1528.

32. Lazarow, P. B., and De Duve, C. (1976): A fatty acyl-CoA oxidation system in rat liver peroxisomes enhancement by clofibrate, a hypolipidemic drug. *Proc. Natl. Acad. Sci. USA*, 73:2043–2046.

33. Mayer, A. J., and Hübscher, G. (1971): Mitochondrial hexokinase from small intestinal mucosa and brain. *Biochem. J.*, 124:491–500.

34. Mc Dougal, D. B., Little, K. D., and Crane, R. K. (1960): Studies on the mechanism of intestinal absorption of sugars. IV. Localization of galactose concentration within the intestinal wall during active transport *in vitro*. *Biochim. Biophys. Acta*, 45:483–489.

35. Miller, D., and Crane, R. K. (1960): The concept of a digestive surface in the small intestine: cellular nature of disaccharide and phosphate ester hydrolysis. *J. Lab. Clin. Med.*, 56:928–929.

36. Mowbray, J., and Ottaway, J. H. (1973): The effect of insulin and growth hormone on the flux of tracer from labelled lactate in perfused rat heart. *Eur. J. Biochem.*, 36:369–379.

37. Murer, H., Hopfer, U., Kinne-Saffran, E., and Kinne, R. (1974): Glucose transport in isolated brush border and lateral-basal plasma membrane vesicles from intestinal epithelial cells. *Biochim. Biophys. Acta*, 345:170–179.

38. Novikoff, P. M., and Novikoff, A. B. (1972): Peroxisomes in absorptive cells of mammalian small intestine. *J. Cell Biol.*, 53:532–560.

39. Oldendorf, W. H. (1973): Carrier-mediated blood-brain barrier transport of short-chain monocarboxylic organic acids. *Am. J. Physiol.*, 224:1450–1453.

40. Porteous, J. W. (1979): Intestinal metabolism. *Environ. Health Perspect.*, 33:25–35.

41. Porteous, J. W. (1980): Glutamate, glutamine, aspartate asparagine, glucose and ketone-body metabolism in chick intestinal brushborder cells. *Biochem. J.*, 188:619–632.

42. Saunders, D. R., and Sillery, J. (1979): Effect of calcium on absorption of fatty acid by rat jejunum *in vitro*. *Lipids*, 14:703–706.

43. Schultz, S. G., and Curran, P. F. (1970): Coupled transport of sodium and organic solutes. *Physiol. Rev.*, 50:637–718.

44. Srivastava, L. M., Shakespeare, P., and Hübscher, G. (1968): Glucose metabolism in the mucosa of the small intestine: a study of hexokinase activity. *Biochem. J.*, 109:35–42.

45. Van Berkel, Th. J. C., De Jonge, H. R., Koster, J. F., and Hülsmann, W. C. (1974): Kinetic evidence for the presence of two forms of M_2 type pyruvate kinase in rat small intestine. *Biochem. Biophys. Res. Commun.*, 60:398–405.

46. Van den Berg, J. W. O., and Hülsmann, W. C. (1971): Insoluble hexokinase in the brushborder region of rat small intestinal epithelial cells. *FEBS Lett.*, 12:173–175.

47. Vodovar, N., Desnoyers, F., and Flanzy, J. (1972): Absorption intestinale de l'huile de colza. Aspect ultrastructurel. *CR Acad. Sci. Paris*, 274(D):1743–1745.

48. Watford, M., Lund, P., and Krebs, H. A. (1979): Isolation and metabolic characteristics of rat and chicken enterocytes. *Biochem. J.*, 178:589–596.

49. Watts, D. J., and Randle, P. J. (1967): Evidence for the existence of a pyruvate permease in heart muscle. *Biochem. J.*, 104:51P.

50. Wieland, O. (1957): Eine enzymatische Methode zur Bestimmung von Glycerin. *Biochem. Z.*, 329:313–319.

51. Windmueller, H. G., and Spaeth, A. E. (1978): Identification of ketone bodies and glutamine as the major respiratory fuels *in vivo* for postabsorptive rat small intestine. *J. Biol. Chem.*, 253:69–76.
52. Windmueller, H. G., and Spaeth, A. E. (1980): Respiratory fuels and nitrogen metabolism in vivo in small intestine of fed rats. *J. Biol. Chem.*, 255:107–112.

Intestinal Toxicology, edited by C. M. Schiller.
Raven Press, New York © 1984.

Intestinal Digestion and Absorption of Fat-Soluble Environmental Agents

A. Kuksis

*Banting and Best Department of Medical Research, University of Toronto,
Toronto, Ontario, M5G 1L6 Canada*

The intestinal mucosa is the main contact area for a host of both natural and synthetic fat-soluble substances, which are ingested along with solid foods and liquids, or are taken as drugs. Before absorption, these chemicals may become modified by the enzymes secreted into the alimentary tract or by the microorganisms residing there. Of special concern is the micellarization of the dietary fats during the course of normal digestion and absorption, and the passive nature of the absorption process, involving a membrane transfer of partially degraded lipid esters in the form of surface-active materials. It is reasonable, therefore, to assume that the interaction of the foreign substances with the absorbing cell surface will depend on the quantity and concentration of the agents ingested, the amount of food accompanying them, as well as on the metabolic state of the mucosa. At present few factual data exist about the digestion and absorption of foreign substances by the intestinal mucosa. It is believed, however, that many of the fat-soluble environmental agents and drugs are absorbed by mechanisms similar to those responsible for the uptake of micronutrients, such as the fat-soluble vitamins, although the latter mechanisms also are not well understood.

The following chapter briefly summarizes the current understanding of the digestion and absorption of fats and other lipids and points out how this knowledge may help in the rationalization of the uptake and plasma transport of the lipid-soluble environmental pollutants and toxic agents.

GENERAL FEATURES OF LIPID DIGESTION AND ABSORPTION

The intestinal digestion and absorption of fat consists of a multistep process that is characterized by an active involvement of the salivary and pancreatic lipases and the biliary detergents, the intestine, and the lymphatics. Through an integrated function of these organs the dietary fat is extensively hydrolyzed, absorbed, and delivered to the peripheral blood for subsequent metabolism. The dietary fat also serves as a vehicle for the entry of the fat-soluble vitamins as well as other fat-soluble substances into the body, and the fatty digestion products facilitate their uptake by the mucosal cells from which they are transferred to the bloodstream in the form of chylomicrons and lipoproteins.

The following sections summarize the major steps of the fat digestion and absorption process with special emphasis on the mechanisms that may facilitate the solubilization and absorption of the fat-soluble environmental agents. In this connection, attention may be called to previous reviews on dietary fat digestion and absorption (86,196,226,253) and on the absorption of the fat-soluble vitamins (106), drugs (228), and environmental agents (115,201).

Digestion

The dietary fats consist largely of triacylglycerols and glycerophospholipids, with smaller amounts of free fatty acids, steryl esters, free sterols, and of still smaller amounts of fat-soluble vitamins and any other fat-soluble additives or contaminants of the food. To be absorbed, these lipids must be first converted to the free acids, monoacylglycerols, lysophospholipids, and free alcohols, by processes that take place primarily in the lumen of the small intestine under the influence of pancreatic lipases and bile salts (86,196,226,253). Certain hydrolytic steps may take place, however, also at other sites, such as the mouth and the stomach (96,97).

Gastric Stage

The dietary fats are first acted upon by the enzymes of the mouth. The lingual lipase secreted by the lingual serous glands of the tongue is a potent enzyme that hydrolyzes long-chain triacylglycerols (97). *In vitro* studies have shown that in the absence of a fatty acid acceptor, the reaction products are mainly diacylglycerols and free fatty acids, and only small amounts of monoacylglycerols and glycerol are formed. In the presence of excess fatty acid acceptor (albumin), the triacylglycerol is completely hydrolyzed to glycerol and free fatty acids.

The production of diacylglycerols by lingual lipase has been shown to be stereospecific. The enzyme hydrolyzes the sn-3-position of triacylglycerols twice as fast as the sn-1-position (119,191). This was established in the rat (191) by subjecting racemic mixtures of alkyldiacylglycerols, consisting of equimolar amounts of 1-0-octadecyl-2,3-dioctadecenoyl-sn-glycerol (labeled with either ^{3}H in the alkyl moiety or with ^{14}C in both acyl groups) and 3-0-octadecyl-1,2-dioctadecenoyl-sn-glycerol (labeled with either ^{14}C in the alkyl moiety or with ^{3}H in the acyl groups) to lingual lipase. The lingual lipase of a premature human infant was shown (119) to hydrolyze the sn-3-position of synthetic triacylglycerols about four times faster than the sn-1-position.

Although early studies suggested that the stomach was an important site of fat digestion, it was generally believed that hydrolysis of dietary fat did not start until the fat passed through the duodenum (33). Studies with dogs (67) and ruminants (254) have given evidence of marked intragastric lipolysis after diversion of the pancreatic secretions. This lipolytic activity appears to be due to swallowed lingual lipase. Hamosh and Scow (97) observed a 50 to 90% decrease in intragastric lipolysis after diversion of the oral secretions from the stomach of the rats. Toothill et al. (254) observed a complete absence of lipase from the stomach of ruminants after a similar treatment. Hamosh et al. (96) showed that lingual lipase has several characteristics in common with gastric lipase, including the apparent molecular weight, pH optimum, the mixtures of reaction products formed, as well as the acid and heat inactivation (59). The broad pH range of 2.2 to 6.0 has been claimed to permit the digestion of dietary fat by lingual lipase immediately after food enters the stomach as well as during and after the meal (96). Others have reported (99) that an enzyme present in homogenates of gastric mucosa and secreted in the stomach lumen during lipid meal hydrolyzes the short- and medium-chain triacylglycerols preferentially. However, Staggers et al. (239) demonstrated that the lingual lipase of the weaning rat hydrolyzes the medium chain-length fatty acids from the milk fat triacylglycerols preferentially, in addition to possible specificity for the sn-3-position. Hence, it is possible that the latter lipolytic activity toward the short and medium chain-length fatty acids in the stomach is also due to the lingual lipase.

Hernell and Olivecrona (102) pointed out that a lipase in primate milk also would not be denatured at the acid pH of the stomach and on reaching the infant duodenum could act after it had been activated by bile salts. Wang et al. (266) purified this enzyme from human milk and determined its fatty acid and positional specificity. It was found that the enzyme had no significant stereospecificity, but that it attacked the short-chain fatty acids faster than the long-chain acids, regardless at which position they were found. The fatty acids in the secondary position, however, were generally released at a lower rate than those at the primary positions. Furthermore, there was no demonstrable requirement for bile salt activation in the hydrolysis of short-chain triacylglycerols, but long-chain triacylglycerols were not attacked in the absence of bile salts. The bile salt-activated milk lipase also hydrolyzes other esters, such as *p*-nitrophenylacetate and other simple esters (265).

Intestinal Stage

Triacylglycerol hydrolysis is higher in the small intestine than in the stomach because of the action of pancreatic lipase and bile. Pancreatic lipase acts on triacylglycerols at the oil-water interface of the intraluminary lipid particles. The enzyme releases the fatty acids from the primary positions of the glycerol molecule and does not attack the secondary position directly (29,150). Stereospecific analyses have shown (1,38,170,251) that pancreatic lipase attacks the acids in the sn-1- and sn-3-positions at equal rates to yield the sn-1,2- and sn-2,3-diacylglycerols as intermediates in equal quantities. Paltauf et al. (192) and Akesson et al. (1) showed that pancreatic lipase hydrolyzes the outer bonds in the sn-3-position of 1-alkyl-2,3-diacyl-sn-glycerol and in the sn-1-position of 1,2-diacyl-3-alkyl-sn-glycerol at equal rates. Unexpectedly, pancreatic lipases attacked the 2-acyl-3-alkyl-sn-glycerol faster than the 1-alkyl-2-acyl-sn-glycerol (1). This study also demonstrated that 1-acyl-3-alkyl-sn-glycerol was degraded faster than its enantiomer by pancreatic lipase. Akesson and Michelsen (2) showed that a triacylglycerol analog, X-1,2-diacyl-3-S-alkyl-3-thioglycerol-S-oxide also is deacylated in the intestinal tract. The sulfoxide analog was suitable for optical rotatory dispersion (ORD) and circular dichroism (CD) analysis, and in chyle the 2,3-diacyl-1-S-tetradecyl-1-thio-sn-glycerol-S-oxide clearly dominated over the 1,2-diacyl-3-S-tetradecyl-3-thio-sn-glycerol-S-oxide for both diastereoisomers. Although several mechanisms for this selectivity can be advanced, it is most probably explained by stereospecificity at the acyltransferase level, since Paltauf (191) has found that 1-0-alkyl-sn-glycerol is acylated in the intestinal mucosa but not 3-O-alkyl-sn-glycerol.

The rate of long-chain (12–18 carbon atoms having 0, 1, and 2 double bonds) fatty acid hydrolysis is similar, but when the triacylglycerols are composed of fatty acids of 10 carbon atoms or less, these acids are released faster than the long-chain ones, regardless of their positional location in the original triacylglycerol molecule (57,74). According to Sampugna et al. (215), however, the short- and long-chain fatty acids are released at equal rates from the same triacylglycerol molecule, although the shorter chain triacylglycerols as a class are attacked faster than the longer chain triacylglycerols. The dependence of the activity of pancreatic lipase on the structure of the fatty acid (double-bond location, geometry, and chain lengths greater than 18 carbons) has been studied by Brockerhoff (38). Noda et al. (180) found that 2,3-dioleoyloxybutane and 1-hexadecyloxy-3-oleoyloxybutane were degraded more slowly by pancreatic lipase and that 1-hexyloxy-2-octanoyloxypropane resisted hydrolysis.

The 2-monoacylglycerols are also hydrolyzed into fatty acids and glycerol, but this apparently takes place following a prior isomerization to the sn-1- or sn-3-monoacylglycerols (31,183). The released glycerol follows the portal route and is hardly reused for glycerolipid synthesis in the intestinal mucosa, although some glycerokinase activity has been demonstrated there (148). Sklan (231) has claimed that the chicken intestine can utilize free glycerol in the formation of monoacylglycerols.

The pancreatic lipase also catalyzes the reverse reaction, and the fatty acids located at positions 1 and 3 of the triacylglycerol molecules and the intraluminal free fatty acids are readily exchanged (30,206).

The pancreatic lipase is activated by bile salts and by a colipase (159,168). The action of the colipase has been attributed to the need for establishing effective contact with the substrate (43). Bile salts at concentrations exceeding the critical micellar concentration (CMC) usually found in the bile and in the intestinal lumen inhibit the lipase by preventing its contact with the triacylglycerol substrate when colipase is absent. If colipase is present and associated with the lipase, the enzyme system may be adsorbed at the triacylglycerol-water interface and the lipase is active. The lipase is quickly denatured in the absence of bile salts (34). Recent studies (136) indicate that phospholipids and bile cholesterol might transport the lipase-colipase complex to the triacylglycerol-water interface.

The pancreatic juice also contains a nonspecific carboxylic ester hydrolase. This enzyme is responsible for the hydrolysis of the cholesteryl esters, which cannot be absorbed in the ester form (113). In addition, this enzyme catalyzes the hydrolysis of a variety of esters, such as *p*-nitrophenylacetate, β-naphthol acetate and laurate, and the long-chain monoacylglycerols (156,169), including the 2-monoacylglycerols (225). The enzyme requires bile salts for activation, except for the more water-soluble substrates, which, however, are also more rapidly hydrolyzed in the presence of the bile salts (75). It is believed that this enzyme is responsible for the hydrolysis of the esters of vitamins A, D, and E (17,91).

Dietary glycerophospholipids are converted to the corresponding lysophospholipids by pancreatic phospholipase A_2 (221). This enzyme is present in the pancreatic juice in an inactive zymogen form. The complete structure of phospholipase A_2 from the porcine pancreas has been determined and the mechanism of activation elucidated (64,65). According to de Haas et al. (65), the pancreatic phospholipase A_2, unlike the snake venom phospholipase A_2, shows a marked preference for anionic phospholipids, such as phosphatidic acid, cardiolipin, and phosphatidylglycerol. The enzyme has a requirement for calcium ions and bile salts. The pancreas does not secrete a specific phospholipase A_1, which attacks the sn-1-position of glycerophospholipids to yield the corresponding 2-lysoglycerophospholipids (8), but a phospholipase A_1 type of activity has been demonstrated for purified pancreatic lipase (233).

Phospholipids from the bile have been shown to be more resistant to phospholipase A_2 hydrolysis than dietary phospholipids (35). However, several variables, particularly lipid components, may modify the organization of luminal micelles and consequently the lipid absorption process (207,234). Direct comparisons are therefore difficult to make. There appears to be no firm evidence for the recirculation of intact biliary phosphatidylcholines (207).

Mansbach et al. (149) have isolated a novel phospholipase from the intestine with a narrow enzymatic substrate specificity. Its activity was demonstrated by the surface barostat technique with phosphatidylglycerol as substrate. It was not found to be active with phosphatidylcholine in either the barostat assay or in a conventional assay. In the gut, the activity was found with both phosphatidylcholine and with phosphatidylglycerol as substrates. Since the enzymatic activity increased with pancreatic disease, it was obvious that the enzyme activity was not due to pancreatic phospholipase. Bacterial origin of the phospholipase was excluded by showing that the enzyme activity was present in germ-free rats. Likewise, gastric and salivary gland origins were excluded in that significant phospholipase activity was found in rats with gastric fistulae. It was proposed that the intestinal phospholipase may be important in gut bacterial control, in digestion of vegetable matter (phosphatidyl glycerol is a major lipid in both bacteria and plants), and in digestion of phospholipids in lumen. The latter activity would be in addition to that of pancreatic phospholipases, which are subject to proteolytic degradation (207). A comparison of the novel phospholipase and the purified lipase from pancreas (233) suggests that they are different enzymes. The intestinal mucosal enzyme requires Ca^{2+} for activity, whereas the pancreatic enzyme works even in the presence of ethylenediaminetetraacetate (EDTA).

The sphingomyelins are attacked by two other phospholipases active in the intestinal lumen, one of which releases the ceramide moiety of the sphingomyelin and another one that degrades the ceramide to free nitrogenous base and free fatty acid (178,179). Only limited studies have been performed with the latter enzymes.

Micellarization

As a result of the action of pancreatic lipase and the phospholipases, the tri-acylglycerols and glycerophospholipids are converted into the monoacylglycerols, lysophospholipids, and free fatty acids. Analyses of intestinal contents after a fatty meal have shown (93) that the bile salt concentration is around 10 mM in normal subjects, whereas the total fatty acid concentration is at least twice as high. Cholesterol and phospholipids contribute only small amounts of lipid to the total lipid mass, but they are important in the structure of micelles and phase equilibria (202).

Formation of Mixed Micelles

The lipolysis products along with any other fat-soluble substances, such as free sterols, vitamins A, D, E, and K, are subject to the process of micelle formation in which the lipid components interact with bile salts to form mixed aggregates or micelles. According to Hofmann and Borgstrom (104) the lipolytic products are dispersed as if there were two phases in the intestinal lumen. One of these is an emulsion phase of lipid particles in the 2,000 Å to 50,000 Å range suspended in an aqueous medium; the other is a micellar phase made up of particles 20 Å to 30 Å, which is formed in the presence of bile salts. The bile salts are characterized by the presence of hydrophobic and hydrophilic parts, which enable the amphipathic molecules to interact with both the lipids and the aqueous environment.

Patton and Carey (197) have observed that during fat digestion a sequence of physicochemical events occurs in which product phases are formed that are readily dispersed under physiological conditions. With both foreign and native components, two not just one distinct and reversible product phases are formed sequentially from the oil phase in the presence of micellar bile salt solutions. Both are presumably substrates that can be dispersed by bile salts to form a mixed micellar phase. In previous attempts to isolate the phases of fat digestion from intestinal contents either ultracentrifugation or ultrafiltration were used. Prolonged ultracentrifugation is necessary to obtain a clear micellar phase. However, this treatment produces a marked gradient and only a small fraction becomes clear (202). Patton and Carey (197) suggest that a clear micellar phase in the supernatant may not occur during fat digestion because of a continuous production of the viscous isotropic phase. The so-called micellar phase would therefore always be a two-phase system. Obviously the rate of formation relative to the rate of solubilization and absorption will determine the phase relationship occurring *in vivo* during fat digestion. It is not known if the liquid crystalline phases are substrates from which fat absorption occurs. Lindstrom et al. (139) recently reexamined the occurrence of the various lipid-water phases in the intestinal contents during fat absorption in man. They identified the cubic, reversed hexagonal, lamellar and L2 phases, along with mixed micelles. They also pointed out that the nature and properties of the lipid phases found depend on the lipid composition of intestinal contents. Thus, Lutton (143) demonstrated that fats made up predominantly of C_{12} chain-length fatty acids (coconut oil) form monoacylglycerols which only yield a lamellar liquid crystalline phase. Addition of a triacylglycerol oil to this phase, however, directly gives an L2 phase (276).

The fat-soluble vitamins are similar in their physical characteristics to cholesterol, free fatty acids, lipid-soluble drugs, and to many of the lipid-soluble environmental agents (106). The solubilization of the fat-soluble vitamins is accomplished by interaction with the biological detergents, bile acids, phospholipids, and the lipolysis products of neutral fats. It is believed that the fat-soluble vitamins are dissolved within the nonpolar interior of the micellar particles, but an interaction with the surface monolayer of the micelle cannot be excluded. The mixed micelles penetrate the unstirred water layer where the fat-soluble vitamins become partitioned into the monomeric phase and penetrate the lipid cell membrane. Therefore the formation of bile salt micelles is very important for the solubilization of fat-soluble vitamins. Hollander (106) has pointed out that doubling the normal bile salt concentration leads to increased absorption of fat-soluble vitamins, but this phenomenon is likely due to an injury to the cell membrane (77,219).

Impaired Micelle Formation

Any condition that results in a reduced concentration of bile salts within the intestinal lumen (below critical micelle concentration) will result in impaired micellar solubilization of lipids. Thus, drugs affecting bile salt concentration affect micelle formation and lipid absorption. Comai and Sullivan (60) have reported on the effects of cholestyramine, colestipol, and Pluronic L-101 (1% dietary supplement maximum) on the solubilization and absorption of cholesterol and triacylglycerols from a standard meal over a 2-hr period at 72 hr and 5 days in the meal model. Lipid absorption during a 72-hr period was significantly reduced by all compounds. The percent excretion of glycerol tri(1-^{14}C)oleate was increased significantly by Pluronic L-101 (10-fold), cholestyramine (5.7-fold) and colestipol (2.7-fold). The excretion of (^{3}H) cholesterol was enhanced significantly by cholestyramine (1.6-fold) and colestipol (1.3-fold). Cholestyramine and colestipol are hypocholesterolemic agents that act by sequestration of luminal bile salts, leading to enhanced bile salt synthesis (hepatic) from cholesterol. Removal of bile salts from the lumen of cholestyramine or colestipol markedly disrupts micelle formation and leads to the significant reduction in dietary cholesterol absorption and to the milder but significant reduction in triacylglycerol absorption (60,194). The bile salt sequestering resins may also bind free fatty acids, which would further decrease the micelle formation that is necessary for the solubilization and absorption of cholesterol and other lipids.

The Pluronic L-101 contains 10% hydrophilic units and 90% hydrophobic units, and possess good wetting characteristics. It is insoluble in water and has a molecular weight of 3,600. It is a nonabsorbable polymeric compound of polyoxyethylene (hydrophilic) units and polyoxypropylene (hydrophobic) units, whose physical properties depend on the proportion of the hydrophilic and hydrophobic groups. Recently several Pluronics (L-31, L-61, L-81, and L-121) were shown to reduce significantly but nonselectively the absorption of triacylglycerols and cholesterol and to reduce serum cholesterol levels in rats made hypercholesterolemic by dietary excess cholesterol (28). The mechanism of reduction of triacylglycerol absorption by Pluronic L-101, shown in the study by Comai and Sullivan (60), appeared not to involve bile salt sequestering. The intestinal contents of rats treated with Pluronic L-101 contained a higher percentage of triacylglycerols and a lower percentage of free fatty acids than the controls, indicating an inhibition of pancreatic lipase. Tso et al. (259) demonstrated that Pluronic L-81 impairs the lymphatic transport of fatty acids when infused together with trioleoylglycerol. The effect was not due to either impaired digestion or reesterification. The block seemed to be at a step subsequent to reesterification. It was removed when the infusion of the detergent was interrupted.

Rogers et al. (211) have reported that the activities of microsomal acyl-coenzyme A (CoA) synthetases are restored to normal levels in bile fistula rats by the infusion of sodium taurocholate and phosphatidylcholine, although infusion of sodium taurocholate alone results in some increase in specific enzyme activities. Thus bile salts and phosphatidylcholine appear to be necessary for the lymphatic transport of intraluminally administered fat.

Sklan (231) has presented evidence to indicate that a lack of monoacylglycerol in the lumen may also lead to decreased micelle formation and impaired fat absorption. This is a practical problem when feeding acidified soapstocks, a byproduct of edible oil refining, to poultry. Absorption of fatty acids was about 9% less from acidified soapstocks containing mainly free fatty acids, free from neutral oil. Significantly increased absorption resulted following the addition of glycerol, which resulted in the synthesis of monoacylglycerols.

Absorption

Preceding sections have dealt with the digestion of triacylglycerols and steryl esters and with the solubilization of digestion products in the form of mixed micelles. On reaching the brush border, the micelle may enter the cell intact, or the individual components may first dissociate from the micelle and enter the cell separately. It is not certain which of these processes occurs or if both occur. It is also not certain if the lipids pass through the plasma membrane by simple diffusion or by more complex processes including protein binding. The rate of uptake of nutrients from the bulk phase of the intestinal lumen into the mucosal cells is determined by the characteristics of two consecutive barriers, the unstirred water layer and the mucosal membrane. For many solutes—such as fatty acids, monoacylglycerols, and cholesterol—the step limiting the rate of uptake is the unstirred water layer.

Concept of Unstirred Water Layer

Wilson et al. (275) proposed the idea of an unstirred water layer adjacent to the epithelial cells as a rate-limiting factor for intestinal fat absorption on the basis of discrepancies between the measured and expected uptake of bile acids and free fatty acids by the cell membranes. The unstirred water layer is believed to be an unequilibrated area along the luminal surface of the small intestine with a thickness estimated to be in the range of 50 to 500 μm, depending on the experimental conditions (271). It is thinnest at the tip of the microvilli (50 μm). Clement (58) pointed out that this layer has no morphological basis. It is neither the mucus nor the glycocalyx. However, it allows the understanding of the intestinal uptake of the luminal lipids in physicochemical terms. The unstirred water layer presents a lower resistance to small molecules, and the rate of diffusion of long-chain fatty acid monomers is greater than that of the aggregates of mixed micelles. The unstirred water layer can therefore be visualized to promote the breakup of mixed micelles, and the dissociation of the free fatty acids and monoacylglycerols from the bile salts and other micellar components (58); however, the factors governing this dissociation have not been clearly defined.

More recent studies have shown that the unstirred water layer is rate-limiting for the passage of small, hydrophobic substances, whereas the enterocyte membrane forms a permeability barrier for more hydrophilic compounds (242). Thompson (252) investigated the effect of age on the rate of uptake of a homologous series of saturated fatty acids. At each rate of stirring, the unstirred water layer was lowest in the suckling and the mature rather than in the old animals. The values for the rate of uptake were corrected for differences in the unstirred water layer to yield estimates of the true passive permeability properties of the membrane. From these values the increment for energy change associated with the addition of each methylene group to the fatty acid chain was 50% higher in the suckling and in the mature animals than in the old animals. The estimated surface area of the jejunal membrane was also higher in the suckling and the mature animals. These results suggest that discrepancies in uptake of fatty acids (and possibly of other solutes) in animals of different ages can be explained by differences in the passive permeability properties and functional surface area of the membrane and by differences in the overlaying unstirred water layer. The short-chain acetic acid showed a higher rate of uptake than expected from a linear extrapolation of the relation from the longer chain fatty acids in mature animals. A similar finding was made for *n*-butyric and *n*-hexanoic acids in mature animals. This has been attributed in the past to a carrier-mediated difference (165). On the basis of measurements of the uptake of (^{14}C)inulin into the intervillar space in luminally lavaged canine jejunum, Riu and Grim (209) have concluded that essentially all lipid absorption must take place via the villous tips, the crypt region appearing to be totally impenetrable.

There is considerable evidence that the mixed micelles do not remain intact during the uptake by the mucosal cell. Thus, when the jejunum is perfused with a mixed micellar solution, some of the micellar solutes, such as fatty acids and monoacylglycerols, are taken up very rapidly, while cholesterol is taken up more slowly and the conjugated bile salts are excluded (229). Uptake of different solutes at independent rates has also been demonstrated with everted sacs (272). Comparisons of the uptake of oleic acid and of a monooleoylglycerol, which is a nonhydrolyzed analog of monooleoylglycerol, have shown that the ratio of lipid uptake was different from the ratio in the micelles. However, the uptake ratio was predictable from the independent uptake ratios and from the micellar concentrations of the co-solutes. Since the micelle supposedly does not penetrate the cell membrane, it must be concluded that the lipid is taken up as simple molecules. In such a case the maximum rate of uptake would occur when the monomer solution at the interface was saturated. Thus, the micellar solubilization would increase the driving force for transport across the unstirred layer and would indirectly increase the driving force for penetration of the cell membrane (229).

Uptake of Lipolysis Products

The potential energy utilized for the uptake of the lipids is a function of concentration. Hoffman (103) showed that a linear relationship exists between uptake and concentration of fatty acids in the micellar phase using everted sacs of the intestine. Likewise, Lee et al. (137) reported that the uptake is determined by the concentration of the solubilized fatty acid and not by the volume of the oil phase or the concentration of the bile acids. Uptake of the solubilized fatty acid is about 2.7 times faster from bile acid micelles than from non-ionic micelles. This compares well with the diffusibility measured in a diffusion cell, which is about 2.2 times faster for bile acid micelles (229).

Competition between long-chain (trioleoylglycerol) and medium-chain (trioctanoylglycerol) fatty acids has been shown to occur during steady state intestinal absorption in anaesthetized rats (56), but interpretation of the study is complicated by the markedly increased acidity of the luminal contents found during medium-chain fatty acid absorption. Clark (53) demonstrated that the inhibition of uptake did not occur at 0°C, when triacylglycerol synthesis was blocked. Incubation of slices at low pH (5.8) or in the presence of dimethylsulfoxide also reduced uptake of oleic acid and its incorporation into triacylglycerols. However, when everted sacs of jejunum were similarly incubated, octanoate, dimethylsulfoxide, or low pH caused no inhibition of oleic acid uptake or esterification. These results indicate that the significance of kinetic data describing intestinal fatty acid absorption, which were obtained from *in vitro* experiments, is highly questionable and that suitable models for *in vivo* uptake kinetics have yet to be developed. Experiments by Hyun et al. (114) had suggested that 2-ethyl-caproic acid suppressed esterification or uptake of oleic acid in lymphatic and portally cannulated rats and diverted unesterified fatty acids to the portal route, mucosal uptake not being affected.

Parsons et al. (195) demonstrated that stearic, oleic, elaidic, and linoleic acids are absorbed at equal rates when administered to volunteers by a duodenal perfusion in a micellar solution with taurocholate but excluding 2-monoacylglycerols. These measurements were based on examination of both the duodenal contents and the plasma at various times during and following the perfusion. Mishkin et al. (166) showed a uniform uptake and esterification of micellar (^{3}H) oleate and (^{14}C)palmitate along the entire length of the small intestine *in vivo*. He and his co-workers (166) also used monooleoylglycerol along with the free fatty acids in the bile salt micelles.

Chow and Hollander (50) demonstrated a dual, concentration-dependent absorption mechanism for linoleic acid by rat jejunum *in vitro*. At low concentrations (42–1,260 μM), the relationship between linoleic acid concentration and its absorption rate best approximated to a rectangular hyperbola. At high concentration (2.5–4.2 mM) the relationship between the two parameters was linear. The separate administration of 2,4-dinitrophenol, cyanide, or azide, or a decrease in the incubation temperature from 37 to 20 °C did not change the absorption rate of linoleic acid. Linoleic acid absorption rate was decreased after the addition of phosphatidylcholine, oleic, linoleic, and arachidonic acids or the substitution of taurocholate with the non-ionic surfactant Pluronic F-68. It was concluded that facilitated diffusion was the predominant mechanism for absorption at low concentrations, whereas at high concentrations simple diffusion was predominant. Chow and Hollander (51) have confirmed the above *in vitro* findings in the unanaesthetized rat *in vivo*. A similar mechanism had been demonstrated earlier by less extensive studies with arachidonic acid (49).

The effect of phosphatidylcholine on jejunal absorption of fatty acids and 1-monooctadecenoylglycerol was studied in healthy volunteers by Ammon et al. (6) using the jejunal perfusion system which excluded pancreatic and biliary secretions from the test segment. Phosphatidylcholine was found to reduce significantly the absorption of oleic acid and the 1-monooctadecenoylglycerol, while it had no effect on the absorption of ricinoleic acid. *In vitro* phosphatidylcholine reduced the monomer activities of all these lipids.

Mattson et al. (154) measured the absorbability of the fatty acid component by the fat balance technique. They determined the absorbability of fats containing various amounts of stearic acid esterified to the glycerol backbone. The triacylglycerols were sn-1-stearoyl-2,3-dioleoyl (SOO); sn-2-stearoyl-1,3-dioleoyl (OSO); 2-oleoyl-1,3-distearoyl (SOS); 1-oleoyl-2,3-distearoyl (OSS), and 1,2,3-trioleoyl (OOO). The following values for the absorbability of the stearate component in the presence and in the absence of divalent cations were obtained: OSO, 98, and 99%; SOO, 55 and 96%; SOS, 37 and 70%; OSS, 59 and 60%. It is apparent that 18:0 esterified at the sn-2-position of the glycerol is well absorbed, as the 2-monostearoylglycerol is well absorbed. If it is esterified at the sn-1- and sn-3-positions, it is released as free stearic acid, which, in the presence of Ca^{2+} and Mg^{2+}, is poorly absorbed.

The plant sterols campesterol and sitosterol are not absorbed as readily as cholesterol by the mammalian intestine, but the mucosal components and interactions responsible for this absorptive discrimination are unknown. Attempts to obtain definitive evidence *in vitro* have resulted in a failure of several well-characterized intestinal tissue preparations (246,247) to distinguish between cholesterol and sitosterol during the uptake from solutions containing physiological concentrations of bile salts. Likewise, Child and Kuksis (44) found that the use of simple sterol-bile salt micelles did not allow demonstration of a preferential uptake of cholesterol (over sitosterol) in rat enterocytes. However, addition of phospholipid to the incubation medium reduced the damage to the cell membranes induced by bile salts and reestablished a preferential cholesterol uptake (45). In a follow-up study Child and Kuksis (46) demonstrated that a similar discrimination is obtained for the corresponding 7-dehydro derivatives of cholesterol and sitosterol in the villous cell and in the brush border vesicles prepared from the villous cells. The latter membranes were markedly superior to the villous cells in selectively absorbing 7-dehydrocholesterol and displayed a level of discrimination comparable to that found with the parent sterols in the intestinal wall following feeding.

In order to elucidate further the basis of mucosal discrimination between cholesterol and plant sterols, Child and Kuksis (47) compared the selectivity of absorption among the 7-dehydro derivatives of cholesterol, campesterol, and sitosterol and the corresponding derivatives with modified ring structures. Following conversion of the 7-dehydrosterols to the calciferol derivatives, the C_{27} sterol was absorbed only 1.4 times faster than the C_{29} sterol by brush border membranes. Complete oxidation of the calciferol derivatives to the des-AB-8 ones resulted in a total loss of discrimination among the various side-chain homologs during absorption from micellar solution. It was therefore concluded that the selective absorption of animal and plant sterols depends on the presence of a complete ring system, although not necessarily a rigid or planar one.

The maximum transport of cholesterol to the lymph depends on the solubility of cholesterol in the triacylglycerol fat fed (244). Lymph transport studies in the rat have shown that the chain length of the carrier triacylglycerol is important for the absorption and transport of the cholesterol (246). Sylven and Borgstrom (246) have shown that the longer the fatty chain, the higher the rate of cholesterol transport to the chyle and the higher the amount of cholesterol taken up by the intestinal mucosa. The presence of the lipolytic products of dietary triacylglycerols in the bile salt micellar phase greatly increases the concentration of cholesterol in this phase compared with the solubility in pure bile salt micelles (32,230). The shorter the fatty chain, the less cholesterol is absorbed, and if the oil phase is made up by a hydrocarbon, cholesterol absorption is decreased to almost zero (246).

Klauda and Quackenbush (124) reported that cholesterol is equally well absorbed from a variety of fats and oils by lymph duct cannulated rats. Of these only hydrogenated coconut oil depressed the absorption rate. In subsequent experiments it was found that ethyl oleate also depressed cholesterol absorption compared with the triacylglycerol. The difference appears to reflect a need for monoacylglycerol, since addition of 2-monooleoylglycerol to ethyl oleate improved cholesterol absorption (125).

The absorption of the various micellar components is greatly influenced by the composition of the mixed micelle. Hollander and Morgan (107) showed that unsaturated long-chain fatty acids, oleic, linoleic, linolenic, and arachidonic, inhibit cholesterol absorption. Likewise, addition of phosphatidylcholine in the range of 0.1 to 1.5 mM caused a progressive, dose-related inhibition of cholesterol absorption. It was speculated that the inhibitory effect of these components on cholesterol absorption was likely to have been caused by changes in cholesterol solubility in these micelles and shifts in the partition coefficient of cholesterol away from the cell membrane to the micelles. Child and Kuksis (44) also have noted that addition of phosphatidylcholine to bile salt micelles containing cholesterol results in a decreased overall uptake of sterols, although the discrimination between cholesterol and plant sterols is enhanced.

Grundy and Mok (94) recently reported studies suggesting the occurrence in man of significant isotope exchange between intraluminal radiolabeled cholesterol and unlabeled mucosal cholesterol. If significant isotope exchange does occur during intestinal transit, any results obtained by absorption tests using radioisotopic cholesterol would necessarily be inaccurate. Samuel and McNamara (216) have obtained evidence that currently available methods for the measurement of cholesterol absorption (most of which are based on the use of radioisotopic sterols for differentiating exogenous from endogenous sterols) reliably quantitate the absorption of cholesterol and that the results of such tests are not significantly confounded by *in vivo* isotopic exchange (94). Zilversmit (280) recently discussed a model for cholesterol absorption that allows the contrasting of mass and isotopic measurements and of single-dose and constant-infusion administration methods. The results show that when absorption is calculated from the amount of lymph or fecal isotopically labeled cholesterol after constant infusion or after a single dose, one obtains a measure of exogenous cholesterol absorption that is in very good agreement with that derived from the increment of cholesterol (lymph) mass. Since the amount of cholesterol label appearing in lymph also appears to be a good measure of the increment in lymph cholesterol mass, it would appear that methods based on the measurement of labeled cholesterol in plasma may give equally valid measures of exogenous cholesterol absorption. In rats and in humans, a dual isotope plasma ratio method has been found to correspond closely to values obtained from fecal analysis (280).

Uptake of Fat-Soluble Vitamins

Much information about the mechanism of absorption of fats and other lipids has been gained from studies of the uptake of the fat-soluble vitamins by various preparations of intestinal mucosa. Hollander and Muralidhara (108) determined the rate of absorption of vitamin A by the everted gut sac technique. When the retinol concentration of the infusate, which was kept within the physiological range (30 to 300 μM), was comapred with the rate of retinol absorption, the relationship delineated apparent saturation kinetics. Since the retinol absorption remained unchanged upon addition of metabolic uncouplers and inhibitors such as 2,4-dinitro-phenol, oligomycin, or potassium cyanide to the infusate, it was concluded that retinol absorption in this range of concentration is a carrier-mediated passive absorption process. When the relationship between retinol absorption rate and its concentration was explored at the pharmacological range of luminal concentration, the transport process occurred by simple passive diffusion. Passive diffusion of retinol at high intraluminal concentrations masks the coexisting carrier-mediated transport that was dominant in the physiological range of concentration (108).

Noguchi et al. (182) demonstrated that lymphatic transport of Sudan Blue and vitamin A acetate is very small in the absence of bile. When sodium taurocholate and egg phosphatidylcholine were coadministered with emulsions, lymphatic trans-port of lipid-soluble compounds was normal even in bile fistula rats. The addition of one of them could not recover completely the lymphatic transport of lipid-soluble compounds. It was concluded that both bile salts and phosphatidylcholine were necessary for the lymphatic transport of fat and lipid-soluble compounds, which interact with oil administered intraluminally. However, overall contribution of lymphatic pathway to the disappearance from the intestinal lumen was very small, and the main route of the absorption was thought to be the portal pathway. The phosphatidylcholine did not affect the lymphatic transport of Sudan Blue and vitamin A acetate at all in the absence of sodium taurocholate.

Absorption of the tocopherols likewise is dependent on the animal's ability to digest and absorb fat. Bieri and Farrell (24) have presented a brief review on the absorption of vitamin E, with emphasis on the physical form in which it reaches the intestine, the efficiency of absorption, and the effect of dietary fat unsaturation on absorption from the intestine. Most tocopherol enters the bloodstream via lymph where it is associated with chylomicrons and low-density lipoproteins. With mixed micelles α-tocopherol is absorbed via the lymph to the extent of 43% (160). When the bile duct is cannulated, absorption from the mixed micelles is reduced to 20%. A similarly high lymphatic absorption of α- and γ-tocopherol (46%) is found (199) with emulsions containing Tween, lard, and serum albumin. Hollander and Mur-alidhara (108) have shown that the fat-soluble vitamin uptake is progressively decreased in proportion to the concentration of the added polyunsaturated fatty acid. Nakamura et al. (175) demonstrated that hydrolysis of α-tocopherol esters may not be necessarily a prerequisite for intestinal absorption. However, the per-centage of absorption of slowly hydrolyzed esters of lymph was relatively lower than that of moderately or easily hydrolyzable esters.

Hollander and Rim (109) studied the lymphatic appearance rate of [³H]phylloquinone in rats with cannulated bile and lymph ducts. Addition of short-chain fatty acids (butyrate) to the infusate enhanced total absorption of vitamin K, into the bile and lymph, whereas addition of polyunsaturated fatty acids inhibited the total absorption of the vitamin.

Resynthesis of Dietary Fat

The process of digestion and absorption of dietary fat is completed by reesteri-fication of the fatty acids and alcohols by the intestinal mucosa. This helps to maintain an effective gradient for the passive uptake of the products of lipolysis and to prevent the mucosal cell from potential injury from the surface active acids and monoacylglycerols. The reesterification takes place in the microsomal fraction, where the fatty acids are activated to acyl-CoA and transesterified to appropriate alcohol acceptors. Both 2-monoacylglycerol and sn-glycerol-3-phosphate derived from glucose metabolism can serve as acceptors for acyl-CoA and normally do so in a ratio of about 70 to 30, respectively (33,86,196).

Stereochemical Course of Acylglycerol Synthesis

The phosphatidic acid pathway of triacylglycerol formation proceeds via the exclusive formation of the sn-1,2-diacylglycerols, which are further esterified at the sn-3-position utilizing a different pool of acyl-CoA, and may yield enantiomeric products. The sn-2,3-diacylglycerols cannot be formed by this route. The stereochemical course of reacylation of the sn-2-monoacylglycerols is controversial, both complete specificity for sn-1,2-enantiomer formation as well as complete absence of specificity resulting in rac-1,2-diacylglycerol formation having been claimed in addition to various intermediate proportions of the products (133). Recently, Bugaut et al. (39) reexamined the stereochemical course of the 2-monoacylglycerol esterification by means of 2-monolauroylglycerol and deuterated palmitic acid in combination with stereospecific enzymic hydrolyses and gas chromatography with mass spectrometry. It was observed that the sn-1,2- and sn-2,3-diacylglycerol enantiomers were formed in approximately 70:30 ratio, respectively. This clearly showed that the 2-monoacylglycerol acyltransferase, if a single enzyme, possessed only a partial stereospecificity. Alternatively, the result could have been explained by the presence of two stereospecific acyltransferases operating at unequal rates or present in unequal concentrations. Further resolution of the problem awaits the isolation of the pure monoacylglycerol acyltransferases.

The medium- and short-chain fatty acids that are produced by lipolysis either in the lumen or following absorption in the cell are not activated and esterified and secreted into the lymph in the form of chylomicrons (208). Instead, they pass directly into the portal vein as free fatty acids, bind physically to the plasma albumin, and are delivered to the liver as fatty acid by the portal circulation. This is in contrast to the synthesis of milk fat triacylglycerols in which the short-chain fatty acids are found to be specifically esterified to the sn-3-position of the triacylglycerol molecule.

Reesterification of Sterols

The absorption of dietary cholesterol in the intestine has been extensively studied with regard to the delivery of free cholesterol to the mucosal membrane and its reesterification within the mucosal cell. Two roles for pancreatic cholesterol esterase in this process have been proposed. It catalyzes the hydrolysis of dietary cholesteryl ester and may catalyze cholesterol reesterification after being taken up by the villus cell (255). Bhat and Brockman (20,21) observed that pancreatic cholesterol esterase shows an affinity for free fatty acids, a product of lipolysis.

These workers (22,23) also found that the rate of accumulation of cholesteryl ester in rat intestinal sacs is enhanced up to threefold by adding porcine cholesterol esterase to the uptake medium. The enzyme must be catalytically active and does not exert its effect via its activity in the medium. These workers have proposed a plausible mechanism. Once adsorbed in the luminal surface of the membrane, the enzyme catalyzes a small percentage of the cholesterol esterification in the membrane (22). Being highly non-polar, this ester readily partitions to the hydrocarbon region of the bilayer from where it can return or partition to the inner surface of the membrane. On the inner surface the intestinal cholesterol esterase, perhaps of pancreatic origin (90,255), again catalyzes the free/esterified cholesterol equilibrium which favors hydrolysis. Thus, cholesterol esterases on each surface of the membrane can catalyze the flip-flop of cholesterol (via the ester) from one leaflet of the membrane to the other. This is in agreement with the conclusion of Chow and Hollander (48), namely, that uptake of cholesterol has a free energy of activation equal to 20 kcal/mol, which argues against diffusion of cholesterol to the villous membrane as the sole rate-determining step. The pathway proposed by Bhat and Brockman (22) is consistent with the known properties of cholesterol absorption, such as its specificity, and with the source requirement for fatty acids such as triacylglycerol, and for cholesterol esterase. Klein and Rudel (126) have shown that in the nonhuman primate during high cholesterol infusion, dietary cholesterol is esterified preferentially, as previously observed in lower animals on high cholesterol diets.

Swell et al. (243) postulated that sitosterol was not absorbed by the intestinal mucosa because it was not readily esterified in the intestinal wall of lymph fistula rats. Evidence has been accumulating that acyl-coA:cholesterol acyltransferase (ACAT) is the enzyme responsible for catalyzing cholesterol esterification in the enterocyte (80,101). The ability of this enzyme to catalyze the esterification of sitosterol and the degree to which sitosterol competes with and/or interferes with cholesterol esterification are matters of importance in understanding the metabolism of cholesterol in the gut. Field and Mathur (81) have demonstrated that the CoA-dependent esterification rate of cholesterol is at least 60 times greater than that of β-sitosterol. Membrane β-sitosterol does not interfere with nor compete with cholesterol esterification. Inadequate esterification of plant sterol may play a role in the poor absorption of β-sitosterol by the gut.

The lack of esterification of sitosterol by ACAT in the intestinal mucosa is consistent with the finding of virtually all of the plant sterols in the free form in the chyle of dogs with thoracic duct fistula (132).

Biosynthesis of Membranes and Lipoproteins

It has long been recognized that absorption of fat and its transport as chylomicrons into lymph is accompanied by an increased turnover of mucosal phospholipid (95). Some are exported as coating for chylomicrons (210,221), and some are utilized for increased membrane turnover associated with exocytosis (213). There is some evidence that the phospholipid synthesis is limiting the clearance if not the absorption of neutral fat even under normal physiological conditions. Thus, Clark (53) has shown that phosphatidylcholine enhances triacylglycerol output in the lymph even in rats with bile ducts intact. Shaikh and Kuksis (223) have shown that there is an expansion of the total phospholipid pool of the intestinal mucosa during fat absorption, which is proportional to the fat load, when assayed in isolated cells of rat intestinal mucosa. This expansion of the phospholipid pool size is accompanied by an increase in the total phospholipid and individual phospholipid turnover, which exceeds that anticipated on the basis of the known lipid composition of the chylomicron surface coat (224). It was suggested that all the phospholipids were subject to increased turnover during fat absorption, not just those involved in chylomicron assembly. Obviously all or most membranes of the villous cell were turned over at increased rate during the process of fat absorption.

In addition to the apparent protection of the integrity of the microvillar membranes, luminal phosphatidylcholine may have an important role in fat transport by providing the necessary surfactant for chylomicron coating and by supporting protein biosynthesis. O'Doherty et al. (186) found that the addition of choline, lysophosphatidylcholine, or phosphatidylcholine to a gastric test meal consisting of lipid and bile salts markedly reduced the mucosal accumulation of absorbed lipid in bile fistula rats. The appearance of the fatty gut was associated with the recovery of decreased amounts of radioactive fatty acids in the liver and adipose tissue of these animals. All of these effects were readily cleared by the inclusion of choline, lysophosphatidylcholine, or phosphatidylcholine in the meal. These observations have been since confirmed in isolated villous cells of rat intestinal mucosa with essentially identical results (187,188). Similar findings in the bile fistula rats have been obtained by Clark (54) and Tso et al. (260), who analyzed the lymph. In a parallel study Tso et al. (262) attempted to evaluate the relative importance of choline chloride, lysophosphatidylcholine, and phosphatidylcholine as sources of the luminal choline. The addition of choline chloride to the meal increased lymphatic output of triacylglycerols and phospholipid but to lesser degree than found in bile fistula rats supplemented with phosphatidylcholine or in rats with intact bile ducts. The addition of dioleoylphosphatidylcholine was as effective as that of biliary phosphatidylcholine. Hence it was concluded that a luminal supply of 1-palmitoyllysophosphatidylcholine from the bile was not essential. Apparently, the essential structure was the lysophosphatidylcholine, which was reesterifed in the intestinal mucosa to phosphatidylcholine before incorporation into the chylomicron surface, as also suggested by the work of O'Doherty (185). Tso et al. (261) have extended these observations further using rats with bile and thoracic duct lymph fistulae and a bile salt stabilized emulsion of trioleoylglycerol as the source of the lipid. Greater than 95% uptake of fat was realized in all groups. However, the presence of supplemental phosphatidylcholine in the infusate greatly enhanced the lymphatic triacylglycerol and phosphatidylcholine output in the bile-diverted rats as compared with rats without phosphatidylcholine supplementation. In the absence of luminal phosphatidylcholine there was increased accumulation of mucosal triacylglycerol, as originally shown by O'Doherty et al. (186).

However, Mansbach (147) and Ng and Holt (176) were unable to observe enhanced lymphatic transport of infused trioleoylglycerol in the presence of added luminal phosphatidylcholine. Although the data from these studies are difficult to interpret because of differences in experimental design and lack of experimental detail, it would appear that in all these instances the infused loads of micellar lipid were so small as not to tax the available endogenous phosphatidylcholine mass or the capability of its biosynthesis. This possibility finds support in the early studies of Tso and Simmonds (263) where no difference could be found in mucosal lipid content in bile fistula rats, with or without phosphatidylcholine supplementation, when the lipid loads were kept low.

Barnes et al. (12) and Snipes (236) have suggested that fat malabsorption is present in animals fed essential fatty acid (EFA)-deficient diets. Clark et al. (55) reinvestigated the absorption of fat in EFA deficiency and demonstrated that EFA deficiency does not reduce the absorptive capacities for trioleoylglycerol or for a medium-chain trioctanoylglycerol measured 3 and 2 hr after maximal-rate duodenal infusion. The specific activities of the microsomal esterifying enzymes acyl-CoA:monoacylglycerol acyltransferase and fatty acid CoA ligase in jejunal mucosa were 30% lower in EFA-deficient rats. Accumulation of lipid in the intestinal wall was increased in the deficient rats. Because more than 90% of the absorbed mucosal fat was present as triacylglycerol, EFA deficiency appeared to affect the synthesis of or release of chylomicron lipid from the intestine. In EFA deficiency it is possible that changes occur in the availability of appropriate phospholipids for chylomicron formation or that the membranes of the endoplasmic reticulum or Golgi apparatus (where chylomicron formation and assembly is thought to occur) may be affected. Thus, current evidence suggests that the defective transport of large molecules in EFA deficiency is due to abnormalities of exit, not of uptake.

The formation and secretion of chylomicrons also require protein biosynthesis. This was first suggested by the observation that in the absence of apoprotein B (abetalipoproteinemia), the intestine is not able to synthesize triacylglycerol-rich lipoprotein particles, a condition that is partially mimicked by puromycin poisoning of the intact animal (214) or of the isolated villous cells (188). Glickman et al. (92) have used an immunofluorescent staining technique to demonstrate that fluorescent stain appears at the apical portion of the absorptive cells, and the density of the stain increases during active fat absorption. The intestine also synthesizes other lipoproteins (226), including apoprotein A-I, which serves as an activator of lecithin-cholesterol acyltransferase. The functional significance of the various intestinal apoproteins is not known.

Furthermore, few details are known about the mechanism of lipoprotein and chylomicron secretion from the cell, although it has been demonstrated that the lipoproteins from the microsomal or Golgi vesicles travel toward the basolateral membranes, where they appear to fuse with the membrane and discharge their contents into the intercellular space by reverse pinocytosis (208,253). Riley and

Glickman (208) have presented evidence, suggesting that the intracellular movement depends, in part, on intact microtubular function.

INTERACTION WITH FAT-SOLUBLE ENVIRONMENTAL AGENTS

The fat-soluble environmental agents include both noxious and relatively harmless substances, which are derived from natural (66) and synthetic (201) sources. For the present purpose these materials have been grouped according to their general physicochemical properties, with the specific origin and metabolic basis of any toxicity being mentioned only in passing. In most instances the potential absorbability of these compounds has been implied from studies of their partition between organic solvents and water, which has been demonstrated to be closely related to the actual appearance of the chemicals in lymph, blood, and tissues. There is evidence that the lipophilic xenobiotics are absorbed in a similar fashion to the trace nutrient lipids and fat-soluble vitamins, the uptake of which is intimately dependent on the normal processes of fat digestion and absorption (106). Since lipid absorption is passive, sufficient quantities of lipid in monomolecular solution must exist close to the enterocyte membrane to create the diffusion gradient responsible for absorption. Patton (196) has suggested a scheme of fat digestion which provides a continuous hydrocarbon domain for the transfer of lipids from the lumen to the enterocyte and which may be pertinent to the assimilation of various lipophilic compounds by the villous cells. A nondispersible mixed triacylglycerol phase containing the fat-soluble foreign substances is hydrolyzed by the action of pancreatic lipase to monoacylglycerols and free fatty acids. These form a viscous isotropic phase that is subsequently solubilized by bile salts, producing a aqueous micellar solution. Trace lipids are able to flow from the bulk dietary oil into the viscous isotropic phase to be eventually solubilized in the hydrophobic interiors of the mixed micelles. The micelles serve to carry the products of fat digestion and trace lipids through the aqueous phase to the absorbing villous cell membrane. Upon breakup of the mixed micelles in the unstirred water layer, the lipophilic xenobiotics are partitioned from the aqueous phase to the lipid phase of the plasma membrane of the villous cell.

Hydrocarbons

The intestinal absorption of the neutral hydrocarbons has challenged the imagination of physiologists and biochemists for many decades and has served as proof of both absorbability and nonabsorbability of a given lipid form. Work with isotopic tracers has demonstrated that relatively large amounts of aliphatic hydrocarbons may be metabolized during absorption, while the polycyclic hydrocarbons are subject to much more limited metabolic transformation.

Paraffins

These are relatively harmless compounds widely distributed in nature and extensively employed in various commercial products including food packaging materials. Channon and Collinson (42) first demonstrated the absorption of liquid paraffin from the alimentary tract of rats and pigs. These findings were confirmed and extended by others (84,240). Stetten (240) fed deuterated hexadecane to rats and found that it was taken up by the intestinal tract of rats to a considerable degree and converted to fatty acids. Systematic studies of the absorption of deuterium labeled normal C_8-C_{18} hydrocarbons were reported by Bernhard (18). When a 20% solution of hydrocarbons was fed in olive oil, about 20% was recovered in the lymph lipids. The chain length did not seem to have any effect on the extent of absorption. McWeeny (161) administered intragastrically to rats a 2% solution of $(1-^{14}C)n$-hexadecane in olive oil and found that 13 to 16% of the alkane was absorbed over a period of 15 hr with 20 to 30% of the absorbed radioactivity appearing in the lymph lipids as fatty acids. Kollatukudy and Hankin (128) found that nonadecane was absorbed in the rat and converted to the corresponding fatty acid. Although a great variety of bacteria are known to oxidize alkanes to fatty acids, a rigid exclusion of intestinal bacteria was not always achieved in the above experiments.

The need for the simultaneous administration of triacylglycerols for the hydrocarbon absorption appears to have been firmly established, although the mechanism of action is not well understood. Elbert et al. (71) reported that administration of pure mineral oil to rats resulted, at most, in 3% absorption, whereas feeding of equimolar amounts of octadecane and trioleoylglycerol led to the absorption of about 50% of the octadecane, which was recovered in the lymph partly as fatty acid. Krabisch and Borgstrom (129) have demonstrated that the effect of trioleoylglycerol on hydrocarbon absorption is paralleled by a largely increased solubility of the paraffin in the mixed bile salt micelle compared with the pure bile salt micelle. Thus, using a turbidity method, Krabisch and Borgstrom (129) found the solubility of octadecane in 8 mM sodium taurocholate to be less than 0.2 μmol/ml. If 7.2 μmol of 1-monooleoylglycerol was included in the solution, the solubility of octadecane increased more than 10-fold. The ready absorption of hydrocarbons in the presence of the lipolytic products of triacylglycerols favors the idea that the absorption of the nonpolar lipids takes place via a mixed micellar phase, which may be taken up intact by the mucosal membrane (however, see below).

It is possible that dispersion of lipolytic product phases, with better solubilization properties for nonpolar lipids compared with mixed micelles, might provide additional route for uptake of nonpolar lipids. The observation that latex dispersions are taken up (218) indicates that absorption of colloid particles larger than micelles might be possible.

Consumption of diets rich in squalene has clearly increased the squalene concentration in lymph (220) or serum (140). Absorption of the saturated analog, squalane, however, was insignificant (220). Feeding squalene has increased squalene and sterol concentration in serum and liver of the rat and enhanced fecal excretion of bile acids (140), suggesting that squalene absorbed from the diet participated in the overall cholesterol synthesis. Tilvis and Miettinen (256) recently demonstrated that ^{3}H-squalene is, like cholesterol-4-^{14}C, absorbed through the lymphatic route and that approximately 20% of absorbed ^{3}H-squalene is cyclized to sterols during the transit through the intestinal wall. An increase in dietary squalene load (8–48 mg) decreased the absorption percentage of ^{3}H-squalene (46%–26%), but did not affect the absorption of ^{14}C-cholesterol (47%). The more rapid appearance of dietary ^{3}H-squalene than of ^{14}C-cholesterol in chyle and serum was rationalized by the fairly high difference in squalene concentration between the test mixture and intestinal mucosal cells, which was not the case for the dietary ^{14}C-cholesterol.

Polycyclics

The aromatic polycyclic hydrocarbons in the environment have received close attention ever since benzo(a)pyrene was first demonstrated to be carcinogenic. To date about 100 polycyclic hydrocarbons have been identified in the environment and in foods (141). It is believed that the bulk of these materials is formed during pyrolysis of organic substances by a series of reactions involving the combination of free radicals (9), although some are formed biosynthetically or are of geochemical origin. These compounds possess extremely low solubility in water, whereas most of them are very soluble in organic solvents. Their solubility in water, however, can be increased greatly in the presence of other organic compounds. This characteristic, along with their absorption on surfaces, as well as micelle formation in the presence of surface-active agents, is pertinent to their appearance in foods and to their absorption by the intestine. The absorption of polycyclic hydrocarbons in experimental animals has been studied extensively (264). In most instances, however, the test compounds were administered by peritoneal routes (injection), and the results may not have much relevance to the evaluation of orally ingested polycyclics. The data obtained from the oral administration of several radioactive polycyclics indicate that they are rapidly absorbed and eliminated through biliary excretion in the feces and in urine. Some of the absorbed material is retained in the adrenals, the ovaries, and in body fat, where it could be detected after 8 days. Extensive testing (41,141) indicates that only a few of the known carcinogenic polycyclic aromatic hydrocarbons are capable of inducing cancer in animals when administered orally. Furthermore, the cancers induced orally were restricted to leukemia, stomach tumors, hepatoma, and pulmonary adenoma, whereas nonoral administration routes led to skin tumor formation. Mammary gland tumors were induced by both routes of administration. From an extensive review of the literature, Lo and Sandi (141) have concluded that most foods contain low levels of polycyclic aromatic hydrocarbons, unless pyrolytic reactions, curing at high temperatures, or the smoking processes contribute directly or indirectly to such compounds. The possible roles of dietary fats in polycyclic hydrocarbon carcinogenesis have been reviewed by Hopkins and West (110).

To determine the physicochemical behavior of xenobiotic hydrocarbons in simulated intestinal content, Laher and Barrowman (135) examined the partition of 7,12-dimethylbenzanthracene (DMBA), 3-methylcholanthrene (MC), and benzo-

(a)pyrene between an emulsified oil phase and a mixed micellar solution. In a mixed lipid-bile salt system, negligible amounts of hydrocarbon were present in aqueous solution below the critical micellar concentration of sodium taurocholate. Once the critical concentration was reached, the hydrocarbons exhibited nearly identical partitions from the lipid into the micellar system, which was enhanced by increased concentrations of bile salt, reduction of triacylglycerol concentration, and the formation of mixed rather than pure bile salt micelles. The partition of DMBA and MC into micelles was optimized by long-chain monounsaturated (oleic) acid and monooleoylglycerol as compared with their octanoic and linoleic acid counterparts. This is consistent with the observation of Borgstrom (32), who found that cholesterol partitioned more in favor of an aqueous phase when the fatty acid species was oleic rather than linoleic. In contrast (see below), the polychlorinated biphenyls appeared to favor the aqueous phase when the polyunsaturated rather than the monounsaturated fatty acid was present. In a mixed micellar system, excluding the oil phase and an excess of DMBA, a molar saturation ratio (mol hydrocarbon/mol bile salt) was calculated by regression analysis to be 0.162.

Early studies by Ekwall et al. (70) showed several polycyclic aromatic hydro-carbon carcinogens to undergo aqueous solubilization in the presence of high concentrations of bile salt (in excess of 100 mM). Norman (184) demonstrated MC solubilization in solutions of conjugated and unconjugated bile salts beginning at 12 mM.

The simulated intestinal system of Laher and Barrowman (135) was modeled after that used by El-Gorab and Underwood (72) in their studies on the solubilization of β-carotene and retinol. It contains concentrations of fatty acids, monoacylgly-cerol, triacylglycerol, phospholipid, and sodium ion likely to be found postpran-dially in the small intestine. Since Laher and Barrowman (135) have estimated that approximately six molecules of bile salt can solubilize one molecule of hydrocarbon when allowed to form mixed fatty acid-monoacylglycerol-bile salt micelles, it appears that a true micellar solubilization is occurring, and the principle of at least one molecule of solute per micelle is maintained. As hydrolysis proceeded, increas-ing quantities of DMBA partitioned into the aqueous phase, reaching a maximum of 13% of the hydrocarbon in the aqueous phase at 40% hydrolysis. It was evident that depletion of the triacylglycerol content at fixed fatty acid and monoacylglycerol concentration significantly promoted the partition of the polycyclic aromatic hy-drocarbons from an oil phase into an aqueous micellar phase. Triacylglycerol hydrolysis is, therefore, necessary for an effective partition of hydrocarbon from an oil phase into a water-dispersible bile salt solution.

From the studies of Laher and Barrowman (125) and the above discussion it can be supposed that the polycyclic aromatic hydrocarbons following ingestion will participate in the same digestive and dispersive processes as trace nutrient lipids in the intestinal lumen. Because of the requirement for mixed bile salt micelles to promote the solubilization of hydrocarbons in an aqueous medium simulating lu-minal conditions, it is probable that mixed micelles are the vehicles responsible for delivery of hydrocarbons to the absorptive villous cells of the small bowel.

Biphenyls and Triphenyls

The polychlorinated biphenyls and triphenyls have been used for many years as heat-transfer agents, sealants, adhesives, and as dielectric fluids in electrical transformers and capacitors. Polychlorinated polycyclics have been found to contaminate cereals, milk fat, poultry products, fish products and have been detected in human adipose tissues. The polychlorinated biphenyls can induce vomiting, diarrhea, weakness, nail pigmentation, and skin eruptions in human subjects. Allen and Norback (4) have shown that these agents, when administered orally, induce gastric hyperplasia and dysplasia in rhesus monkeys. Although histopathological changes resembling precarcinomatous lesions have been shown in the gastric submucosa of animals receiving these agents, their effect on the human alimentary tract has remained uncertain.

Laher and Barrowman (135) have examined the partition of a polychlorinated biphenyl mixture (Arochlor 1242), containing 42% chlorine, from an oil phase into an aqueous micellar phase and have found it to be promoted by free fatty acid and monoacylglycerols. As for the transfer of polycyclic aromatic hydrocarbons, hydrolysis of triacylglycerol was necessary for an appreciable partition of the biphenyl from the oil phase into the aqueous bile salt solution. The polychlorinated biphenyls appeared to favor aqueous solubilization when the polyunsaturated rather than monounsaturated fatty acid and monounsaturated acylglycerol were present. This behavior contrasted with that of the polycyclic aromatic hydrocarbons, which partitioned into the aqueous phase more readily in the presence of the monounsaturated fatty acid and monoacylglycerol. The polychlorinated biphenyls are excreted in breast milk (273) and residues have been detected in human adipose tissue (162).

These contradictory observations, in spite of otherwise similar behavior in the simulated intestinal system, are difficult to interpret, but Laher and Barrowman (135) have suggested that they could be explained by a stereochemical fit into the lipid cores of the mixed micelles, if a true micellar solubilization was occurring. It was speculated that the various polycyclic aromatic hydrocarbons studied might have a better fit when the oleic acid lipids were incorporated into the micelles rather than linoleic acid and monolinoleoylglycerol. The polychlorinated biphenyl might be better accommodated in the mixed micelles when linoleic rather than oleic acid and monooleoylglycerol are present.

Laher and Barrowman (135) showed that fatty acids and monoacylglycerols of medium-chain length form micelles with a lower capacity to solubilize the hydrocarbons than the corresponding long-chain lipids. This is in agreement with the work of Takahashi and Underwood (250), who found that aqueous solubilization of α-tocopherol was increased when lipids of medium-chain length were incorporated into bile salt micellar system but that this effect was threefold to sevenfold less than for a corresponding long-chain mixture. It was further speculated that a greater expansion of the hydrophobic interior by long-chain lipids might be responsible for the observed difference, if the hydrocarbons do undergo solubilization in the lipid cores of the mixed bile salt micelles.

From these studies it is obvious that the polychlorinated biphenyls following ingestion will participate in the same digestive and dispersive processes as trace nutrient lipids in the intestinal lumen. The nondiscriminating hydrocarbon continuum necessary for the efficient absorption of essential micronutrients, such as the fat-soluble vitamins, may therefore become readily compromised by the fat-soluble environmental agents, regardless of their actual toxicity to the absorptive cell.

Other polychlorinated aromatic hydrocarbons are produced industrially as organic pesticides. These substances have widely contaminated the environment ever since their widespread use was introduced in agriculture. Thus, dichlorodiphenyltrichloroethane (DDT) and dichlorodiphenyldichloroethylene (DDE) residues have been found in small quantities in body fat of normal human beings. The extent of food contamination by these pesticides is variable and may be considerable at certain times in certain geographic areas, although, generally, the amounts detectable in food substances are low (164,274). Food products of animal origin usually contain larger quantities of DDT and DDE than vegetables and fruit. Durham (68) and Lo and Sandi (141) have prepared extensive reviews of pesticide residues in foods. Studies (267) on human subjects occupationally exposed to pesticides, however, have not yielded significant adverse clinical findings. The chlorinated hydrocarbon type of pesticides are not readily degraded in the environment and accumulate in various food chains (141).

Absorption of the fat-soluble pesticides by the gastrointestinal tract is influenced by both the nature of the pesticide ingested and the type and quantity of food and bacteria present. The gastrointestinal absorption of dieldrin, one of the chlorinated hydrocarbon insecticides, has been studied by Heath and Vanderkar (98) in the rat. These workers observed that radioactively labeled dieldrin appeared in the lymph in a 7:1 ratio to portal vein after oral administration. The absorption varied with the vehicle of administration of the dieldrin. The mechanism of transport of pesticides from the gastrointestinal tract has been studied by several investigators with conventional *in vitro* techniques. Shah and Guthrie (222) reported that absorption of several fat-soluble insecticides through the proximal small intestine is a passive process. While the trichlorobis(p-chlorophenyl)ethane family of compounds (DDT) have been banned from use in some countries, they are still widely used in many other countries, and thus their continued use can constitute a serious problem for the global population. The urinary excretion of bis(p-chlorophenyl) acetic acid (DDA), a metabolite of DDT, can be used as an indicator of exposure to DDT (277). The current Environmental Protection Agency (EPA) procedure available for the determination of DDA involves chemical derivatizaton and GLC using an electron capture detector. Ingestion, even in trace amounts, results in storage and concentration of DDT in fatty tissues, where it is slowly dehydrochlorinated to DDE and/or dichlorodiphenyldichloroethane (DDD) and ultimately excreted as DDA in urine (222).

Long-Chain Acids and Esters

This group of compounds includes both naturally occurring and synthetic compounds. The long-chain aliphatic carboxylic acids occur naturally as glycerol esters, and the synthetic aromatic carboxylic acids are produced industrially in the form of short-chain alcohol esters. The alkyl and aryl sulphonates represent mainly soaps. All these compounds are widely encountered in the environment, but their physiological effects, with notable exceptions, are relatively mild.

Aliphatic Acids

These include the naturally occurring long-chain saturated and monounsaturated fatty acids, the positional and geometric isomerization products of natural unsaturated fatty acids arising from industrial hydrogenation of natural fats and oils, some hydroxy fatty acids, as well as the brominated fatty acids used in various foods, drinks, and industrial products (66).

Several laboratories have reported that the consumption by weanling rats of triacylglycerols containing 22 carbon monounsaturated acids, erucate or cetoleate, results in a marked accumulation of lipids in the heart (14). Similar results were obtained with partly hydrogenated rapeseed oil, which, however, still contained significant amounts of erucic acid. Mattson and Streck (155) showed that the consumption of fat containing behenic acid resulted in no accumulation of lipids in the heart. This was true whether the dietary fat was completely hydrogenated rapeseed oil, in which the erucic acid had been converted to behenic acid, or a mixture of mono-, di-, and triacylglycerols prepared from the completely hydrogenated rapeseed oil. A similar lack of increase in heart lipids was observed when the dietary fat was 2-behenoyldilinoleoylglycerol. These observations may be due to either the inability of behenic acid to cause an accumulation of heart lipids or the inability of the animal to absorb a significant amount of behenic acid. The impaired absorption of behenic acid was demonstrated in thoracic duct cannulated rats: Following the feeding of 2-behenoyldilinoleate, only 24% of the behenate moiety was found in the lymph. Results obtained by Tomarelli et al. (257) and Filer et al. (82) have shown that a saturated fatty acid attains maximum absorbability when it is esterified at the sn-2-position of a triacylglycerol that contains unsaturated fatty acids in the sn-1- and sn-3-positions. However, behenic acid was still poorly absorbed.

Hülsmann et al. (112) have observed that feeding rapeseed oil, rich in erucic acid, for 4 days results in a significant increase in the lipoprotein lipase activities of heart and adipose tissue. The authors speculate that the increased lipase activity of heart may contribute to lipid accumulation in this organ. Blomstrand and Svensson (26) have shown that erucic acid is incorporated into several phospholipids of the rat heart but that erucic acid seems to have a specific affinity to be incorporated into the cardiolipin molecule of the rat heart mitochondria. Reports from other laboratories (e.g., ref. 52) indicate that erucic acid inhibits the oxidation of other long-chain fatty acids in the mitochondria, with an increased triglyceride synthesis in the heart tissue as a consequence. The specific effect of erucic acid on the cardiolipin is associated with a specific inhibitory effect on the mitochondrial fatty acid catabolism, as well as on the mitochondrial respiration and the energy supply of the heart. Szlam and Sgoutas (248) have studied the absorption of 20:1

and 22:1 acids in the form of rapeseed oil by rats. The results show that the accumulation of dietary 20:1 and 22:1 acids in serum, lipoproteins, and their lipid subfractions is highly dependent on the alimentary condition of the animal. Unfasted rats incorporated 20:1 and 22:1 acids in all lipoproteins and their lipid subclasses, whereas starved rats had 20:1 and 22:1 acids only in high-density lipoprotein (HDL) triacylglycerols.

Kritchevsky et al. (131) have reported that native peanut oils are more atherogenic than randomized oils of the same fatty acid composition. Manganaro et al. (146) have shown that the natural peanut oils contain the long-chain fatty acids largely in the sn-3-position and have discussed the possible effect of this structural feature of the oil upon its absorption. Ammon et al. (5) have reported adverse effects of long-chain fatty acids on solute absorption by the intestinal mucosa of man during perfusion of the jejunum.

Fatty acids with *trans*-double bonds occur in some natural oils from leaves and seeds of plants and ruminant fats, but the main source in our diets is from partial hydrogenation of vegetable and marine oils. During this process, a wide variety of geometrical and positional isomers of fatty acids arise, depending on the original composition of the oils (69). Recent studies of Canadian margarines showed that most of the *trans*-isomers were monoenes and only small or negligible amounts of *trans*-dienes were present (15). Thus, *trans*-isomers in average processed fats are composed primarily of *trans*-octadecenoic (*t*-18:1) acid. A report submitted to the U.S. Food and Drug Administration in 1976 concluded (see ref. 241) that hydrogenated soybean oil is not hazardous to the public as far as dietary levels that are now current or that might reasonably be expected in the future are concerned. An epidemiological survey, however, claimed a significant positive correlation between dietary *trans*-fatty acid components and cancer causation (73), though there are a number of criticisms against the concept (7,10,174). Since dietary fat is thought to enhance the development of bowel tumors, presumably by stimulating production of bile acids (110,205), attempts have been made to determine if dietary *trans*-fatty acids might affect the biliary and fecal excretion of steroids. Sugano et al. (241) have shown that dietary hydrogenated fats influence neither the concentration nor composition of biliary bile steroids, irrespective of the presence or absence of cholesterol in the diet. The increased fecal steroid excretion corresponded to an increase in total excreta. The results suggested that dietary *trans*-fatty acids, in relation to *cis*-polyunsaturated fatty acids, provoke demonstrable change in steroid homeodynamics.

Blomstrand and Svensson (27) studied the incorporation of dietary isomeric fatty acids derived from different partially hydrogenated marine oils into individual phospholipids of mitochondrial membranes of rat heart. The ability of rat cardiac mitochondria to oxidize palmitoylcarnitine and to synthesize adenosine triphosphate (ATP) was depressed after feeding partially hydrogenated herring oil and rapeseed oil. Dietary *cis*-isomers of 22:1 seem to have a specific ability to interface with cardiac ATP synthesis and also to alter the fatty acid composition of cardiolipin of rat heart.

Brominated vegetable oils have been widely used in the soft drink industry as dispersing agents for the flavoring citrus oils (138). They give the drink a cloudy appearance simulating the natural fruit juice. Although the brominated oils were originally classified as safe by the FDA and were permitted by the Canadian Food and Drug Directorate, subsequent studies in several laboratories (89,121,171,172) have indicated the toxicity of brominated vegetable oils when fed to rats. More recently the brominated vegetable oils have been used as flame retardants (134) and thus still represent a potential contaminant of the environment.

Conacher et al. (62) investigated the hydrolysis of brominated vegetable oils by pancreatic lipase. It was shown that brominated olive, sesame, corn, and cottonseed oils were hydrolyzed with the same specificity as the nonbrominated oils. There was a decrease in the activity of the enzyme. Under conditons that gave 50% hydrolysis of corn oil, approximately 20% hydrolysis was obtained with brominated olive oil, 16% hydrolysis with brominated sesame oil, and 12% hydrolysis with brominated corn and cottonseed oils. As the content of tetrabromostearate increased, resulting in a higher melting point of the substrate, the activity of the lipase decreased. Since the brominated oils were degraded in the same manner as the common vegetable oils, they were assumed to be absorbed and deposited in a similar fashion. The 9,10-dibromo- and 9,10; 12,13-tetrabromostearates were detected in the livers and hearts of rats after administration of brominated cottonseed oils.

Lipid-bound bromine has been demonstrated in rat tissues following consumption of brominated vegetable oils by several investigators (89,120,121). Animals fed brominated corn oil had higher lipid bromine concentration than those fed either the dibromo- or tetrabromostearates (89). Maximum concentration of lipid in heart and liver was observed at 5 days. Perhaps brominated monoacylglycerols are better absorbed than brominated fatty acids. Whether the increase in tissue lipids involves increased levels of triacylglycerols or simply an increase in lipid mass from the substitution of brominated fatty acids for nonbrominated fatty acids has not been determined (120).

In another experiment Jones et al. (121) compared the effects of feeding rats for 25 days diets containing 2% of either brominated corn oil, monoacylglycerol of tetrabromostearate, monoacylglycerol of bromostearate, or a mixture of the two monoacylglycerols, which provided proportions of brominated acids comparable to that found in the brominated corn oil. All diets produced an increase in lipid content of heart. The tetrabromostearate appeared to be the more active in producing the changes, particularly serious intracellular fatty degeneration. Although the concentrations of brominated acids in the heart and liver lipids were comparable in rats fed brominated corn oil or brominated monoacylglycerol, brominated corn oil provided the more pronounced effects. It was speculated that this was due to the presence of small amounts of other brominated sterol or the small amounts of hexabromostearate (1%) derived from linolenic acid. Another consideration was the position of the brominated acid on the glycerol molecule. In corn oil, the majority of the linoleic acid is found in the sn-2-position and therefore the majority of the tetrabrominated stearate would be present largely in the 2-monoacylglycerols following pancreatic lipolysis, whereas the synthetic monoacylglycerols would be largely of the sn-1- and sn-3-type.

It has been reported (167) that dibromopalmitate is not oxidized by the β-oxidation system of mitochondria. James and Kestell (118) identified 5,6-dibromsebacic acid as an excretion product following dosing of rats with 9,10-dibromostearic acid. It could have been formed by a combination of β-oxidation and ω-oxidation followed by β-oxidation. Earlier work has shown that α-halogenated acids inhibit fatty acid oxidation (40,193). Machulla et al. (144) have made a comparative evaluation of Cl-34m, Br-77, and I-123 labeled fatty acids for metabolic studies of the myocardium.

Castor oil is an effective purgative when taken in sufficiently high doses. Myer (173) showed that its activity is due to ricinoleic acid. The specific reasons for this purgative action have not been elucidated, although most textbooks of pharmacology suggest that it is due to the intestinal release of ricinoleic acid, which is irritant to the bowel mucosa inducing vigorous peristalsis. Watson and Gordon (268) have reported that this effect may be due to the poor absorbability of ricinoleic acid, which would then accumulate in the intestine and form soaps or soap solution, which may also lead to purgation, diarrhea, or sprue. Although castor oil is easily and rapidly hydrolyzed in the small bowel, the activation and absorption of the free acid is not efficient. The result is a rapid accumulation of ricinoleic acid and its mineral salts. Nevertheless, some 5 to 10% of the fatty acids in the carcass triacylglycerols can be shown to be ricinoleic acid, when ricinoleic acid or triricinoleoylglycerol is fed to rats (200,268,269). Despite the rather heavy accumulation in triacylglycerols, no ricinoleic acid is incorporated into tissue phospholipids. On the basis of these results, Watson and Murray (269) suggest that the incorporation of ricinoleate into triacylglycerols may proceed via the acylation of monoacylglycerols rather than via the *de novo* formation of phosphatidic acid. Barber et al. (11) have shown that ricinoleoyl-CoA is essentially inactive with 1-acyl or 2-acyl-sn-glycerol-3-phosphorylcholine as acceptors. However, it can serve as acyl donor when glycerol-3 phosphate or 1-acyl-sn-glycerol-3-phosphate are available to yield di- and monoricinoleoyl-3-glycerophosphates, respectively. However, the possibility remains that ricinoleic acid could have become esterified to the sn-1,2-diacylglcyerols to yield sn-3-ricinoleoyl-1,2-diacylglycerols. This concept is supported by the appearance of butyrate and other unusual fatty acids in the sn-3-position of many natural triacylglycerols and of long-chain unsaturated acids at that position in liver triacylglycerols (36). Therefore, the acylation at the sn-3-position may be the principal site of entry of ricinoleate into the triacylglycerols *in vivo*. The potential opportunity for randomization of the acids at the sn-1- and sn-3-positions during exchange in tissue deposits prevents a clear understanding of biosynthetic selectivity for simple assessment of these lipid structures. Ricinoleic acid can induce fluid and electrolyte accumulation in several species (37). In addition, Racusen and Binder (203) have demonstrated that ricinoleate can induce active secretion of anions across the rat colon. This effect occurred along with an increase in mucosal cell cyclic AMP levels. Exposure of rat colon to ricinoleate causes the release of prostaglandin E, which may be responsible for increased cyclic adenosine monophosphate (AMP) concentrations (19). However, the mechanisms for prostaglandin E production by ricinoleate and the contribution of this process to the induction of active secretion are not known. Binder (25) has speculated that ricinoleate and dihydroxy bile acids act to induce an active anion secretion simultaneous to the increase in mucosal permeability and that it is the active anion secretion process that is primarily responsible for the net fluid and electrolyte accumulation. Maenz and Forsyth (145) have shown that in the brush border vesicles the secretory effects caused by ricinoleate are expressed at concentrations significantly below levels that have been associated with detergent effects or altered epithelial morphology. It was concluded that ricinoleate is a calcium ionophore in the jejunal brush border vesicles and that ricinoleate could have a significant intestinal secretory activity due to this Ca^{2+} ionophore property. Ganginella et al. (88) have reported cytotoxic effects of ricinoleic acid and other surfactants on isolated intestinal epithelial cells.

Aromatic Acids

Sodium benzoate is widely used as a preservative in foods. All commercial drinks analyzed by Conacher et al. (16) contained sodium benzoate as a preservative. Because of the acidity of the drinks, sodium benzoate was apparently present as benzoic acid, which was extracted with diethyl ether. The extensive studies by Hogben (105) on the absorption of organic acids from the rat intestine *in vivo* failed to reveal any specificity with respect to chemical structure other than a dependence on pK_a and the lipid solubility of the non-ionized form. Jackson et al. (116) presented evidence for the transport of the aromatic acids, benzoic and phenylacetic acids. Competitive interactions were demonstrated between benzoic and phenylacetic acids, and benzoic and pentanoic acids (117), but the interpretation of these interactions is complex. Transport of benzoic acid was observed only in rat jejunum and not in rat ileum or the hamster intestine. Spencer and Brody (237) have shown that the hamster intestine accumulated a number of aromatic acids, including phenylacetic acid, and Spencer et al. (238) showed that several benzoic acid derivatives were accumulated by the intestine of the mouse.

The widespread use of organic plasticizers and stabilizers has increased the hazard of environmental contamination by various aromatic acid esters, which have a variety of metabolic effects. Nikinorow et al. (177) have studied the oral toxicity of several of these compounds, such as di-*n*-butyl phthalate, di(2-ethylhexyl)phthalate, di(*n*-octyl) tin-*S*,*S'*-bis (isooctylmercaptoacetate), dibenzyl tin *S*,*S'*-bis(isooctylmercaptoacetate), and have shown in the rat that these agents can induce congestion of the small intestine and mucosal sloughing in the stomach and intestines. Di(2-ethylhexyl)phthalate (DEHP) is the most widely used commercial plasticizer, with global production of approximately 4×10^9 lb annually (198). In recent years there has been rising concern over the safety of phthalate esters. This concern emanates from a wide variety of biological studies indicating that phthalate esters are mutagenic, teratogenic, display cytotoxicity, alter lipid metabolism, inhibit various enzymes, and alter the ultrastructure of tissues (16,198). Additionally, DEHP contaminates virtually all ecosystems (198) and has been found in human tissue (190) and in the food supply of man (258). In view of what has just been stated, there has been an interest in using less toxic substitutes of DEHP in certain applications such as in the production of polyvinylchloride plastic medical devices (e.g., plastic blood storage bags, catheters, etc.). Di(2-ethylhexyl)adipate, also known as dioctyladipate or DOA, is a plasticizer that is gaining attention as a DEHP-substitute in certain applications. Bell (16) has determined the effects of DOA feeding on lipid metabolism in the rat. Male rats weighing 150 to 160 g were fed a stock diet supplemented with 0.5 to 1.0% (wt/wt) DOA, which was mixed with the diet following dissolving in diethyl ether. The studies indicate that DOA shares similar biological properties with DEHP in that DOA is an inhibitor of hepatic cholesterogenesis, possesses plasma cholesterol-lowering activity, and modifies hepatic phospholipid metabolism.

In the case of the rat, DOA is metabolized in the gut and other tissues to yield the monoester, adipic acid (249), and presumably 2-ethylhexanol (3). Whereas 2-ethylhexanol is unlikely to generate acetate (3), there is evidence that adipate can undergo β-oxidation to some extent (249) and might, therefore, contribute to the endogenous acetate pool.

Sulfonic Acids

Wetting agents, such as alkyl and aryl sulfates, and sulfonates generally induce only a low order of toxicity in human beings, although they have been associated with irritation of the stomach and intestines. Early studies by Freeman et al. (85) demonstrated that oral ingestion (4 months, 100 mg/day) of a mixture of alkyl aryl sodium sulfonates in human subjects did not significantly alter digestion and absorption of other foodstuffs, as determined by body weight changes and analysis of fecal fat and nitrogen. However, larger doses given to dogs irritated the gastrointestinal tract and resulted in loose stools and increased fecal mucus.

Other surface-active agents also may become ingested, because they are used for cleaning and disinfecting, as in bottling plants, canneries, dairies, and restaurants. These agents include alkyl dimethyl benzyl ammonium chloride, sodium dioctyl sulfosuccinate, sodium lauryl sulfate, polyethyleneglycol monoisoctyl phenol ether, and sulfoethyl methyl oleylamide. Chronic toxicity studies incorporating oral feeding regimens of these agents in rats have shown that all of the detergents except polyethyleneglycol monoisooctyl phenyl ether induced diarrhea, gastrointestinal mucosal irritation, intestinal bloating, and small hemorrhages of the gastric mucosa (83). More recently Weaver and Griffith (270) tested dogs with a variety of detergents, including sodium alkylbenzene-sulfonate and showed that all of these are potent emetic agents. Linear alkylbenzene sulfonate, which is currently the most widely used surfactant in detergent formulations, is readily absorbed in the intestinal tract of rats and enters the portal venous blood (163) and has been observed to induce histopathology of the rat gastrointestinal tract after long-term feeding (0.02 to 0.5% of diet).

It is well established that decyl sulfate, as well as natural detergents such as bile and sodium taurocholate, alters the gastric mucosal barrier with consequent changes in permeability, resulting in increased influx of hydrogen ions and increased efflux of sodium and potassium ions from the mucosa (63). Smyth and Calandra (258) studied the toxicity of 22 alkylphenol polyoxyethylene surfactants administered orally to rats. They noted only negligible toxic effects, but did report congested gastrointestinal tracts of animals given high doses. The absorption of the surfactants, cetyltrimethylammonium bromide and sodium lauryl sulfate, into rat intestinal tissue was studied *in vitro* from the standpoint of absorption kinetics above and below the critical micelle concentration (181). It was found that these agents were transported into the gut mucosa by first-order kinetics below the critical micelle concentration and at zero-order kinetics above it.

Feldman et al. (79) and Feldman and Reinhard (7) demonstrated that sodium taurocholate accelerates the release of total phosphorus, lipid phosphrous, and protein from the everted rat small intestine at concentrations above CMC. Those studies indicate the direct action of surfactants on the intestinal membrane resulting in an alteration in the membrane permeability. Feldman and Reinhard (78) examined the effects of a series of anionic detergents (surfactants) and showed a loss of protein from the everted rat intestine at surfactant concentrations above the CMC. These studies indicate the direct action of surfactants on the small intestinal membrane, resulting in an alteration in the membrane permeability. Kirkpatric et al. (123) have examined the differential solubilization of protein, phospholipid, and cholesterol of erythrocyte membranes by detergents.

Surfactants are one of the most important group of adjuvants in pharmaceutical preparations and their effect on the absorption of various drugs has been studied extensively (228). Surfactants can influence overall critical determinants of the rate and extent of drug absorption—*viz* drug solubility and dissolution rate, gastric emptying and membrane permeation. These complications prevent formulation of conclusions concerning the general nature of the influence of surfactants on the absorption of drugs from the gastrointestinal tract. Various surfactants are known to inhibit the intestinal absorption of inorganic electrolytes and water-soluble nutrients, i.e., compounds considered to be transported by active and carrier-mediated processes.

Yasuhara et al. (279) have investigated the intestinal absorption mechanism of nonlipophilic low molecular weight drugs that are not in accordance with pH-partition theory. As a result of these investigations, it has been suggested that the components of brush border membrane, i.e., glycocalyx, phospholipids, glycolipids, protein, etc., play an important role in the absorption processes of ionic drugs. Furusawa et al. (87) have shown that a reasonable correlation exists between the absorption and percentage transfer of *p*-aminobenzoic acid to lecithin-containing chloroform. Recently, Hori et al. (111) have reported that free fatty acids in the intestinal mucosa increase the permeability of *p*-aminobenzoic acid across bilayer lipid membrane. Yasuhara et al. (279) have reinvestigated the absorption of *p*-aminobenzoic acid by the intestine and have concluded that it involves a specific absorption mechanism and the contribution of the protein components, in addition to the lipids, to the absorption of *p*-aminobenzoic acid from the rat small intestine. Specifically, protein and sulfhydryl groups within the brush border membrane are involved in the absorption process of *p*-aminobenzoic acid.

Yasuhara et al. (278) have determined the effect of surfactants on the absorption of *p*-aminobenzoic acid from the rat small intestine. The surfactants tested were Tween 80, Triton X-100, cetyltrimethylammonium chloride (CTAB), and sodium dodecyl sulfate (SLS). The absorption of acetyl *p*-aminobenzoic acid from the small intestine was increased by these four surfactants. The order of magnitude of the absorption-enhancing effect was as follows: Triton X-100>SLS>CTAB>Tween 80. The exsorption of the *p*-aminobenzoic acid to the small intestinal lumen was greatly increased by the addition of SLS to the perfusate. In spite of such a general increase in the membrane permeability, the absorption of *p*-aminobenzoic acid from the small intestine was significantly inhibited by these four detergents. The extent of inhibition was dependent on the concentration of surfactants and the exposure time of intestine to surfactants. SLS greatly accelerated the release of protein from the small intestine, and an inverse correlation was found between the amount of released protein and the absorption of *p*-aminobenzoic acid in the presence of SLS. The specific inhibitory effect of surfactants may be attributed to the solubilization and following release of protein, which is responsible for the absorption of *p*-aminobenzoic acid. The magnitude of each surfactant effect was found to be somewhat different from every other surfactant tested. It was suggested that this quantitative difference may be dependent on the solubilizing potency of biological membranes. For non-ionic surfactants there is a strong correlation between structure and solubilizing potency. Studies with mitochondria, microsomes, and bacterial membranes have shown that almost all effective surfactants are in the 12.5 to 14.5 hydrophile-lipophile balance (HLB) range (100). Those with higher HLB values (such as Tween) failed in solubilization of membrane. These findings are in good agreement with the results of Yasuhara et al. (278) that Triton X-100 (HLB, 13.5) is much more potent than Tween 80 (HLB, 15.0) for the effect on the permeability of the intestinal membrane. Further quantitative investigations are necessary to elucidate the exact mechanism of action of surfactants in altering the membrane permeability to drugs.

During the course of a detailed biochemical investigation into the mechanism of action of the hypolipidemic agent, 4-benzyloxybenzoate (BRL 14280), Fears et al. (76) showed that this acid behaves as a fatty acid and participates in glycerolipid metabolism. With the aromatic acid in the diet of rats, similar compounds accumulated in the adipose tissue. Chemical characterization of the material synthesized *in vivo* showed that the metabolite was a triacylglycerol in which one of the fatty acid moieties was substituted by the 4-benzyloxybenzoate. There is no evidence for the participation in glycerolipid turnover of naturally occurring acids containing aryl groups in animals, but a recent identification has been reported (189) of ω-cyclohexyl fatty acids in acidophilic, thermophilic bacteria. The unusual fatty acids were esterified in a triacylglycerol type of material and accounted for between 74% to 93% of the total fatty acids. Participation of an unnatural acid in the formation of triacylglycerols presumably necessitates prior activation of the acyl-CoA derivative. It is of relevance to note that benzoyl-CoA and phenacetyl-CoA can be produced *in vivo* (142) and medium-chain fatty acid:CoA ligase is active with a variety of aliphatic and aromatic carboxylic acids. The use of synthetic fatty acids to obtain information about normal lipid metabolism was, in fact, started by Knoop (127), who derived the principles of fatty acid β-oxidation with phenyl-substituted and odd-number carbon fatty acids.

Polyglycerol Esters

Polyglycerol esters have been used for more than 50 years as food emulsifiers and are known to be well absorbed in the rat. Recent investigations by King et al. (122) have demonstrated that 2.5 to 10% polyglycerol ester (deca-glycerol deca-oleate) added to the diet of rats is relatively nontoxic but nevertheless interferes with the absorption of dietary fat. This effect is mediated through an undefined biochemical mechanism; morphological changes such as villus flattening were not observed.

The acylation of mono- and diacylglycerols of fat-forming acids with adipic acid produces a series of viscous compounds with a number of potentially useful properties. Thus, polymers of saturated fatty acids, adipic acid, and glycerol tend to be relatively low melting, possess a resistance to oxidation, and have been considered for use in the food industry. Shull et al. (227) determined the digestibility, absorption, and *in vivo* oxidation of the two types of adipic acid esters of glycerides, an sn-1,3-diacyl-2-adipate and polymers of fatty acids, adipic acid, and glycerol. In female rats these products were absorbed as readily as ordinary fats. The digestibility coefficient of 93% correlated well with the degree of absorption of the (^{14}C)stearic acid moiety of both diacylglyceroladipate and the polymeric fat. However, the absorbed (^{14}C) material that expired during the 8-hr experimental period differed markedly for the two fats. In one experiment, four times as much radioactivity from stearic acid appeared in the expired carbon dioxide when the diacylglyceroadipate was fed than when the polymeric fat was given.

Industrial glycols, such as ethylene glycol (ethanediol) or 1,3-butanediol, are commonly encountered in the environment and are frequently ingested in small amounts along with the diet. Several laboratories have examined the effects of these materials on the growth and metabolism of the rat. Romsos et al. (212) recently showed that body weight gain and energy intake of both pigs and chicks were depressed when the dietary energy derived from butanediol exceeded approximately 20%. Butanediol feeding increased circulating β-hydroxybutyrate and acetoacetate levels. Blood lactate levels were also increased by dietary butanediol. Plasma triacylglycerol levels were increased in pigs and unchanged in chicks fed butanediol-containing diets. The addition of 18% butanediol to the diet had no effect on glucose conversion to fatty acids. The study showed that the pig and chicken can effectively utilize dietary butanediol for body weight gain provided the butanediol level in the diet does not exceed 15 to 20% of dietary energy. Because the initial steps of butanediol metabolism are similar to those of ethanol metabolism, it is of interest that Rawat (204) has shown that hepatic glucose conversion to carbon monoxide is markedly depressed in the rat but not in the guinea pig when ethanol is added to the buffer. These diols occur at relatively low levels in normal mammalian tissue, a fact that can be rationalized on the basis of the strong biophysical activity of diol-derived phosphatidylcholine and phosphatidyl-serine analogs (13).

The sucrose polyester (SPE) is a mixture of the hexa-, hepta-, and octa-esters that are formed by esterification of sucrose with long-chain fatty acids. It has the appearance and physical properties of triacylglycerols, but differs from them in being neither degraded nor absorbed (153,157,158). The consumption of diets containing SPE results in a decrease in the absorption of dietary cholesterol in rats (152) and in man (130). Mattson et al. (151) showed that sucrose polyester also interferes with the absorption of vitamin A. The effect of SPE on vitamin A metabolism was determined by measuring the amount of the vitamin that was stored in the liver of rats following the ingestion of a known amount of vitamin A. In one study, vitamin A was administered as an oral dose in a vehicle consisting of various proportions of cottonseed oil and SPE. Each 1% replacement of cottonseed oil by SPE resulted in a 0.26% decrease in the amount of vitamin A found in the liver. In a second study, vitamin A was incorporated into diets in which the fat component consisted of various proportions of cottonseed oil and SPE. When these diets were consumed for 1 week each 1% replacement of cottonseed oil by SPE resulted in a 0.8% decrease in the storage of vitamin A by the liver. It is proposed that in the lumen of the intestine, vitamin A distributes between the customary micellar phase and the unhydrolyzed oil phase of SPE. Vitamin A in the latter phase is eliminated in the feces.

Sklan et al. (232) showed that raw soybean meal interfered with fat absorption (presumably by binding free fatty acids and making them unavailable for micelle formation). Raw soybean meal had been previously shown to bind bile acids (217).

SUMMARY AND CONCLUSIONS

Fat-soluble environmental agents have become a source of much concern for public health because of their widespread distribution, high resistance to biodegradation, and potential toxic or carcinogenic properties. These compounds range from the relatively harmless simple paraffins and alcohols to the more complex polychlorinated polycyclics and aromatic acids and their esters, with well-established adverse physiological effects. Although some of the higher molecular weight esters are subject to lipolysis, most of the environmental agents undergo little luminal transformation and are subject to micellarization and assimilation in the native form. These compounds appear to be absorbed via the pathways normally involved in the uptake of fat-soluble vitamins and other lipophilic micronutrients. The appearance of fat-soluble compounds in the lymph and tissues closely parallels their solubility in organic solvents, and the relative absorbability of many foreign substances has been deduced from their partition between organic solvents and appropriate aqueous buffers. Such simple physicochemical measurements, however, fail to take into account detailed structural differences among the solutes, which affect their subsequent metabolism in the intestinal mucosa.

The absorption of the different foreign lipophiles is affected by the nature of the dietary lipids and their lipolysis products. This suggests that the environmental agents form mixed micelles that are either taken up intact or that facilitate the transport of the foreign substances through the unstirred water layer, which constitutes a barrier to their absorption.

The mixed micelles formed from the bile salts and the lipolysis products of dietary triacylglycerols and glycerophospholipids readily incorporate appropriately shaped and/or charged lipophilic substances into their interior or between the amphipathic molecules making up the micelles. The solubilized molecules are capable of exchanging rapidly between the micelles and a true molecular solution from which they are believed to be taken up by the brush border membrane of the villous cells. The solubilization in the micelle is competitive, and the extent to which a given compound will be incorporated depends on the nature of the accompanying lipids in the medium. Since the fat-soluble vitamins remain largely unabsorbed in the absence of bile salts, the bile salts may be essential also for the absorption of the fat-soluble environmental agents and drugs. The result of the micellar solubilization is to increase the concentration gradient many fold and thus to favor the passive absorption of these substances. There is no evidence for the participation of specific membrane receptors or carrier proteins in the absorption process, although a thorough investigation of this aspect of the assimilation of the lipophilic foreign substances has not been made.

On the basis of studies with the normal lipolytic products of dietary fats and bile salts it has been shown that different solutes are taken up at different rates, hence it must be concluded that micelles are not taken up intact. However, the region where dissociation occurs and the factors affecting it have not been established, although the unstirred water layer would appear to be a likely site. Uptake of the foreign lipophiles would therefore be expected to depend on their monomer activity in a true molecular solution. The uptake of the monomer presumably would be further influenced by the lipid composition of the brush border membrane, which varies with the dietary fat composition and the metabolic state of the villus cell. The composition of the dietary fat also affects the structure of the lipoproteins that the intestinal villous cell forms and that serve as a vehicle for the transfer of the fat-soluble environmental agents to the bloodstream. On the basis of the above considerations and from studies of the absorption of natural fats and fat-soluble vitamins, it is possible to make shrewd guesses about the digestion and absorption of various fat-soluble environmental agents, but a full understanding of the mechanism involved requires detailed biochemical studies with individual agents, which have not yet been performed.

ACKNOWLEDGMENTS

The studies of the author and his collaborators referred to in this review were supported by grants from the Medical Research Council of Canada and the Ontario Heart Foundation, Toronto, Canada.

REFERENCES

1. Akesson, B., Gronovitz, S., Herslof, B., Michelsen, P., and Olivecrona, T. (1983): Stereospecificity of different lipases. *Lipids*, 18:313–318.
2. Akesson, B., and Michelson, P. (1981): Digestion and absorption of a sulphoxide analogue of triacylglycerol in the rat. *Chem. Phys. Lipids*, 29:341–349.
3. Albro, D. W. (1975): The metabolism of 2-ethylhexanol in rats. *Xenobiotica*, 5:625–636.
4. Allen, J. R., and Norback, D. H. (1973): Polychlorinated biphenyl- and triphenyl-induced gastric mucosal hyperplasia in primates. *Science*, 179:498–499.
5. Ammon, H. V., Thomas, P. J., and Phillips, S. F. (1977): Effect of long-chain fatty acids on solute absorption: perfusion studies in the human jejunum. *Gut*, 18:805–813.
6. Ammon, H. V., Thomas, P. J., and Phillipis, S. F. (1979): Effect of lecithin on jejunal absorption of micellar lipoids in man and on their monomer activity *in vitro*. *Lipids*, 14:395–400.
7. Applewhite, T. H. (1979): Statistical "correlations" relating trans fats to cancer: a commentary. *Fed. Proc.*, 38:2435.
8. Arnesjo, B., Nilsson, A., Barrowman, J., and Borgstrom, B. (1969): Intestinal digestion and absorption of cholesterol and lecithin in the human. *Scand. J. Gastroenterol.*, 4:653–665.
9. Badger, G. M. (1962): Mode of formation of carcinogens in human environment. *Nat. Cancer Inst. Monogr.*, 9:1.
10. Bailar, J. C. (1979): Dietary fats and cancer trends—further critique. *Fed. Proc.*, 38:2435–2439.
11. Barber, E. D., Smith, W. L., and Lands, W. E. M. (1971): Incorporation of ricinoleic acid into glycerolipids. *Biochim. Biophys. Acta*, 248:171–179.
12. Barnes, R. H., Miller, E. S., and Burr, G. O. (1941): Fat absorption in essential fatty acid deficiency. *J. Biol. Chem.*, 140:773–778.
13. Baumann, W. J., Schupp, E., and Lin, J-T., (1975): Diol Lipids of rat liver. Quantitation and structural characteristics of neutral lipids and phospholipids derived from ethanediol, propanediols, and butanediols. *Biochemistry*, 14:841–847.
14. Beare-Rogers, J. L. (1983): Trans and positional isomers of common fatty acids. *Adv. Nutr. Res.*, 5:172–200.
15. Beare-Rogers, J. L., Gray, L. M., and Hollywood, R. (1979): The linoleic acid and trans fatty acids of margarines. *Am. J. Clin. Nutr.*, 32:1805–1809.
16. Bell, F. P. (1983): Effect of the plastisizer di(2-ethylhexyl)adipate (dioctyl-adipate, DOA) on lipid metabolism in the rat: I. Inhibition of cholesterogenesis and modification of phospholipid synthesis. *Lipids*, 18:211–215.
17. Bell, N. H., and Ryan, P. (1969): Absorption of vitamin D oleate in the rat. *Am. J. Clin. Nutr.*, 22:425–430.
18. Bernhard, K. (1953): Absorption of aliphatic hydrocarbons, caratene and vitamin A in the rat. *Fette Seifen Anstrichmittel*, 55:160–166.
19. Beubler, E., and Juan, H. (1977): The function of prostaglandins in transmucosal water movement and blood flow in the rat jejunum. *Naunyn-Schmiedeberg's Arch. Pharmacol.*, 299:89–94.
20. Bhat, S. G., and Brockman, H. L. (1981): Enzymatic synthesis/hydrolysis of cholesteryl oleate in surface films. *J. Biol. Chem.*, 256:3017–3023.
21. Bhat, S. G., and Brockman, H. L. (1982): Lipid hydrolysis catalyzed by pancreatic cholesterol esterase. Regulation by substrate and product phase distribution and packing density. *Biochemistry*, 21:1547–1552.
22. Bhat, S. G., and Brockman, H. L. (1982): The role of cholesteryl ester hydrolysis and synthesis

in cholesterol transport across rat intestinal mucosal membrane. A new concept. *Biochem. Biophys. Res. Commun.*, 109:486–492.

23. Bhat, S. G., and Brockman, H. L. (1983): Effects of cholesterol esterase on intestinal uptake of cholesterol. Evidence for cholesteryl ester-mediated movement of cholesterol across membranes. *Fed. Proc.*, 42:1256. Abs. No. 5648.

24. Bieri, J. G., and Farrell, P. M. (1976): Vitamin E. *Vitam. Horm.*, 34:31–75.

25. Binder, J. H. (1980): Pathophysiology of bile acid- and fatty acid-induced diarrhea. In: *Secretory Diarrhea*, edited by M. Field, J. S. Fordtran, and G. G. Schultz, pp. 154–178. American Physiological Society, Bethesda.

26. Blomstrand, R., and Svensson, L. (1974): Studies on phospholipids with particular emphasis on cardiolipin of rat heart after feeding rapeseed oil. *Lipids*, 9:771–780.

27. Blomstrand, R., and Svensson, L. (1983): The effect of partially hydrogenated marine oils on the mitochondrial function and membrane phospholipid fatty acids in rat heart. *Lipids*, 18:151–170.

28. Bochenek, W. J., and Rodgers, J. B. (1979): Effect of polyol detergents on cholesterol and triglyceride absorption. Hypolipidemic action of chronic administration of hydrophobic detergent. *Biochim. Biophys. Acta*, 489:503–506.

29. Borgstrom, B. (1952): On the action of pancreatic lipase on triglycerides *in vivo* and *in vitro*. *Acta Physiol. Scand.*, 25:328–347.

30. Borgstrom, B. (1954): On the mechanism of pancreatic lipolysis of glycerides. *Biochim. Biophys. Acta*, 13:491–504.

31. Borgstrom, B. (1964): Influence of bile salt, pH and time on the action of pancreatic lipase; physiological implications. *J. Lipid Res.*, 5:522–531.

32. Borgstrom, B. (1967): Partition of lipids between emulsified oil and micellar phases of glyceride-bile salt dispersions. *J. Lipid Res.*, 8:598–608.

33. Borgstrom, B. (1974): Fat Digestion and Absorption. In: *Intestinal Absorption, Vol. 4B, Biomembranes*, edited by D. H. Smyth, pp. 555–620. Plenum Press, New York.

34. Borgstrom, B. (1977): Physico-chemical characteristics of the lipase-colipase-bile salt system. *Exp. Ann. Biochim. Med.*, pp. 173–182. Masson, Paris.

35. Boucrot, P., and Clement, J. (1971): Resistance to the effect of phospholipase A of the biliary phospholipids during incubation of bile. *Lipids*, 6:652–656.

36. Breckenridge, W. C. (1978): Stereospecific analysis of triacylglycerol. In: *Handbook of Lipid Research. Vol. 1, Fatty Acids and Glycerides*, edited by A. Kuksis, pp. 197–232. Plenum Press, New York.

37. Bright-Asare, P., and Binder, H. J. (1973): Stimulation of colonic secretion of water and electrolytes by hydroxy fatty acids. *Gastroenterology*, 64:81–88.

38. Brockerhoff, H. (1970): Substrate specificity of pancreatic lipase. Influence of the structure of fatty acids on the reactivity of the esters. *Biochim. Biophys. Acta*, 212:92–101.

39. Bugaut, M., Myher, J. J., Kuksis, A., and Hoffman, A. G. D. (1984): An examination of the stereochemical course of acylation of 2-monoacylglycerols by rat intestinal villus cells using d_3-palmitic acid. *Biochim. Biophys. Acta (in press)*.

40. Burgess, R. A., Butt, W. D., and Baggaley, A. (1968): Some effects of alpha-bromo-palmitate, an inhibitor of fatty acid oxidation, on carbohydrate metabolism in the rat. *Biochem. J.*, 109:38P–39P.

41. Campbell, A. D., Korwitz, W., Burke, J. A., Jelinek, C. F., Rodricks, J. V., and Shibko, S. I. (1977): In: *Handbook of Physiology, Section 9, Reactions to Environmental Agents*, edited by D. H. K. Lee, pp. 167–179. American Physiological Society, Bethesda, MD.

42. Channon, H. J., and Collinson, G. A. (1929): LXXVII. The unsaponifiable fraction of liver oils. V. The absorption of liquid paraffin from the alimentary tract of the rat and pig. *Biochem. J.*, 23:676–688.

43. Chapus, C., Sari, H., Semeriva, M., and Desnuelle, P. (1975): Role of colipase in the interfacial adsorption of pancreatic lipase at hydrophobic interfaces. *FEBS Lett.*, 58:155–158.

44. Child, P., and Kuksis, A. (1980): Uptake and transport of sterols by isolated villus cells of rat jejunum. *Can. J. Biochem.*, 58:1215–1222.

45. Child, P., and Kuksis, A. (1982): Differential uptake of cholesterol and plant sterols by rat erythrocytes *in vitro*. *Lipids*, 17:748–754.

46. Child, P., and Kuksis, A. (1983): Uptake of 7-dehydro derivatives of cholesterol, campesterol and

sitosterol by rat erythrocytes, jejunal villus cells, and brush border membranes. *J. Lipid Res.*, 24:552–564.

47. Child, P., and Kuksis, A. (1983): Critical role of the ring structure in the differential uptake of cholesterol and the plant sterols *in vitro*. *J. Lipid Res.*, 24:1196–1209.

48. Chow, S., and Hollander, D. (1977): Intestinal cholesterol uptake by everted sacs of rat small intestine: kinetic and thermodynamic aspects. *Lipids*, 13:239–245.

49. Chow, S. L., and Hollander, D. (1978): Arachidonic acid intestinal absorption: Mechanism of transport and influence of luminal factors on absorption *in vitro*. *Lipids*, 13:768–776.

50. Chow, S. L., and Hollander, D. (1979): A dual, concentration-dependent absorption mechanism of linoleic acid by rat jejunum *in vitro*. *J. Lipid Res.*, 20:349–356.

51. Chow, S. L., and Hollander, D. (1981): Linoleic acid absorption in the unanesthetized rat: mechanism of transport and influence of luminal factors on absorption. *Lipids*, 14:378–385.

52. Christopherson, B. O., and Bremer, J. (1972): Erucic acid—an inhibitor of fatty acid oxidation in the heart. *Biochim. Biophys. Acta*, 280:506–514.

53. Clark, S. B. (1971): The uptake of oleic acid by rat small intestine: a comparison of methodology. *J. Lipid Res.*, 12:43–55.

54. Clark, S. B. (1978): Chylomicron composition during duodenal triglyceride and lecithin infusion. *Am. J. Physiol.*, 235:E183–E190.

55. Clark, S. B., Enkers, T. E., Singh, A., Balint, J. A., Holt, P. R., and Rodgers, J. B., Jr. (1973): Fat absorption in essential fatty acid deficiency: a model experimental approach to studies of the mechanism of fat malabsorption of unknown etiology. *J. Lipid Res.*, 14:581–588.

56. Clark, S. B., and Holt, P. R. (1969): Inhibition of steady state intestinal absorption of long-chain triglycerides by medium-chain triglyceride in the rat. *J. Clin. Invest.*, 48:2235–2243.

57. Clement, J. (1980): Intestinal absorption of triacylglycerols. *Reprod. Nutr. Develop.*, 20(4B):1285–1307.

58. Clement, G., Clement, J., and Bezard, J. (1962): Action of human pancreatic lipase on synthetic mixed symmetrical triglycerides of long-chain acids and butyric acid. *Biochem. Biophys. Res. Commun.*, 8:238–242.

59. Cohen, M., Morgan, R. G. H., and Hoffman, A. F. (1971): Lipolytic activity of human gastric and duodenal juice against medium and long chain triglycerides. *Gastroenterology*, 60:1–15.

60. Comai, K., and Sullivan, A. C. (1980): *In vivo* meal model for the evaluation of agents which affect the absorption of triglyceride and cholesterol. *Biochem. Pharmacol.*, 29:1475–1482.

61. Conacher, H. B. S., Chadha, R. K., and Sahasrabudhe, M. R. (1969): Determination of brominated vegetable oils in soft drinks by gas-liquid chromatography. *J. Am. Oil Chem. Soc.*, 46:558–560.

62. Conacher, H. B. S., Hartman, D. K. J., and Chadka, R. K. (1970): Pancreatic lipolysis of some brominated vegetable oils. *Lipids*, 5:497–498.

63. Davenport, H. W. (1968): Destruction of the gastric mucosal barrier by detergents and urea. *Gastroenterology*, 54:175–180.

64. De Haas, G. H., Postema, N. M., Nieuwenhuizen, W., and Van Deenen, L. L. M. (1968): Purification and properties of an anionic zymogen of phospholipase A from porcine pancreas. *Biochim. Biophys. Acta*, 159:118–129.

65. De Haas, G. H., Postema, N. M., Nieuwenhuizen, W., and Van Deenen, L. L. M. (1968): Purification and properties of phospholipase A from porcine pancreas. *Biochim. Biophys. Acta*, 159:103–117.

66. Dhopeshwarkar, G. A. (1981): Naturally occurring food toxicants: toxic lipids. *Progr. Lipid Res.*, 19:107–118.

67. Douglas, G. J., Jr., Reinauer, A. J., Brooks, W. C., and Pratt, J. H. (1953): The effect on digestion of excluding the pancreatic juice from the intestine. *Gastroenterology*, 23:452–459.

68. Durham, W. F. (1963): Pesticide residues in foods in relation to human health. *Residue Rev.*, 4:33–81.

69. Dutton, H. J. (1979): Hydrogenation of fats and its significance. In: *Geometrical and Positional Fatty Acid Isomers*, edited by E. A. Emken and H. J. Dutton, pp. 1–16. American Oil Chemists Society, Champaign, IL.

70. Ekwall, P., Setala, K., and Sjoblom, L. (1951): Further investigations on the solubilization of carcinogenic hydrocarbons by association colloids. *Acta Chem. Scand.*, 5:175–180.

71. Elbert, A. G., Schleifer, C. R., and Hees, S. M. (1966): Absorption, digestion and excretion of ^{3}H-mineral oil in rats. *J. Pharm. Sci.*, 55:923–929.

72. El-Gerab, M., and Underwood, B. A. (1973): Solubilization of β-carotene and retinol into aqueous solutions of mixed micelles. *Biochim. Biophys. Acta*, 306:58–66.
73. Enig, M. G., Munn, J., and Keeney, M. (1978): Dietary fat and cancer trends—a critique. *Fed. Proc.*, 37:2215–2220.
74. Entressangles, B., Pasero, L., Savary, P., Sarda, L., and Desnuelle, P. (1961): Influence de la nature des chaines grasses sur la vitesse de leur hydrolyze par la lipase pancreatique. *Bull. Soc. Chim. Biol.*, 43:581–591.
75. Erlanson, C., and Borgstrom, B. (1970): Purification and further characterization of co-lipase from porcine pancreas. *Biochim. Biophys. Acta*, 271:400–412.
76. Fears, R., Baggaby, K. H., Alexander, R., Morgan, B., and Hindley, R. M. (1978): The participation of ethyl 4-benzyloxybenzoate (BRL 10894) and other aryl-substituted acids in glycerolipid metabolism. *J. Lipid Res.*, 19:3–11.
77. Feldman, S., and Gibaldi, M. (1969): Bile salt induced permeability changes in the isolated rat intestine. *Proc. Soc. Exp. Biol. Med.*, 132:1031.
78. Feldman, S., and Reinhard, M. (1976): Interaction of sodium alkyl sulfates with everted rat small intestinal membrane. *J. Pharm. Sci.*, 65:1460–1462.
79. Feldman, S., Reinhard, M., and Wilson, C. (1973): Effect of sodium taurodeoxycholate on biological membranes. Release of phosphorus, phospholipid, and protein from everted rat small intestine. *J. Pharm. Sci.*, 62:1961–1964.
80. Field, F. J., Cooper, A. D., and Erickson, S. K. (1982): Regulation of rabbit intestinal acyl coenzyme A-cholesterol acyltransferae *in vivo* and *in vitro*. *Gastroenterology*, 83:873–880.
81. Field, F. J., and Mathur, S. N. (1983): Beta-sitosterol:esterification by intestinal acyl coenzyme A:cholesterol acyltransferase (ACAT) and its effect on cholesterol esterification. *J. Lipid Res.*, 24:409–417.
82. Filer, L.·J., Jr., Mattson, F. H., and Fomon, S. J. (1969): Triglyceride composition and fat absorption by the human infant. *J. Nutr.*, 99:293–298.
83. Fitzhugh, O. G., and Nelson, A. A. (1948): Chronic toxicities of surface-active agents. *J. Am. Pharm. Assoc.*, 37:29–32.
84. Frazer, A. C. (1946): The absorption of triglyceride fat from the intestine. *Physiol. Rev.*, 26:103–119.
85. Freeman, S., Burrill, M. W., Li, T. W., and Ivy, A. C. (1945): The enzyme inhibitory action of an alkyl aryl sulfonate and studies of its toxicity when ingested by rats, dogs and humans. *Gastroenterology*, 4:332–343.
86. Friedman, H. I., and Nylund, B. (1980): Intestinal fat digestion, absorption and transport. *Am. J. Clin. Nutr.*, 33:1108–1139.
87. Furusawa, S., Okumura, K., and Sezaki, H. (1972): Enhanced migration of the ionized forms of acidic drugs from water into chloroform in the presence of phospholipids. *J. Pharm. Pharmacol.*, 24:272–276.
88. Gaginella, T. S., Phillips, S. F., Dozois, R. R., and Go., V. L. M. (1978): Stimulation of adenylate cyclase in homogenates of isolated intestinal epithelial cells from hamsters. *Gastroenterology*, 74:11–15; *Fed. Proc.* (1976), 35:764.
89. Gaunt, I. F., Grosso, P., and Gangoli, S. D. (1971): Brominated maize oil. I. Short-term toxicity and bromine storage studies in rats fed brominated maize oil. *Fed. Cosmet. Toxicol.*, 9:13–19.
90. Galeo, L. L., Clark, S. B., Myers, S., and Vahouny, G. V. (1983): Cholesterol absorption in rat intestine: role of cholesteryl ester and acyl coenzyme A-cholesterol acyltransferase. *Fed. Proc.*, 42:1256. Abs. 5647.
91. Gallo-Torres, H. E. (1970): Obligatory role of bile for the intestinal absorption of vitamin E. *Lipids*, 5:379–384.
92. Glickman, R. M., Green, P. H. R., Lees, R. S., Lux, S. E., and Kilgore, A. (1979): Immunofluorescence studies of apolipoprotein-B in intestinal mucosa. Absence in abetaliproteinemia. *Gastroenterology*, 76:288–292.
93. Go, V. L. M., Poley, J. R., Hoffman, A. F., and Summerskill, W. H. J. (1970): Disturbances in fat digestion induced by acidic jejunal pH due to gastric hypersection in man. *Gastroenterology*, 58:638–646.
94. Grundy, S. M., and Mok, H. Y. I. (1977): Determination of cholesterol absorption in man by intestinal perfusion. *J. Lipid Res.*, 18:263–271.
95. Gurr, M. I., Pover, W. F. R., and Hawthorne, J. N. (1963): Phospholipid composition and turnover in rat intestinal mucosa during fat absorption. *Nature*, 197:79.

96. Hamosh, M., Ganot, D., and Hamosh, P. (1979): Rat lingual lipase. Characteristics of enzyme activity. *J. Biol. Chem.*, 254:12121–12125.
97. Hamosh, M., and Scow, R. O. (1973): Lingual lipase and its role in the digestion of dietary lipid. *J. Clin. Invest.*, 52:88–95.
98. Heath, D. F., and Vandekar, M. (1964): Toxicity and metabolism of dieldrin in rats. *Brit. J. Ind. Med.*, 21:269–279.
99. Helander, H. F., and Olivecrona, T. (1970): Lipolysis and lipid absorption in the stomach of the suckling rat. *Gastroenterology*, 59:22–35.
100. Helenius, A., and Simons, K. (1975): Solubilization of membranes by detergents. *Biochim. Biophys. Acta*, 415:29–79.
101. Helgerud, P., Saarem, K., and Norum, K. R. (1981): Acyl CoA:cholesterol acyl-transferase in human small intestine: its activity and some properties of the enzymic reaction. *J. Lipid Res.*, 2:271–277.
102. Hernell, O., and Olivecrona, T. (1974): Human milk lipases. II. Bile salt-stimulated lipase. *Biochim. Biophys. Acta*, 369:234–244.
103. Hoffman, N. E. (1970): The relationship between uptake *in vitro* of oleic acid and micellar solubilization. *Biochim. Biophys. Acta*, 196:193–203.
104. Hoffman, A. F., and Borgstrom, B. (1964): The intraluminal phase of fat digestion of man: The lipid content of the micellar and oil phases of intestinal content obtained during fat digestion and absorption. *J. Clin. Invest.*, 43:247–257.
105. Hogben, C. A. M. (1960): The alimentary tract. *Ann. Rev. Physiol.*, 22:381–406.
106. Hollander, D. (1981): Intestinal absorption of vitamins A, E, D and K. *J. Lab. Clin. Med.*, 97:449–462.
107. Hollander, D., and Morgan, D. (1980): Effect of plant sterols, fatty acids and lecithin on cholesterol absorption *in vivo* in the rat. *Lipids*, 15:395–400.
108. Hollander, D., and Muralidhara, K. S. (1977): Vitamin A-1 intestinal absorption *in vivo*. Influence of luminal factors in transport. *Am. J. Physiol.*, 232:E471–E477.
109. Hollander, D., and Rim, E. (1978): Effect of luminal constituents on vitamin K absorption into thoracic duct lymph. *Am. J. Physiol.*, 234:E54–E59.
110. Hopkins, G. J., and West, C. E. (1976): Possible roles of dietary fats in carcinogenesis. *Life Sci.*, 19:1103–1116.
111. Hori, R., Kagimoto, Y., Kamiya, K., and Inui, K. (1978): Effects of free fatty acids as membrane components on permeability of drugs across bilayer lipid membranes. A mechanism for intestinal absorption of acidic drugs. *Biochim. Biophys. Acta*, 509:510–518.
112. Hulsmann, W. C., Geelhoed-Mieras, M. M., Jansen, H., and Houtsmuller, U. M. T. (1979): Alteration of the lipase activities of muscle, adipose tissue and liver by rapeseed oil feeding to rats. *Biochim. Biophys. Acta*, 572:183–187.
113. Hyun, J., Kothari, H., Herm, E., Mortenson, J., Treadwell, C. R., and Vahouny, G. V. (1969): Purification and properties of pancreatic juice cholesterol ester hydrolase. *J. Biol. Chem.*, 244:1937–1945.
114. Hyun, S. A., Vahouny, G. V., and Treadwell, C. R. (1967): Portal absorption of fatty acids in lymph and portal vein-cannulated rats. *Biochem. Biophys. Acta*, 137:296–305.
115. Jackson, M. J., and Cohn, V. H. (1977): Determinants of xenobiotics transport at biological barriers. In: *Handbook of Physiology*, edited by D. H. K. Lee, pp. 397–418. American Physiological Society, Bethesda.
116. Jackson, M. J., Shiau, Y-F., Bane, S., and Fox, M. (1974): Intestinal transport of weak electrolytes. Evidence in favor of a three compartment system. *J. Gen. Physiol.*, 63:187–213., *Fed. Proc.*, 29:595.
117. Jackson, J. M., and Shiau, Y-F., and Morgan, B. N. (1971): Mutations in transport of weak acids across rat jejunum. *Fed. Proc.*, 30:538., Abs. 1915.
118. James, S. P., and Kestell, P. (1978): The fate of brominated soya oil in the animal body. *Xenobiotica*, 8:557–564.
119. Jensen, R. G., DeJong, F. A., Clark, R. M., Palmgren, L. G., Liao, T. H., and Hamosh, M. (1982): Stereospecificity of premature human infant lingual lipase. *Lipids*, 17:570–572.
120. Jones, B. A., Tinsley, I. J., and Lowrey, R. R. (1983): Bromine levels in tissue lipids of rats fed brominated fatty acids. *Lipids*, 18:319–326.
121. Jones, B. A., Tinsley, I. J., Wilson, G., and Lowrey, R. R. (1983): Toxicology of brominated fatty acids: metabolite concentration and heart and liver changes. *Lipids*, 18:327–334.

122. King, W. R., Michael, W. R., and Coots, R. H. (1971): Subacute oral toxicity of polyglycerol ester. *Toxicol. Appl. Pharmacol.*, 20:327–333.
123. Kirkpatrick, F. H., Gordesky, S. E., and Marinetti, G. V. (1974): Differential solubilization of proteins, phospholipids and cholesterol of erythrocyte membranes by detergents. *Biochim. Biophys. Acta*, 345:154–161.
124. Klauda, H. C., and Quackenbush, F. W. (1970): Cholesterol absorption with different fats following thoracic duct cannulation of the rat. *Lipids*, 5:142–144.
125. Klauda, H. C., and Quackenbush, F. W. (1971): 2-Monoglyceride as an aid to the absorption of cholesterol into the thoracic lymph. *Lipids*, 6:964–965.
126. Klein, R. L., and Rudel, L. L. (1983): Cholesterol absorption and transport in thoracic duct lymph lipoproteins of non-human primates. Effect of dietary cholesterol level. *J. Lipid Res.*, 24:343–356.
127. Knoop, F. (1905): Der Abbau aromatischer Fettsäuren im Tier Körper Beitr. *Chem. Physiol. Pathol.*, 6:150–162.
128. Kolattukudy, P. E., and Hankin, L. (1966): Metabolism of plant wax paraffin (n-nonacosane) in the rat. *J. Nutr.*, 90:167–174.
129. Krabisch, L., and Borgstrom, B. (1974): Cited in Borgstrom, B. Fat digestion and absorption. In: *Biomembranes 4B, Intestinal Absorption*, edited by D. H. Smith, pp. 55–620. Plenum Press, New York.
130. Krause, J. R., and Grundy, S. M. (1978): Effects of sucrose polyester (SPE) on cholesterol metabolism in man. *Circulation*, 58:170. Part II, Abs. No. 659.
131. Kritchevsky, D., Tepper, S. A., Vasselinovitch, D., and Wissler, R. W. (1973): *Atherosclerosis*, 17:225–243.
132. Kuksis, A., and Huang, T. C. (1962): Differential absorption of plant sterols in the dog. *Can. J. Biochem. Physiol.*, 40:1493–1504.
133. Kuksis, A., Shaikh, N. A., and Hoffman, A. G. D. (1970): Lipid absorption and metabolism. *Environ. Health Perspect.*, 33:45–55.
134. Kuryla, W. C. (1973): In: *Flame Retardance of Polymeric Materials, Vol. 1*, edited by W. C. Kuryla and A. J. Papa, pp. 3–31. Marcel Dekker, New York.
135. Laher, J. M., and Barrowman, J. A. (1983): Polycyclic hydrocarbon and polychlorinated biphenyl solubilization in aqueous solutions of mixed micelles. *Lipids*, 18:216–222.
136. Lairon, D., Nalbone, G., Lafont, H., Leonardi, J., Domingo, H., Hauton, J. C., and Verger, R. (1978): Possible roles of bile lipids and colipase in lipase adsorption. *Biochemistry*, 17:52–63.
137. Lee, K. Y., Simmonds, W. J., and Hoffman, N. E. (1971): The effect of partition of fatty acid between oil and micelles on its uptake by everted intestinal sacs. *Biochim. Biophys. Acta*, 249:548–555.
138. Lehman, A. J. (1958): Brominated olive oil and carbonated beverages. Assoc. Food and Drug Off. of U.S. Quart. Bull., 20:71.
139. Lindstrom, M., Ljusberg-Wahren, H., Larsson, K., and Borgstrom, B. (1981): Aqueous lipid phases of relevance to intestinal fat digestion and absorption. *Lipids*, 16:749–754.
140. Liu, G. C. K., Ahrens, E. H., Jr., Schreibman, P. H., and Crouse, J. R. (1976): Measurement of squalene in human tissues and plasma: validation and application. *J. Lipid Res.*, 17:38–45.
141. Lo, M-T., and Sandi, E. (1978): Polycyclic aromatic hydrocarbons (polynuclears) in foods. *Residue Rev.*, 69:35–86.
142. Londesborough, J. C., and Webster, L. T., Jr. (1974): Fatty acyl CoA synthesis. *Enzymes*, 10:469–488.
143. Lutton, S. S. (1965): Phase behaviour of aqueous solutions of monoglycerides. *J. Am. Oil Chem. Soc.*, 42:1068–1070.
144. Machulla, H-H., Stoecklin, G., Kupfernagel, C. H., Freundlief, C. H., Hoeck, A., Vyska, K., and Feinendegen, L. E. (1978): Comparative evaluation of fatty acids labelled with C-11, C1-34m, Br-77 and I-123 for metabolic studies of the myocardium: concise communication. *J. Nuclear Med.*, 19:292–302.
145. Maenz, D. D., and Forsyth, G. W. (1982): Ricinoleate and deoxycholate are calcium ionophores in jejunal brush border vesicles. *J. Membrane Biol.*, 70:125–133.
146. Manganaro, F., Myher, J. J., Kuksis, A., and Kritchevsky, D. (1981): Acylglycerol structure of genetic varieties of peanut oils of varying atherogenic potential. *Lipids*, 16:508–517.
147. Mansbach, C. M. (1977): The origin of chylomicron phosphatidylcholine in the rat. *J. Clin. Invest.*, 60:411–420.

148. Mansbach, C. M., II, and Parthasarathy, S. A. (1982): II. Reexamination of the state of glyceride glycerol in neutral lipid absorption and transport. *J. Lipid Res.*, 23:1009–1019.
149. Mansbach, C. M., II, Pieroni, G., and Verger, R. (1968): Intestinal phospholipase. A novel enzyme. *J. Clin. Invest.*, 69:368–376.
150. Mattson, F. H., and Beck, L. W. (1956): The specificity of pancreatic lipase for the primary hydroxyl groups of glycerides. *J. Biol. Chem.*, 219:735–740.
151. Mattson, F. H., Hollenbach, E. J., and Kuehlthau, C. M. (1979): The effect of an non-absorbable fat, sucrose polyester, on the metabolism of Vitamin A by the rat. *J. Nutr.*, 109:1688–1693.
152. Mattson, F. H., Jandrack, R. J., and Webb, M. R. (1976): The effect of a nonabsorbable lipid, sucrose polyester, on the absorption of dietary cholesterol by the rat. *J. Nutr.*, 106:747–752.
153. Mattson, F. H., and Nolen, G. A. (1972): Absorbability by rats of compounds containing from one to eight ester groups. *J. Nutr.*, 102:1171–1176.
154. Mattson, F. H., Noller, G. A., and Webb, M. R. (1979): The absorbability by rats of various triglycerides of stearic and oleic acid and the effect of dietary calcium and magnesium. *J. Nutr.*, 109:1682–1687.
155. Mattson, F. H., and Streck, J. A. (1974): Effect of the composition of glycerides containing behenic acid on the lipid content of the heart of weanling rats. *J. Nutr.*, 104:483–488.
156. Mattson, F. H., and Volpenhein, R. A. (1968): Hydrolysis of primary and secondary esters of glycerol by pancreatic juice. *J. Lipid Res.*, 9:79–84.
157. Mattson, F. H., and Volpenhein, R. A. (1972): Rate and extent of absorption of the fatty acids of fully esterified glycerol, erythritol, xylitol and sucrose as recovered in thoracic duct cannulated rats. *J. Nutr.*, 102:1177–1180.
158. Mattson, F. H., and Volpenhein, R. A. (1972): Hydrolysis of fully esterified alcohols containing from one to eight hydroxyl groups by the lipolytic enzymes of rat pancreatic juice. *J. Lipid Res.*, 13:325–328.
159. Maylie, M. F., Charles, M., Gache, C., and Desnuelle, P. (1971): Isolation and partial identification of a pancreatic colipase. *Biochim. Biophys. Acta*, 229:286–289.
160. McMahon, M. T., and Thomson, G. R. (1970): Comparison of the absorption of a polar lipid, oleic acid, and a non-polar lipid, α-tocopherol, from mixed micellar solutions and emulsions. *Eur. J. Clin. Invest.*, 1:161–166.
161. McWeeny, D. J. (1968): Ph.D. Thesis. University of Birmingham. 1957. Cited in M. P. Mitchell and G. Hubscher: Oxidation of n-hexadecane by subcellular preparations of guinea pig small intestine. *Eur. J. Biochem.*, 7:90–95.
162. Mes, J., Davies, D. J., and Turton, D. (1982): Polychlorinated biphenyls and other chlorinated hydrocarbon residues in adipose tissues of Canadians. *Bull. Environ. Contam. Toxicol.*, 28:97–104.
163. Michael, W. R. (1968): Metabolism of linear alkylate sulfonate and alkyl benzene sulfonate in albino rats. *Toxicol. Appl. Pharmacol.*, 12:473–485.
164. Mills, A. P. (1963): Pesticide residue content. *J. Assoc. Offic. Agr. Chemists*, 46:762–767.
165. Mishkin, S., Yalovsky, M., and Kessler, J. I. (1972): Stages of uptake and incorporation of micellar palmitic acid by hamster proximal intestinal mucosa. *J. Lipid Res.*, 13:155–168.
166. Mishkin, S., Yalovsky, M., and Kessler, J. I. (1975): Uptake and compartmental distribution of fatty acid by rat small intestine *in vivo*. *Am. J. Physiol.*, 228:1409–1414.
167. Mohamed, H. F., Andreone, T. L., and Dryer, R. L. (1980): Mitochondrial metabolism of D,L-threo-9-,10-dibromopalmitic acid. *Lipids*, 15:255–262.
168. Morgan, R. G. H., Barrowman, J., and Borgstrom, B. (1969): The effect of sodium taurodeoxycholate and pH on the gel filtration behaviour of rat pancreatic protein and lipases. *Biochim. Biophys. Acta*, 175:65–75.
169. Morgan, R. G. H., Barrowman, J., Filipek-Wender, H., and Borgstrom, B. (1968): The lipolytic enzymes of rat pancreatic juice. *Biochim. Biophys. Acta*, 167:355–366.
170. Morley, N. H., Kuksis, A., and Buchnea, D. (1974): Hydrolysis of synthetic triacylglycerols by pancreatic and lipoprotein lipase. *Lipids*, 9:481–488.
171. Munro, I. C., Hand, B., Middleton, E. J., Heggtveit, H. A., and Grice, H. C. (1972): Toxic effects of brominated vegetable oils in rats. *Toxicol. Appl. Pharmacol.*, 2:432–439.
172. Munro, I. C., Middleton, E. J., and Grice, H. C. (1969): Biochemical and pathological changes in rats receiving brominated cottonseed oil for 80 days. *Fed. Cosmet. Toxicol.*, 7:25–33.
173. Myer, H. (1890): Ueber den wirksamen Bestandtheil des Ricinusöls. *Arch. Exp. Pathol. Pharmakol.*, 28:145–152.

174. Myer, W. H. (1979): Further Comments. *Fed. Proc.*, 38:2463–2437.
175. Nakamura, T., Aoyama, Y., Fujita, T., and Katsui, G. (1975): Studies on tocopherol derivatives: V. Intestinal absorption of several d,1-3-,4-³H-α-tocopheryl esters in the rat. *Lipids*, 10:627–633.
176. Ng, P. Y., and Holt, P. R. (1974): Sources of chylomicron phospholipid. (Abs.) *Clin. Nutr.*, 22:695.
177. Nikonorow, M., Mazyr, H., and Piekaca, H. (1973): Effect of orally administered plasticizers and polyvinyl chloride stabilizers in the rat. *Toxicol. Pharmacol.*, 26:253–259.
178. Nilsson, A. (1968): Metabolism of sphingomyelin in the intestinal tract of the rat. *Biochim. Biophys. Acta*, 164:575–584.
179. Nilsson, A. (1969): The presence of sphingomyelin and ceramide-cleaving enzymes in the small intestinal tract. *Biochim. Biophys. Acta*, 176:339–347.
180. Noda, M., Tsukahara, H., and Ogafa, M. (1978): Enzymic hydrolysis of diol lipids by pancreatic lipase. *Biochim. Biophys. Acta*, 529:270–279.
181. Nogami, H., Hasegawa, J., Hanano, M., and Fuwa, T. (1968): Studies on absorption and excretion of drugs. XIII. The sorption of surface active agents into the intestinal tissue of rat and their effect on the drug absorption *in vitro*. *Chem. Pharm. Bull. (Tokyo)*, 16:2101–2106.
182. Noguchi, T., Jinguji, Y., Kimura, T., Muranishi, S., and Sezaki, H. (1975): Mechanism of the intestinal absorption of drugs from in water emulsions. VI. Role of bile in the lymphatic transport of lipid-soluble compounds from triolein emulsions. *Chem. Pharm. Bull. (Tokyo)*, 23:782–786.
183. Noma, A., and Borgstrom, B. (1971): The acid lipase of castor beans. Positional specificity and reaction mechanism. *Biochim. Biophys. Acta*, 227:106–115.
184. Norman, A. (1960): The beginning solubilization of 20-methylcholantrene in aqueous solutions of conjugated and non-conjugated bile acid salts. *Acta Chem. Scand.*, 14:1295–1299.
185. O'Doherty, P. J. A. (1979): The importance of the steric configuration of lysophosphatidylcholine in the lymphatic transport of fat. *Lipids*, 14:84–87.
186. O'Doherty, P. J. A., Kakis, G., and Kuksis, A. (1973): Role of luminal lecithin in intestinal fat absorption. *Lipids*, 8:249–255.
187. O'Doherty, P. J. A., Yousef, I. M., Kakis, G., and Kuksis, A. (1975): Protein and glycerolipid biosynthesis in isolated intestinal epithelial cells of normal and bile fistula rats. *Arch. Biochem. Biophys.*, 169:252–261.
188. O'Doherty, P. J. A., Yousef, I. M., and Kuksis, A. (1973): Effect of puromycin on protein biosynthesis in isolated mucosal cells. *Arch. Biochem. Biophys.*, 156:586–594.
189. Oshima, M., and Ariga, T. (1975): ω-Cyclohexyl fatty acids in acidophilic thermophilic bacteria. *J. Biol. Chem.*, 250:6963–6968.
190. Overturf, M. L., Druilhet, R. E., Liehr, J. G., Kirkendahl, W. M., and Caprioli, R. M. (1979): Phthalate ester in normal and pathological human kidneys. *Bull. Environ. Contam. Toxicol.*, 22:536–542.
191. Paltauf, F. (1971): Metabolism of the enantiomeric 1-0-alkylglycerol ethers in the rat intestinal mucosa in vivo; incorporation into 1-0-alkyl and 1-0-alk-1-enyl glycerol lipids. *Biochim. Biophys. Acta*, 239:38–46.
192. Paltauf, F., Esfandi, F., and Holasek, A. (1974): Stereospecificity of lipases. Enzyme hydrolysis of enantiomeric alkyl diacylglycerols by lipoprotein lipases, lingual lipase and pancreatic lipase. *FEBS Lett.*, 40:119–123.
193. Pande, S. V., Siddiqui, A. W., and Gatereau, A. (1971): Inhibition of long chain fatty acid activation by α-bromopalmitate and phytanate. *Biochim. Biophys. Acta*, 248:156–166.
194. Parkinson, T. M., Gunderson, K., and Nelsen, N. A. (1970): Effects of colestipol (U-26, 597A), a new bile acid sequestrant, on serum lipids in experimental animals and man. *Atherosclerosis*, 11:531–537.
195. Parsons, H. G., Kuksis, A., and Emken, E. A. (1983): Simultaneous measurement of the assimilation of four long chain fatty acids (LCFAs) in human plasma lipids. *Gastroenterology*, 84:1270.
196. Patton, J. S. (1981): Gastrointestinal lipid absorption. In: *Physiology of the Gastrointestinal Tract*, Vol. 2, edited by L. R. Johnson, pp. 1123–1146. Raven Press, New York.
197. Patton, J. S., and Carey, M. C. (1979): Watching fat digestion. *Science*, 204:145–148.
198. Peakall, D. B. (1975): Phthalate esters: occurrence and biological effects. *Residue Rev.*, 54:1–41.
199. Peake, I. R., Windmuller, H. G., and Bieri, J. G. (1972): A comparison of the intestinal absorption, lymph and plasma transport, and tissue uptake of α- and γ-tocopherols in the rat. *Biochim. Biophys. Acta*, 260:679–688.
200. Perkins, E. G., Endres, J. G., and Kummerow, F. A. (1961): The metabolism of fats. Effect of

dietary hydroxy acids and their triglycerides on growth, carcass, and fecal fat composition in the rat. *J. Nutr.*, 73:291–298.

201. Pfeiffer, C. J. (1977): Gastroenterologic response to environmental agents—absorption and interactions. In: *Handbook of Physiology, Section 9: Reactions to Environmental Agents*, edited by D. H. K. Lee, pp. 349–374. American Physiological Society, Bethesda.

202. Porter, H. P., Saunders, D. R., Tytgat, G., Brunser, O., and Rubin, C. E. (1971): Fat absorption in bile fistula man. *Gastroenterology*, 60:1008–1019.

203. Racusen, L. C., and Binder, H. J. (1979): Ricinoleic acid stimulation of active anion secretion in colonic mucosa of the rat. *J. Clin. Invest.*, 63:743–749.

204. Rawat, A. K. (1972): The red-ox-state in relation to ethanol metabolism by rat and guinea pig liver *in vitro*. *Arch. Biochem. Biophys.*, 151:93–101.

205. Reddy, B. S. (1981): Dietary fat and its relationship to large bowel cancer. *Cancer Res.*, 41:3700–3705.

206. Reiser, R., and Fu, H. C. (1966): Acyl group exchange in the intestinal lumen during fat absorption. *Biochim. Biophys. Acta*, 116:563–569.

207. Reisser, D., and Boucrot, P. (1978): *In vitro* and *in vivo* effects of exogenous lipids on the enzymatic hydrolysis of rat bile phospholipid. *Lipids*, 13:796–800.

208. Riley, J. W., and Glickman, R. M. (1979): Fat malabsorption. Advances in our understanding. *Am. J. Med.*, 67:980–988.

209. Riu, K. H., and Grim, E. (1982): Unstirred water layer in canine jejunum. *Am. J. Physiol.*, 242:G364–G369.

210. Rodgers, J. B., O'Brien, R. J., and Balint, J. A. (1975): The absorption and utilization of lecithin by the rat jejunum. *Am. J. Org. Dis.*, 20:208–213.

211. Rodgers, J. B., Tandon, R., and O'Brien, R. J. (1973): Distribution of lipid reesterifying enzymes in jejunal microsomes of bile fistula rats. Attempts to correlate enzyme activities with microsomal phospholipid content. *Biochim. Biophys. Acta*, 326:345–354.

212. Romsos, D. R., Belo, P. S., Miller, E. R., and Leveille, G. A. (1975): Influence of dietary 1,3-butanediol on weight gain, blood, and liver metabolites and lipogenesis in the pig and chick. *J. Nutr.*, 105:161–170.

213. Sabesin, S. M., and Frase, S. (1977): Electron microscopic studies of the assembly, intracellular transport, and secretion of chylomicrons by rat intestine. *J. Lipid Res.*, 18:496–511.

214. Sabesin, S. M., and Isselbacher, K. J. (1965): Protein synthesis inhibition: mechanism for the production of impaired fat absorption. *Science*, 147:1149–1151.

215. Sampugna, J., Quinn, J. G., Pitas, R. E., Carpenter, D. L., and Jensen, R. G. (1967): Digestion of butyrate glycerides by pancreatic lipase. *Lipids*, 2:397–401.

216. Samuel, P., and McNamara, D. J. (1983): Differential absorption of exogenous and endogenous cholesterol in man. *J. Lipid Res.*, 24:265–276.

217. Sarafin, J. A., and Nesheim, M. C. (1970): Influence of dietary heat labile fractions of soybean meal upon bile acid pools and turnover in the chick. *J. Nutr.*, 100:786–796.

218. Sanders, E., and Ashworth, C. T. (1961): A study of particulate intestinal absorption and hepatocellular uptake. Use of polystyrene latex particles. *Exp. Cell Res.*, 22:137–155.

219. Saunders, D. R. (1975): Regional differences in the effect of bile salt absorption by rat small intestine *in vivo*. *J. Physiol.*, 250:373–383.

220. Schoen, H., and Fahsold, W. (1960): Untersuchungen zur Frage der Resorption von Squalen. *Klin. Wschr.*, 38:177–179.

221. Scow, R. O., Stein, Y., and Stein, O. (1967): Incorporation of dietary lecithin and lysolecithin into lymph chylomicrons in the rat. *J. Biol. Chem.*, 242:4919–4924.

222. Shah, A. H., and Gutrie, F. E. (1970): Penetration of insecticides through the isolated midgut of insects and mammals. *Comp. Gen. Pharmacol.*, 1:391–399.

223. Shaikh, N. A., and Kuksis, A. (1982): Expansion of phospholipid pool size of rat intestinal villus cells during fat absorption. *Can. J. Biochem.*, 60:444–451.

224. Shaikh, N. A., and Kuksis, A. (1983): Further evidence for enhanced phospholipid synthesis by rat jejunal villus cells during fat absorption. *Can. J. Biochem. Cell Biol*, 61:370–377.

225. Shakir, K. M. M., Gabriel, L., Sundaram, S. G., and Margolis, S. (1982): Intestinal phospholipase A and triglyceride lipase: localization and effect of fasting. *Am. J. Physiol.*, 242:G168–G176.

226. Shiau, Y-F. (1981): Mechanisms of intestinal fat absorption. *Am. J. Physiol.*, 240:G1–G9.

227. Shull, R. L., Gayle, L. A., Coleman, R. D., and Alfin-Slater, R. B. (1961): Metabolic studies of glyceride esters and adipic acid. *J. Am. Oil Chem. Soc.*, 38:84–86.

228. Sieber, S. M., Cohn, V. H., and Wynn, W. T. (1974): The entry of foreign compounds into the thoracic duct lymph of the rat. *Xenobiotica*, 4:265–284.
229. Simmonds, W. J. (1976): Uptake of fatty acid and monoglyceride. In: *Lipid Absorption: Biochemical and Clinical Aspects*, edited by K. Rommel, H. Goebell, and R. Bohmer, pp. 51–64. MTP Press Ltd., St. Leonard's House, Lancaster, England.
230. Simmonds, W. J., Hofmann, A. F., and Theodor, E. J. (1967): Absorption of cholesterol from a micellar solution: intestinal perfusion studies in man. *J. Clin. Invest.*, 46:874–890.
231. Sklan, D. (1979): Digestion and absorption of lipids in chicks fed triglycerides or free fatty acids: synthesis of monoglycerides in the intestine. *Poultry Sci.*, 58:855–889.
232. Sklan, D., Hurwitz, S., Budowski, P., and Ascarelli, I. (1975): Fat digestion and absorption in chickens fed raw or heated soybean meal. *J. Nutr.*, 105:57–63.
233. Slotboom, A. J., De Haas, G. H., Bonsen, P. P. M., Burbach-Wetsterhuis, G. J., and Van Deenen, L. L. M. (1970): Hydrolysis of phosphoglycerides by purified lipase preparations—substrate-positional- and stereospecificity. *Chem. Phys. Lipids*, 4:15–29.
234. Slotbom, A. J., Van Dam-Mieras, M. C. E., and De Haas, G. H. (1977): Regulation of phospholipase A activity by different lipid-water interfaces. *J. Biol. Chem.*, 252:2948–2951.
235. Smith, H. F., Jr., and Calandra, J. C. (1969): Toxicologic studies of alkylphenol polyoxyethylene surfactants. *Toxicol. Apl. Pharmacol.*, 14:315–334.
236. Snipes, R. L. (1968): The effect of essential fatty acid deficiency on the ultrastructure and functional capacity of the jejunal epithelium. *Lab. Invest.*, 18:179–189.
237. Spencer, R. P., and Brody, K. R. (1964): Biotin transport by small intestine of rat, hamster and other species. *Am. J. Physiol.*, 206:653–657.
238. Spencer, R. P., Brody, K. R., and Vishno, F. (1966): Species differences in the intestinal transport of p-aminobenzoic acid. *Comp. Biochem. Physiol.*, 17:883–889.
239. Staggers, J. E., Fernando-Warnakulasuriya, J. P., and Wells, M. A. (1981): Studies on fat digestion, absorption and transport in the suckling rat. II. Triacylglycerols: molecular species, stereospecific analysis, and specificity of hydrolysis by lingual lipase. *J. Lipid Res.*, 22:675–679.
240. Stetten, D. W., Jr. (1943): Metabolism of paraffin. *J. Biol. Chem.*, 147:327–332.
241. Sugano, M., Ide, M., Kohno, M., Watanabe, M., Cho, Y-J., and Nagata, Y. (1983): Biliary and fecal steroid excretion in rats fed partially hydrogenated soybean oil. *Lipids*, 18:186–192.
242. Sundqvist, T., Magnusson, K. E., Sjodahl, R., Stjernstrom, I., and Tagesson, C. (1980): Passage of molecules through the wall of the gastrointestinal tract. *Gut*, 21:208–211.
243. Swell, L., Trout, E. C., Jr., Field, H., Jr., and Treadwell, C. R. (1959): Absorption of ³H-beta-sitosterol in the lymph fistula rat. *Proc. Soc. Exp. Biol. Med.*, 100:140–142.
244. Sylven, C., and Borgstrom, B. (1968): Absorption and lymphatic transport of cholesterol in the rat. *J. Lipid Res.*, 9:596–601.
245. Sylven, C., and Borgstrom, B. (1969): Absorption and lymphatic transport of cholesterol and sitosterol in the rat. *J. Lipid Res.*, 10:179–182.
246. Sylven, C., and Borgstrom, B. (1969): Intestinal absorption and lymphatic transport of cholesterol in the rat: influence of the fatty acid chain length of the carrier triglyceride. *J. Lipid Res.*, 10:351–355.
247. Sylven, C., and Borgstrom, B. (1970): Influence of blood supply on lipid uptake from micellar solutions by the rat intestine. *Biochim. Biophys. Acta*, 203:365–375.
248. Szlam, F., and Sgoutas, D. S. (1978): Eicosenoic and Docosenoic acid incorporation in serum lipoproteins in rats fed rapeseed oil. *Lipids*, 13:121–127.
249. Takahashi, T., Tanaka, A., and Yamaha, T. (1981): Elimination, distribution and metabolism of di(2-ethylhexyl)adipate (DEHA) in rats. *Toxicol.*, 22:223–233.
250. Takahashi, Y. I., and Underwood, B. A. (1974): Effect of long and medium chain length lipids upon aqueous solubility of α-tocopherol. *Lipids*, 9:855–859.
251. Tattrie, N. H., Bailey, R. A., and Kates, M. (1958): The action of pancreatic lipase on stereoisomeric triglycerides. *Arch. Biochem. Biophys.*, 78:319–327.
252. Thomson, A. B. R. (1980): Effect of age on uptake of homologous series of saturated fatty acids into rabbit jejunum. *Am. J. Physiol.*, 239:G363–G371.
253. Thomson, A. B. R., and Dietschy, J. M. (1981): Intestinal lipid absorption: major extracellular and intracellular events. In: *Physiology of the Gastrointestinal Tract*, Vol. 2, edited by L. R. Johnson, pp. 1147–1220. Raven Press, New York.
254. Toothill, J., Thomson, S. Y., and Edwards-Webb, J. D. (1976): Studies on lipid digestion in the preruminant calf. The source of lipolytic activity in the abomassum. *Br. J. Nutr.*, 36:439–443.

255. Treadwell, C. R., and Vahouny, G. V. (1968): Cholesterol absorption. In: *Handbook of Physiology, Vol. III, Alimentary Canal*, pp. 1407–1438. American Physiological Society, Washington, D.C.
256. Tilvis, R. S., and Miettinen, T. A. (1983): Absorption and metabolic fate of dietary ^{3}H-squalene in the rat. *Lipids*, 18:233–238.
257. Tomarelli, R. M., Meyer, B. J., Weaber, J. R., and Bernhart, F. W. (1968): Effect of positional distribution of the fatty acids of human milk and infant formulas. *J. Nutr.*, 95:583–590.
258. Tomita, I., Nakamura, Y., and Yagi, Y. (1977): Phthalic acid esters in various foodstuffs and biological materials. *Exotoxicol. Environ. Safety*, 1:275–287.
259. Tso, P., Balint, J. A., and Rodgers, J. B. (1981): Acute inhibition of intestinal lipid transport by Pluronic L-81 in the rat. *Am. J. Physiol.*, 244:G489–G497.
260. Tso, P., Balint, J. A., and Simmons, W. J. (1977): Role of biliary lecithin in lymphatic transport of fat. *Gastroenterology*, 73:1362–1367.
261. Tso, P., Kendrick, H., Balint, J. A., and Simmonds, W. J. (1981): Role of biliary phosphatidylcholine in the absorption and transport of dietary triolein in the rat. *Gastroenterology*, 80:60–65.
262. Tso, P., Lam, J., and Simmonds, W. J. (1978): The importance of the lysophosphatidylcholine and choline moiety of bile phosphatidylcholine in lymphatic transport of fat. *Biochim. Biophys. Acta*, 528:364–372.
263. Tso, P., and Simmonds, W. J. (1976): Importance of luminal lecithin in intestinal absorption and transport of lipid in the rat. *Austr. J. Exp. Biol. Med. Sci.*, 55:355–357.
264. U.S. Environmental Protection Agency. (1972,1975): Scientific and Technical Assessment Report on Particulate Polycyclic Organic Matter. Washington, D.C.
265. Wang, C-S. (1981): Human milk bile salt-activated lipase. Further characterization and kinetic studies. *J. Biol. Chem.*, 256:10198–20202.
266. Wang, C-S., Kuksis, A., Manganaro, F., Myher, J. J., Downs, D., and Bass, H. G. (1983): Studies on substrate specificity of purified human milk bile salt-activated lipase. *J. Biol. Chem.*, 258:9197–9202.
267. Warnick, S. L., and Carter, J. E. (1972): Some findings in a study of workers occupationally exposed to pesticides. *Arch. Environ. Health.*, 25:265–270.
268. Watson, W. C., and Gordon, R. S., Jr. (1962): Studies on the digestion, absorption and metabolism of castor oil. *Biochem. Pharmacol.*, 11:229–236.
269. Watson, W. C., and Murray, E. S. (1965): Triricinolein synthesis *in vivo*. *Biochim. Biophys. Acta*, 106:311–314.
270. Weaver, J. E., and Griffith, J. F. (1969): Induction of emesis by detergent ingredients and formulations. *Toxicol. Appl. Pharmacol.*, 14:214–220.
271. Westergaard, H., and Dietschy, J. M. (1974): Delineation of the dimensions and permeability characteristics of the two major diffusion barriers to passive mucosal uptake in the rabbit intestine. *J. Clin. Invest.*, 174:718–732.
272. Westergaard, H., and Dietschy, J. M. (1976): The mechanism whereby bile acid micelles increase the rate of fatty acid and cholesterol uptake into the intestinal mucosal cell. *J. Clin Invest.*, 58:97–108.
273. Wickizer, T., and Brilliant, L. B. (1981): Testing for polychlorinated biphenyls in human milk. *Pediatrics*, 68:411–415.
274. Williams, S. (1964): Pesticide residues in total diet samples. *J. Assoc. Offic. Agr. Chemists.*, 47:815–821.
275. Wilson, F. A., Sallee, V. L., and Dietschy, J. M. (1971): Unstirred water layer in the intestine: rate determinant for fatty acid absorption from micellar solutions. *Science*, 174:1031–1033.
276. Wingate, D. L., Phillips, S. F., and Hofmann, A. F. (1973): Effect of glycine-conjugated bile acids with and without lecithin on water and glucose absorption in perfused human jejunum. *J. Clin. Invest.*, 52:1230–1236.
277. Wolfe, H. R., Durham, W. F., and Armstrong, J. F. (1970): Urinary excretion of pesticide metabolites. *Arch. Environ. Health.*, 21:711–716.
278. Yasuhara, M., Kobayashi, H., Kurosaki, Y., Kimura, T., Muranishi, S., and Sezaki, H. (1979): Comparative studies on the absorption mechanism of p-amino-benzoic acid and p-acetamidobenzoic acid from the rat intestine. *J. Pharm. Dyn.*, 2:177–186.
279. Yasuhara, M., Yoshino, T., Kimura, T., Muranishi, S., and Sezaki, H. (1979): Effect of surfactants on the absorption of p–aminobenzoic acid from the rat intestine. *J. Pharm. Dyn.*, 2:251–256.
280. Zilversmit, D. B. (1983): A model for cholesterol absorption: isotope versus mass; single dose versus continued infusion. *J. Lipid Res.*, 24:297–302.

Intestinal Toxicology, edited by C. M. Schiller.
Raven Press, New York © 1984.

Sodium Electrochemical Gradients and Intestinal Absorption

George A. Kimmich

Departments of Biochemistry, and Radiation Biology and Biophysics, University of Rochester Medical Center, Rochester, New York 14642

The small intestine is a highly specialized organ with a primary function of capturing nutrient molecules and ions from the dietary constituents and thereby conserving them for supporting the function of the entire organism. As is true for most complex tissues, individual cell types have specific functions that contribute to the overall functional capability of the intact tissue. In the case of the specific absorptive function of the intestine, the luminal epithelial cells represent the locus at which discrimination occurs with respect to whether a particular solute will be captured for the organism or whether it will be ignored and excreted (25).

Absorption by the epithelium is itself a two-part process that involves the sequential transfer of solutes across the luminal-facing brush border membrane of the epithelial cell followed by a second transfer across the basolateral cell membrane into the villous lamina propria. The capillary network of the lamina propria moves absorbed solutes to the general circulation which therefore serves as the nutrient delivery system for all of the other organ systems.

Clearly, each successive membrane transfer could occur simply via a diffusional or facilitated diffusional mechanism. A mechanism of this sort would not be efficient at removing dietary solutes, however, unless the blood flow through the villous capillary system was rapid, and other organs removed nutrients at a rate rapid enough to ensure a sustained downhill concentration gradient from intestinal lumen to blood. For those solutes such as glucose and certain amino acids that have significant plasma concentration levels, a diffusional absorption mechanism would mandate inefficient recovery from the diet. Instead, for most ions and nutrients (including sugar and amino acids) virtually all of the dietary load is conserved by the intestine by transfer to the circulatory system.

Such efficient dietary extraction implies that the intestinal epithelium must have the ability to move solutes against a concentration gradient, and indeed it is now well understood that concentrative transfer is an especially well-developed intestinal function. If concentrative transfer is defined as movement between two compartments against a concentration gradient, one can envision several possible schematic models for epithelial transfer, depending on whether the individual membrane events

115

are uphill ("pump") or downhill ("leak") transfers. Possible combinations therefore include "pump-leak," "leak-pump," or "pump-pump" models as shown schematically in Fig. 1. Examples of each type of transport are known to occur in vertebrate intestinal tissue as will be discussed below.

GENERAL ENERGETIC CONCEPTS

In physiology, as in all other disciplines, it is not possible to get something for nothing. Uphill or concentrative transfer of a solute requires an input of energy that is greater than the gain in energy represented by solute flow against a concentration gradient. Those transfers designated as "pump" in the general transport models shown in Fig. 1 therefore imply some form of energy input. For "pump-leak" systems (i.e., mechanisms in which uphill transfer occurs at the brush-border boundary of the epithelial cell) the energy input for many transport systems is

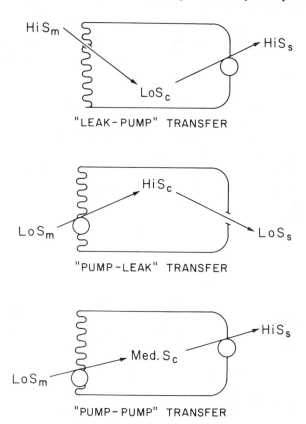

FIG. 1. Schematic representation of three different types of net epithelial solute transfer. The terms "pump" and "leak" in this diagram are used to indicate whether solute is transferred against or down a concentration gradient, respectively. In this sense, a pump transfer is not necessarily against an electrochemical gradient.

provided by the flow of Na+ down a gradient of electrochemical potential. Membrane components exist which can couple the simultaneous flow of Na+ and a particular solute such that the energy provided by Na+ flow down its electrochemical gradient is greater than the energy required by the concomitant flow of solute against its gradient (for reviews see refs. 26 and 27). For some solutes, such as α- or β-methylglucosides, a very high portion of total permeability to the intestinal epithelium is linked to the presence (and simultaneous influx) of Na+ as shown in Table 1.

Transport Thermodynamics

In thermodynamic terms, energy is always the product of an amount times a potential, where the potential term can take different forms such as gravitational, electrical, thermal, chemical, or others. Likewise, the term for amount may be expressed in different ways, including mass, moles of solute or photons, charge or volume among others. For analysis of the energy changes occurring during the function of biological transport systems one therefore needs to consider the number of moles of solute transported and the difference in chemical potential (which is proportional to concentration) through which it moves. For a charged solute it is also necessary to consider the number of moles of electrical charge transferred and the difference in electrical potential through which they move.

The energy released when Na+ flows into a cell is therefore a result of chemical and electrical driving forces when the cell membrane has its usual interior negative electrical polarity. The thermodynamic expression for the energy change is given by:

$$\Delta G_{Na} = n_{Na}\Delta\mu_{Na} + n_c\Delta E$$

where ΔG_{Na} is the change in Gibbs' free energy (energy available to do work), n_{Na} and n_c are the moles of sodium and moles of charge that are transferred, respectively (the two are, of course, equal in the case of monovalent ions), and $\Delta\mu$, ΔE are

TABLE 1. *Effect of Na+ or phlorizin on the unidirectional influx of 3-O-methylglucose (3-OMG) or α-methylglucoside (α-MG) into isolated chicken intestinal epithelial cells*

Sugar	Conc. (μM)	Na+ Conc. (mM)	Phlorizin[a]	Sugar influx[b]	% Control
3-OMG	100	140	−	1.17	100
3-OMG	100	140	+	0.07	6
3-OMG	100	0	−	0.06	5
α-MG	100	140	−	1.55	100
α-MG	100	140	+	0.05	3.5
α-MG	100	0	−	0.02	1.7

[a]Phlorizin concentration = 200 μM.
[b]Values are given in nmol/min · mg protein.

the respective differences in chemical and electrical potential. To add the two terms, a conversion factor, the Faraday, is necessary in order to convert them to the same units. Thus,

$$\Delta G_{\text{Na}} = n_{\text{Na}} \, \Delta\mu_{\text{Na}}{}^+ + n_c F \Delta E$$

For an uncharged solute, the energy change expression involves only a term for the difference in chemical potential:

$$\Delta G_s = n_s \Delta\mu_s$$

If the flow of Na^+ is going to provide sufficient energy to drive the accumulation of an uncharged solute, then the energy change due to solute transfer cannot be greater than the energy change due to Na^+ transfer:

$$n_s \Delta\mu_s \leq n_{\text{Na}}{}^+ \Delta\mu_{\text{Na}}{}^+ + n_c F \Delta E$$

The chemical potential (μ) for a solute is related to its chemical potential in a standard state (μ^o) and is proportional to its concentration (c): $\mu = \mu^o + RT \ln c$. Therefore the difference in chemical potential in moving a solute across a membrane boundary is:

$$\Delta\mu = \mu_1 - \mu_2 \text{ or } \Delta\mu = (\mu^o + RT \ln c_1) - (\mu^o + RT \ln c_2) = RT \ln \frac{c_1}{c_2}$$

where the subscripts 1 and 2 refer to the two different sides of the membrane, R is the ideal gas law constant, and T is the temperature in degrees Kelvin. The full expression for analyzing the energetics of coupled transport between Na^+ and other solutes is therefore:

$$n_S \, RT \ln \frac{(S_i)}{(S_o)} \leq n_{\text{Na}} \, RT \ln \frac{(\text{Na})_o}{(\text{Na})_i} + n_c \, F \Delta E$$

where i and o designate intracellular and extracellular concentrations (or, more properly, chemical activities). Remembering that $n_{\text{Na}+} = n_c$ for sodium, this expression can be rearranged to:

$$\log \frac{(S)_i}{(S)_o} = \frac{n_{\text{Na}+}}{n_S} \left(\log \frac{(\text{Na})_o}{(\text{Na})_i} + \frac{F \Delta E}{2.3 \, RT} \right) = n_r \left(\log \frac{(\text{Na})_o}{(\text{Na})_i} + \frac{F \Delta E}{2.3 \, RT} \right)$$

in which $n_r = n_{Na}/n_S$, or the number of Na^+ ions coupled to the entry of each solute molecule on the Na^+-dependent transport system (coupling stoichiometry). From this expression it is apparent that transport systems that are linked to the entry of Na^+ should establish a solute gradient that is a function of three parameters: (a) the Na^+ concentration gradient which exists across the plasma membrane, (b) the electrical membrane potential across the same boundary, and (c) the Na:solute coupling stoichiometry.

Experimental Analysis of Transport Energetics

Work with isolated intestinal epithelial cells in the past few years has been useful in demonstrating the importance of each of the above elements in the energization of sugar accumulation by the intestinal epithelium (for short reviews, see refs. 25,26,28). Figure 2 shows data for uptake of α-methylglucoside by adenosine triphosphate (ATP)-depleted isolated intestinal epithelial cells in which a gradient of either chemical potential (Na+ concentration) or electrical potential (created by diffusion of a permeable ion) or both were experimentally imposed. Note that an

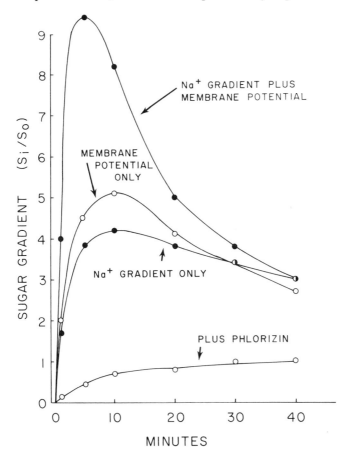

FIG. 2. Transient accumulation of α-methylglucoside by ATP-depleted isolated intestinal epithelial cells driven by experimentally imposed chemical gradients of Na+ or membrane potential or an electrochemical Na+ gradient. A transmembrane Na+ gradient was created by preincubation of the cell population in Tris-acetate and sudden dilution into Na-acetate. For a membrane potential, the cells were preincubated in Na-acetate and diluted into $NaNO_3$ to create a diffusion potential (interior negative) because of the imposed nitrate gradient. The Na+ electrochemical gradient was obtained with cells preequilibrated with Tris-acetate and diluted into $NaNO_3$. Final Na+ concentration in all three test cases was 155 mM. Osmolarity in preincubation media as well as incubation media was 320 mosmolar.

imposed gradient of a chemical potential for Na^+ can induce a transient accumulation of sugar against a four- to fivefold concentration gradient. The sugar gradient is transient because the ATP-depleted cells are unable to maintain the imposed Na^+ gradient, and it dissipates as Na^+ diffuses into the cell. If Na^+ is preequlibrated across the cell membrane, and these cells are then added to a medium with a high NO_3^- concentration, an interior negative membrane potential is created because of the NO_3^--induced diffusion potential, and again the cells establish a transient sugar gradient of about fivefold, which in this case persists until the imposed NO_3^- gradient dissipates. When gradients of chemical potential for Na^+ *and* electrical potential due to NO_3^- diffusion are both imposed, then the cells can establish a transient sugar gradient as high as 9- to 10-fold.

It is important to recognize that the effect of the membrane potential on sugar accumulation capability is absolutely dependent on the presence of Na^+. In the absence of Na^+, the same gradient of NO_3^- used for the experiment shown in Fig. 2 causes no change in sugar uptake by the cells. If a gradient of a different monovalent cation is imposed, there is also no sugar accumulation.

Normally, intestinal epithelial cells, like most other cell types, maintain both an Na^+ gradient and a membrane potential due to the activity of the Na^+ - K^+ ATPase, which utilizes chemical energy in the form of ATP to extrude Na^+ from the cell and to accumulate K^+ against concentration gradients. This "Na^+ pump" is rheogenic (i.e., catalyzes a net charge transfer) and therefore directly acts to create a membrane potential (71). In addition, the ion gradients established will modify the potential owing to differing permeabilities of the ions and consequent development of diffusion potentials.

The gradient of electrochemical potential for Na^+ established by the Na^+ pump is a form of stored energy that can be tapped by Na^+-dependent transport systems and utilized to accumulate specific solutes against concentration gradients. In a sense the limited amount of chemical "money" represented by the cellular pool of ATP is put into "savings" by transformation into a gradient of electrochemical potential for Na^+ via the Na^+ pump, and this "invested" energy can be translated into other kinds of energy investment (i.e., solute accumulation) if appropriate membrane components are present.

The "appropriate" membrane components are the Na^+-dependent transport systems that allow coupling between "downhill" flow of Na^+ into the cell and "uphill" flow of particular solutes. We have already noted that such systems exist for certain sugars, including α-methylglucoside. Other sugars that satisfy this transport system include the important dietary sugars glucose and galactose as well as a variety of nondietary sugars and sugar analogs (11,12). It is noteworthy that mannose, although common in the diet, is not transported by an Na^+-dependent system. In general, those sugars with a six-membered ring as part of their molecular structure and with an OH group at position 2 in the same configuration as in D-glucose will satisfy the Na^+-dependent carrier (10,27). Small chemical substituent groups (e.g., methyl groups) can be tolerated at most positions, with the exception of position 2. The Na^+-dependent sugar carrier can be selectively inhibited by low concentrations of phlorizin, a glycoside produced by various plants in the *Rosaceae* family (1,2).

MOLECULAR MECHANISM OF TRANSPORT

The molecular events involved in the Na-dependent transfer of solutes are thought to involve membrane components that have binding sites for the solute to be transferred as well as for Na^+. Schematically they can be represented as shown in Fig. 3 in which membrane component *c* (carrier) combines with nNa^+ and a solute molecule to form a complex which can undergo a conformational change and deliver Na^+ and solute to the cell. The membrane potential can activate transport in various ways, depending on the net charge on the free and loaded carrier. For one of the cases shown (Fig. 3c), the free carrier is considered to bear a single negative charge and to bind more than one Na^+ ($n = 2$) such that the loaded carrier is cationic. An

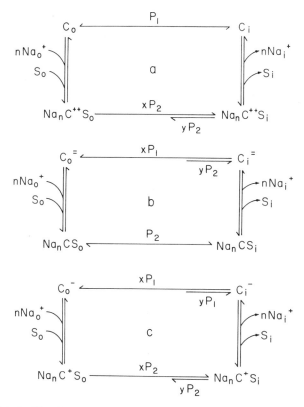

FIG. 3. Models for Na^+-dependent transport systems in which the membrane potential can play different roles dependent on the net charge of the free and loaded carrier forms. The coefficients *x* and *y* are meant to represent potential dependent functions that modify the membrane permeability content *(P)* for each species. Integer *n* represents the number of Na^+ ions moving with each solute *(S)* molecule. For each of the models shown here, *n* is assumed to be 2 (see text), so that the various carrier forms can be assigned the indicated charge.

interior negative membrane potential would help support transport in two ways: (a) by driving the anionic carrier to the outer face of the plasma membrane and (b) by drawing the cationic loaded carrier to the inner membrane face. The x and y coefficients for the rate constants governing membrane transfer events are therefore potential dependent values, and influx kinetics for Na+-dependent transport of solute will be markedly influenced by the magnitude of the membrane potential, as was shown in Fig. 2. Indeed, if the membrane potential is manipulated in a systematic fashion with the aid of NO_3^- gradients, the unidirectional sugar influx can be shown to undergo a corresponding change in rate (Table 2).

If only the free and fully loaded carrier forms can undergo the conformational change necessary to expose binding sites at the two membrane surfaces, then transport of the solute will be totally Na+-dependent, as has been reported for sugar transport (19,33,77). On the other hand, mechanisms can be envisioned in which a partly loaded carrier might deliver one solute only to the cell interior (i.e., either Na+ or sugar). Such models help explain observations indicating that certain transport systems for amino acids might function in the absence of Na+ to admit solute to the cell (14,33). In the latter case, no concentrative accumulation would be possible because in the absence of Na+ there is no energy released by flow of Na+ down a gradient of electrochemical potential. Reports of work with certain neutral amino acid transport systems indicate that such systems may function as facilitated diffusion solute carriers in the absence of Na+ (14).

COUPLING STOICHIOMETRY

No matter what specific model one considers for Na+-dependent transport systems, the concept of Na+-induced transport energization requires that a flow of Na+ is coupled to the flow of solute being transported. For a long time the coupling stoichiometry between Na+ and solute was considered to be 1:1, based in part on

TABLE 2. *Effect of nitrate gradient-induced membrane potentials on the unidirectional influx of α-methylglucoside into isolated intestinal epithelial cells*

$[NO_3^-]$	Calculated $\Delta\psi$[a]	Sugar influx[b]
0 mM	0 mV	0.75
20	− 13	1.42
50	− 25	2.12
80	− 33	2.43
110	− 39	2.70
150	− 44	2.84

[a]Potentials were calculated using the Goldman equation and a permeability ratio of 5 for NO_3^- : Na+.

[b]Values are given in mmol/min · mg protein.

direct measurements (6,19,62) and in part on interpretation of certain kinetic data (14,23,81). Recently, we showed that all of these earlier reports suffer from a systematic error in methodology which leads to an underestimation of the true coupling stoichiometry. The imprecision relates to transport-induced changes in membrane potential which introduce consequent changes in Na^+ fluxes occurring by potential-sensitive routes not related to the Na^+-dependent solute carrier (30,31,37). When appropriate experimental precautions are taken to avoid such changes in potential, the coupling stoichimetry between Na^+ and sugar proves to be 2.0 by direct measurements of carrier-mediated fluxes (Table 3). Phlorizin was utilized in these experiments as a selective inhibitor of the Na^+-dependent sugar carrier in order to identify that part of the Na^+ and sugar fluxes mediated via the Na^+-dependent carrier. Recent kinetic data from another laboratory tend to confirm the 2:1 Na^+:sugar coupling stoichiometry (85).

Other data (81) indicate that a membrane potential is necessary in order for phlorizin binding to the transport system to occur. These observations have been interpreted as indicative of the likelihood that the potential causes a redistribution of the free carrier across the membrane. Comparing this idea with the fact that the initial velocity for Na^+-dependent sugar entry is also strongly potential-dependent, one must conclude that the most likely model for Na^+-dependent sugar transport is the one shown in Fig. 3c in which $n = 2$ and the membrane potential plays a dual role in altering the orientation of two separate carrier species.

TABLE 3. *Coupling stoichiometry ($\Delta Na^+/\Delta S$) for Na^+-dependent transport of 3-O-methylglucose (3-OMG) by isolated intestinal cells measured as the ratio of phlorizin-sensitive Na^+ and 3-OMG fluxes in voltage clamped cells*

Experiment number	[22]Na^+ influx			3-OMG influx[a]			
	Control	+ Phlorizin[b]	ΔNa^+ [c]	Control	+ Phlorizin	ΔS[c]	$\Delta Na^+/\Delta S$
1	46.6	33.7	12.9	12.0	4.8	7.2	1.8
2	67.7	44.5	22.7	17.0	5.2	11.8	1.9
3	76.0	50.3	25.7	19.5	8.4	11.1	2.3
4	101.2	72.8	28.4	28.2	11.5	16.7	1.7
5	81.0	52.0	29.0	24.2	6.8	17.4	1.7
6	50.2	40.0	10.2	8.7	3.2	5.5	1.9
7	44.2	33.0	11.2	8.9	3.9	5.0	2.2
						Mean = 1.93	
8[d]	111.0	68.8	41.2	43.5	10.7	32.2	1.3

[a]Flux values are given in nmol·min^{-1} · mg^{-1} cell protein: $[Na^+] = 112$ mM, $[3\text{-}OMG] = 20$ mM.
[b]Phlorizin was added to a final concentration of 200 μM in order to inhibit the Na^+-dependent sugar transport system.
[c]The Δ values are the differences between control influxes and those observed with phlorizin present. It is, therefore, an estimate of that part of the total flux that is carried by the Na^+-dependent transport system.
[d]This experiment was performed with normally energized cells.
From Kimmich (26), with permission.

OTHER Na+ COUPLED TRANSPORT SYSTEMS

Although the above discussion has focused primarily on intestinal Na^+-dependent sugar transport, this system represents only a special case of a broad spectrum of Na^+-dependent transport systems. Related Na^+-dependent systems have been described in intestinal tissue for neutral (3,4,14,20,63,64), acidic (40,76), and basic amino acids (50,51,66,67,69), imino acids (39,48,49), ascorbic acid (46,78–80), bile salts (18,38,72), phosphate (8,45,52), sulfate (5,44), choline (21), uracil (13), biotin (7), riboflavin (68), thiamine (16), and inositol (9,41).

Neutral Amino Acids

The degree to which each of these systems has been characterized varies widely, but in most cases the general characteristics described for sugars are also true for the other Na^+-dependent systems. The coupling stoichiometry has not been reliably determined for these systems, in part because of the lack of specific inhibitors that can be used to identify carrier-mediated fluxes and in part because the solute-carrier mediated Na^+ flux is often a tiny percentage of total Na^+ flux. The most data have been accumulated for neutral amino acid transport, with the weight of evidence favoring partially loaded carrier forms having permeability to the membrane in addition to the fully loaded form. A model for this likelihood predicts kinetic characteristics in which the K_m for transport is more strongly dependent on Na^+ than the V_{max} (14). These characteristics have, in fact, been reported in some instances. The model described earlier for sugar transport predicts a converse relationship, i.e., Na^+-dependent V_{max} and a K_m that is independent of (Na^+). These kinetic characteristics have also been reported (19,33).

Kinetic data for neutral amino acid influx suggest that the coupling stoichiometry is probably 1:1. Either 2:1 or 1:1 stoichiometry would imply that the membrane potential should play a role in the overall driving force for amino acid transport, and a potential dependence has been described (43,58). Circumstantial evidence drawn from the characteristics of mutual inhibition between Na^+-dependent sugar and amino acid transport systems also suggests that a 1:1 Na^+:amino acid coupling stoichiometry is involved. This conclusion is based on the observation that sugars interfere with amino acid transport more than amino acids interfere with sugar transport, even though the amino acids are transported more rapidly and would be expected to dissipate the membrane potential to a more significant degree if the coupling stoichiometry for the two solutes is equal (32,70). The best explanation for the above observation is that the coupling stoichiometry for amino acids is less than that measured for sugars. On this basis a 1:1 coupling stoichiometry may be predicted.

Acidic Amino Acids

For acidic amino acids, as for sugars, a very high percentage of the total intestinal cellular uptake is absolutely dependent on the presence of Na^+. The best data for this amino acid group have been derived from studies with membrane vesicles prepared from renal tubule epithelium. The intestinal and renal tubule epithelium share a high degree of functional similarity such that properties determined for one tissue often provide an accurate reflection of events which also occur in the other. In this instance, the renal work indicates that aspartate or glutamate transport is not sensitive to changes in the membrane potential (57,73,74,84). It has also been demonstrated that intracellular K^+ stimulates transport in addition to the usual dependence on extracellular Na^+. These observations have been interpreted in terms of the acidic amino acid carrier having a 2 Na^+:1 amino acid stoichiometry, with K^+ moving in the opposite direction to preserve electroneutrality of transport and to account for lack of potential dependence for the system. This concept is pictured schematically in Fig. 4. Another possibility is that K^+ is simply activating the transport system (analogous to allosteric activation of an enzyme) without being transferred across the membrane. This interpretation would imply 1 to 1 coupling between Na^+ and the amino acid.

Inorganic Ions: Phosphate and Sulfate

The transport of several inorganic anions is also thought to be driven by flow of Na^+ into the epithelial cell down a gradient of chemical potential. The best characterized system is one that is operative for inorganic phosphate (8,45,52). Again, work derived from brush-border vesicle preparations has been instrumental in demonstrating a system that is highly Na^+-dependent but not modified by the membrane potential. The transport activity is markedly stimulated by changing pH from 7.0 to 6.0, which suggests that primary phosphate ($H_2PO_4^-$) is the species transported and that the coupling stoichiometry is 1:1, thereby accounting for electroneutral transfer (8). Similar studies using renal tubule epithelial vesicles have demonstrated electroneutral transfer of secondary phosphate ($HPO_4^=$), which suggests that the coupling stoichiometry in renal tubules may be 2 Na^+ per phosphate (22). Other evidence has been reported for Na^+-dependent transport of sulfate (5,44).

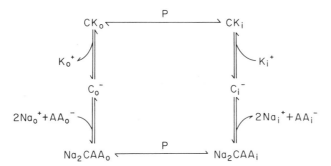

FIG. 4. Schematic representation of a model for acidic amino acid transport that allows a role for cellular K^+ as well as extracellular Na^+. The membrane potential does not provide a part of the driving force for these systems.

Chloride

A great deal of controversy has arisen regarding the role of Na$^+$ in intestinal chloride absorption. It is widely appreciated that there is a high degree of correlation between Na$^+$ and Cl$^-$ absorption, but the mechanistic basis of this apparently coupled set of events is not well understood (for review see ref. 75). One school of thought holds to the idea that fluxes of the two ions are directly coupled via a specific NaCl co-transfer system in a manner which is entirely analogous to the co-transport systems described above for sugars, amino acids, and phosphate (59–61). Such direct coupling implies the existence of Na$^+$-dependent Cl$^-$ fluxes and Cl$^-$-dependent Na$^+$ fluxes, which is the usual way of identifying the existence of co-transport systems. Indeed, ion fluxes with these characteristics have been reported for intact tissue preparations (59,60).

On the other hand, studies with isolated brush-border vesicles have consistently failed to provide confirmatory evidence for the anticipated coupled fluxes (42,54). Because of this and earlier work with intact human intestinal preparations (82,83), it has been suggested that in reality two antiport systems exist, one for Na$^+$/H$^+$ and another for Cl$^-$/OH$^-$ ions. Under weakly buffered conditions, the addition of Na$^+$ to a tissue preparation would initiate an Na$^+$/H$^+$ exchange, formation of a transmembrane pH gradient (elevated interior OH$^-$), and consequent activation of Cl$^-$/OH$^-$ (or Cl$^-$/HCO$_3^-$) exchange. The overall response would be net entry of NaCl and efflux of HOH (or H$_2$CO$_3$) via the two transport systems, which could give the impression of a directly coupled NaCl entry system (82,83). The two alternative models are represented schematically in Fig. 5.

Presumably the way to distinguish between these two ideas is to vary the buffering capacity of the experimental system. A true co-transport between Na$^+$ and Cl$^-$ should be observed independent of the buffering capacity of the cell vesicle interior. Parallel antiport pathways could operate independently of one another if adequate

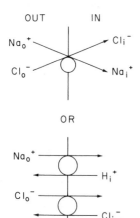

FIG. 5. Alternative models for describing Na$^+$ and Cl$^-$ transport by the intestinal epithelium. In the upper representation, fluxes of Na$^+$ and Cl$^-$ are directly coupled via a co-transport mechanism of the type that has been described for sugars and amino acids. The lower model portrays two antiport systems operating in parallel which are indirectly coupled via transmembrane changes in pH.

buffering capacity was available to provide the required amount of H$^+$ or OH$^-$ ions. This test approach has not been adequately evaluated.

LOCALIZATION OF TRANSPORT COMPONENTS

As mentioned at the outset, the intestinal epithelium exhibits a polarity of function such that nutrient molecules and ions are transferred transcellularly from the luminal to the serosal side of the cell. Thus far, we have only considered events relating to the uptake of solutes into the epithelial cell. It is logical to expect that these concentrative uptake processes might be localized at the brush border or luminal facing end of the epithelial cell. In fact, a great deal of work in recent years has centered on selective preparation of membrane vesicles from either the brush-border or from the basal-lateral boundary of the epithelium. These studies have been instrumental in demonstrating that the Na$^+$-coupled transport systems are localized nearly exclusively in the brush-border membrane (56). The only exception observed to date is for neutral amino acid transport systems, which seem to be Na$^+$-dependent (at least in part) at both cell boundaries (47).

On the other hand, Na$^+$-K$^+$-ATPase, which is responsible for creating cellular gradients of Na$^+$ and K$^+$, is localized in the basal-lateral boundary of the cell (15,17,65). The net result of this distribution of functional activities is a transepithelial transfer of Na$^+$ via a "leak-pump" set of events. Sodium is transferred passively across the brush-border boundary driven by the difference in chemical and electrical potential. This transfer is accomplished by a composite set of paths, in part diffusional, in part coupled to flow of other solutes via co-transport (sugars, amino acids, phosphate, and others as described above), and in part via antiport systems (Na$^+$/H$^+$). Cellular Na$^+$ is extruded via the ATP-driven, basal-lateral localized Na$^+$ pump. The function of this pump maintains a low concentration of cytosolic Na$^+$ as well as the membrane potential, both of which sustain the possibility for continued brush-border Na$^+$ influx.

Those solutes that are driven into the cell against a concentration gradient by Na$^+$ influx must eventually cross the basal-lateral membrane in order to have access to the circulatory system. In general, this is believed to occur via the function of solute carriers, which simply deliver solutes down a concentration gradient (facilitated diffusion). This idea is derived primarily by analogy to sugar transport systems in which facilitated transfer carriers have been well demonstrated for the basal-lateral cell boundary (24,53,55). As one might expect, when the facilitated diffusion carriers are selectively inhibited, the concentrative Na$^+$-dependent transport system can establish a much higher gradient of solute because they are operating against a smaller diffusive "leak" of solute. Indeed, it was the observation of solute gradient enhancement by various agents that provided one of the first clues that serosal-facilitated diffusion transport systems exist (34–36).

For charged solutes such as HPO$_4$$^=$ or Cl$^-$ it seems likely that the serosal transfer event is driven by the interior negative membrane potential such that a step in concentration is involved at *each* pole of the cell. Sodium coupled entry at the brush border would create a cellular concentration of anion which is above the extracellular electrochemical potential for that ion, and the membrane potential would enhance exit across the serosal boundary against a concentration gradient. Whether the latter process is diffusional or via transient association with a membrane component is not understood. Also, it is important to recognize that even though these two-step "pump-pump" systems might move solute at the serosal boundary against a *chemical* concentration gradient, only the brush-border transfer occurs against a gradient of *electrochemical* potential.

SUMMARY

As described above, the small intestine captures a wide variety of ions and nutrients by transport systems that are energized by a fundamentally similar mechanism, namely flow of Na^+ into the cell down a gradient of electrochemical potential. These Na^+-dependent transport systems are themselves specific examples of a broader class of transport systems generally designated as gradient-coupled systems. In mammalian tissues the cation involved is typically sodium, and Na^+-dependent amino acid transport is a characteristic of nearly all animal tissues. Only the intestinal and renal tubule epithelia have developed the capacity for Na^+-dependent transfer of sugars and numerous other solutes.

In contrast, for many species of bacteria, yeast, and other microorganisms, the cation involved in gradient-coupled transport of nutrients is often H^+, and proton-coupled concentrative solute transfer occurs. This presumably reflects the fact that the primary cation transport system in the plasma membrane of these organisms is an H^+ pump rather than the Na^+ pump characteristic of most animal cells. Membrane transport components evolved in each case, which can tap the energy reservoir represented by transmembrane cation gradients. The primary energy capture event in each set of systems is ATP coupled cation extrusion and conversion of a chemical potential in the form of ATP to an electrochemical potential in the form of an ion gradient. Whether or not benefit can be derived from the electrochemical potential gradient depends on the particular membrane constituents present in a given cell type coupling the flow of cation to the flow of other solutes. The amount of energy input to such systems in turn depends on the number of cations coupled to the transfer of each solute molecule, i.e., the coupling stoichiometry. For intestinal tissue, the stoichiometry for sugar transport is 2 Na^+:1 sugar molecule, which undoubtedly helps account for particularly efficient absorption of dietary sugar. Voluminous pancreatic secretions provide the appropriate Na^+ reservoir and the multiple Na^+-dependent transport systems serve to capture dietary nutrients and to conserve body Na^+.

At present, a wealth of information exists which indicates the underlying fundamental similarity for a variety of transport systems that tap the energy of transmembrane electrochemical potential gradients for Na^+ (or H^+) and utilize it for concentrative accumulation of other solutes. Most earlier questions relating to energetic adequacy of the "driving force" have now been resolved (28,30) although molecular details of the transport system remain to be elucidated. Recent evidence raises the tantalizing possibility that the Na^+-dependent transport systems may be reliable *in situ* sensors of chemical or electrochemical potential gradients for Na^+ (29,30). If so, they offer an interesting new method for noninvasive measure of such potentials.

ACKNOWLEDGMENT

The research described in this manuscript was supported, in part, by a grant from the USPHS -AM15365 and in part by the U.S. Department of Energy Contract DE-ACO1-76EV-03490 and has been assigned Report No. UR-3490-2278.

REFERENCES

1. Alvarado, F. (1970): Effect of phloretin and phlorizin on sugar and amino acid transport systems in small intestine. *Fed. Eur. Biochem. Soc. Symp.*, 20:131–135.
2. Alvarado, F., and Crane, R. K. (1982): Phlorizin as a competitive inhibitor of the active transport of sugar by hamster small intestine, *in vitro. Biochim. Biophys. Acta*, 56:170–172.
3. Alvarado, F., and Lherminier, M. (1981): Phenylalanine transport in guinea pig jejunum. A general mechanism for organic solute and sodium transport. *J. Physiol. (Paris)*, 78:131–145.
4. Alvarado, F., and Mahmood, A. (1974): Cotransport of organic solutes and sodium ions in small intestine: A general model. Amino acid transport. *Biochemistry*, 13:2882–2890.
5. Anast, C., Kennedy, R., Volk, G., and Adamson, L. (1965): *In vitro* studies of sulfate transport by the small intestine of the rat, rabbit and hamster. *J. Lab. Clin. Med.*, 65:903–915.
6. Beck, J. C., and Sacktor, B. (1975): Energetics of the Na^+ - dependent transport of D - glucose in renal brush border membranes. *J. Biol. Chem.*, 250:8647–8680.
7. Berger, E., Long, E., and Semenza, G. (1972): The sodium activation of biotin absorption in hamster small intestine *in vitro. Biochim. Biophys. Acta*, 255:873–887.
8. Berner, W., Kinne, R., and Murer, H. (1976): Phosphate transport into brush border membrane vesicles isolated from rat small intestine. *Biochem. J.*, 160:467–474.
9. Caspary, W., and Crane, R. (1970): Active transport of myo - inositol and its relation to the sugar transport system in hamster small intestine. *Biochim. Biophys. Acta*, 203:308–316.
10. Crane, R. K. (1960): Intestinal absorption of sugars. *Physiol. Rev.*, 40:789–825.
11. Crane, R. K. (1965): Na^+ - independent transport in the intestine and other animal tissues. *Fed. Proc.*, 24:1000–1005.
12. Crane, R. K. (1968): Absorption of sugars. In: *Handbook of Physiology, Sec. 6: Alimentary Canal, Volume 3: Intestinal Absorption*, edited by C. F. Cook, pp. 1323–1351. American Physiology Society, Washington, D. C.
13. Csaky, T. (1961): Significance of sodium ions in active intestinal transport *in vitro. Life Sci.*, 10:67–75.
14. Curran, P. F., Schultz, S. G., Chez, R. A., and Fuisz, R. D. (1967): Kinetic relations of the Na^+ - amino acid interaction at the mucosal border of intestine. *J. Gen. Physiol.*, 50:1261–1267.
15. DiBona, D. R., and Mills, J. W. (1979): Distribution of Na^+ - pump sites in transporting epithelia. *Fed. Proc.*, 38:134–143.
16. Ferrari, G., Ventura, U., and Rindi, G. (1971): The Na^+ - dependence of thiamine intestinal transport *in vitro. Life Sci.*, 10:67–75.
17. Fujita, M., Matsui, H., Nagano, K., and Nakao, M. (1971): Assymetric distribution of ouabain sensitive ATP-ase activity in rat intestinal mucosa. *Biochim. Biophys. Acta*, 233:404–408.
18. Gallagher, K., Mauskopf, J., Walker, J. T., and Lack, L. (1978): Ionic requirements for the active ileal bile salt transport system. *J. Lipid Res.*, 17:572–582.
19. Goldner, A. M., Schultz, S. G., and Curran, P. F. (1969): Sodium and sugar fluxes across the mucosal border of rabbit ileum. *J. Gen. Physiol.*, 53:362–383.
20. Hajjar, J. J., and Curran. P. F. (1970): Characteristics of the amino acid transport system in the mucosal border of the rabbit ileum. *J. Gen. Physiol.*, 56:673–691.

21. Herzberg, G. R., and Lerner, J. (1973): Intestinal absorption of choline in the chick. *Biochim. Biophys. Acta*, 307:234–242.
22. Hoffmann, N., Thees, M., and Kinne, R. (1976): Phosphate transport by isolated renal brush border vesicles. *Pflugers Archiv.*, 362:147–156.
23. Hopfer, U., and Groseclose, R. (1980): The mechanism of Na^+ - dependent D - glucose transport. *J. Biol. Chem.*, 255:4453–4462.
24. Hopfer, U., Sigrist, Nelson, K., Ammann, E., and Murer H. (1976): Differences in neutral amino acid and glucose transport between brush - border and basolateral membrane of intestinal epithelial cells. *J. Cell Physiol.*, 89:805–819.
25. Kimmich, G. A. (1979): Intestinal transport: Studies with isolated epithelial cells. *Environ. Health Perspect.*, 33:37–44.
26. Kimmich, G. A. (1981): Gradient coupling in isolated intestinal cells. *Fed. Proc.*, 40:2474–2479.
27. Kimmich, G. A. (1981): Intestinal absorption of sugar. In: *Physiology of the Gastrointestinal Tract*, edited by L. R. Johnson, pp. 1035–1061. Raven Press, New York.
28. Kimmich, G. A. (1982): Intestinal transport of sugar. The energetics of epithelial "pump-leak" systems. In: *Membranes and Transport*, Vol. 2, edited by A. Martonosi, pp. 169–174. Plenum Press, New York.
29. Kimmich, G. A. (1982): The Na^+ - dependent sugar carrier as a sensor of the cellular electro-chemical Na^+ potential. In: *Membrane Biophysics: Structure and Function in Epithelia*, edited by M. Dinno and A. Callahan. pp. 129–142. Alan R. Liss, New York.
30. Kimmich, G. A. (1983): Coupling stoichiometry and the energetic adequacy question. In: *Intestinal Transport — Fundamental and Comparative Aspects*, edited by M. Gilles-Baillien and R. Gilles. Springer-Verlag, New York.
31. Kimmich, G. A. (1983): The Na^+:sugar coupling stoichiometry in chick intestinal cells. *Am. J. Physiol., (in press)*.
32. Kimmich, G. A., and Randles, J. (1973): Interaction between Na^+ - dependent transport systems for sugar and amino acids. Evidence against a role for the sodium gradient. *J. Membr. Biol.*, 12:47–68.
33. Kimmich, G. A., and Randles, J. (1975): Energy coupling to Na^+ - dependent transport systems: Evidence for an energy input in addition to transmembrane ion gradients. *Proc. Fed. Eur. Biochem. Soc.* (Budapest), 9:117–130.
34. Kimmich, G. A., and Randles, J. (1975): A Na^+ - independent phloretin sensitive monosaccharide transport system in isolated intestinal epithelial cells. *J. Membr. Biol.*, 23:57–76.
35. Kimmich, G. A., and Randles, J. (1978): Phloretin - like action of bioflavanoids on sugar accumulation capability of isolated intestinal cells. *Membr. Biochem.*, 1:221–237.
36. Kimmich, G. A., and Randles, J. (1979): Energetics of sugar transport by isolated intestinal epithelial cells: Effects of cytochalasin B. *Am. J. Physiol.*, 237:C56–C63.
37. Kimmich, G. A., and Randles, J. (1980): Evidence for an intestinal Na^+:sugar transport coupling stoichiometry of 2.0. *Biochim. Biophys. Acta*, 596:439–444.
38. Lack, L. (1979): Properties and biological significance of the ileal bile salt transport system. *Environ. Health Perspect.*, 33:79–90.
39. Lerner, J., and Karcher, C. A. (1978): Kinetic properties of imino acid transport systems in the chicken intestine. *Comp. Biochem. Physiol.*, 60A:503–505.
40. Lerner, J., and Steinke, D. L. (1977): Intestinal absorption of glutamic acid in the chicken. *Comp. Biochem. Physiol.*, 57A:11–16.
41. Lerner, J., and Smogula, R. (1979): Myo-inositol transport in the small intestine of the domestic fowl. *Comp. Biochem. Physiol.*, 62A:939–945.
42. Liedke, C. M., and Hopfer, U. (1977): Anion transport in brush border vesicles from rat small intestine. *Biochem. Biophys. Res. Commun.*, 76:579–585.
43. Lucke, H., Haase, W., and Murer, H. (1977): Amino acid transport in brush-border membrane vesicles isolated from human small intestine. *Biochem. J.*, 168:529–532.
44. Lucke, H., Stange, G., and Murer, H. (1978): Sulphate sodium cotransport by brush border membrane vesicles isolated from rat ileum. *Biochem. J.*, 174:951–957.
45. Matsumoto, T., Fontaine, O., and Rasmussen, H. (1980): Effect of 1,25 dihydroxyvitamin D_3 on phosphate uptake into chick intestinal brush border membrane vesicles. *Biochim. Biophys. Acta*, 599:13–23.
46. Mellors, A., Narhwold, D., and Rose, R. C. (1977): Ascorbic acid flux across mucosal border of guinea pig and human ileum. *Am. J. Physiol.*, 233:E374–E379.

47. Mircheff, A. K., Van Os, C. H., and Wright, E. M. (1980): Pathways for alanine transport in intestinal basal lateral membrane vesicles. *J. Membr. Biol.*, 52:83–92.
48. Munck, B. G. (1966): Amino acid transport by the small intestine of the rat. The existence and specificity of the transport mechanism of the imino acids and its relation to the transport of glycine. *Biochim. Biophys. Acta*, 120:97–103.
49. Munck, B. G. (1968): Amino acid transport by the small intestine of the rat. Effect of glucose on the trans-intestinal transport of proline and valine. *Biochim. Biophys. Acta*, 156:192–194.
50. Munck, B. G. (1980): Lysine transport across the small intestine. Stimulating and inhibitory effects of neutral amino acids. *J. Membr. Biol.*, 53:45–53.
51. Munck, B. G., and Schultz, S. G. (1969): Lysine transport across isolated rabbit ileum. *J. Gen. Physiol.*, 53:157–182.
52. Murer, H., and Hildmann, B. (1981): Transcellular transport of calcium and inorganic phosphate in the small intestinal epithelium. *Am. J. Physiol.*, 240:G409–G416.
53. Murer, H., and Hopfer, H. (1977): The functional polarity of the intestinal epithelial cell: Studies with isolated plasma membrane vesicles. In: *Intestinal Permeation*, edited by M. Kramer and F. Lauterbach, pp. 294–312. Excerpta Medica, Amsterdam.
54. Murer, H., Hopfer, H., and Kinne, R. (1976): Sodium proton antiport in brush border membrane vesicles isolated from rat small intestine. *Biochem. J.*, 154:597–604.
55. Murer, H., Hopfer, U., Kinne-Saffran, E., and Kinne, R. (1974): Glucose transport in isolated brush-border and basal-lateral plasma membrane vesicles from intestinal epithelial cells. *Biochim. Biophys. Acta*, 345:170–182.
56. Murer, H., and Kinne, R. (1980): The use of isolated membrane vesicles to study epithelial transport processes. *J. Membr. Biol.*, 55:81–95.
57. Murer, H., Leopolder, A., Kinne, R., and Burckhardt, G. (1980): Recent observations on the proximal tubular transport of acidic and basic amino acids by rat renal proximal tubular brush border vesicles. *Biochemistry*, 12:223–228.
58. Murer, H., Sigrist-Nelson, K., and Hopfer, U. (1975): On the mechanism of sugar and amino acid interaction in intestinal transport. *J. Biol. Chem.*, 250:7392–7396.
59. Nellans, H. N., Frizell, R. A., and Schultz, S. G. (1973): Coupled sodium-chloride influx across the brush border of rabbit ileum. *Am. J. Physiol.*, 225:467–475.
60. Nellans, H. N., Frizell, R. A., and Schultz, S. G. (1974): Brush border processes and transepithelial Na+ and Cl- transport by rabbit ileum. *Am. J. Physiol.*, 226:1131–1141.
61. Nellans, H. N., Frizell, R. A., and Schultz, S. G. (1975): Effect of acetazolamide on Na+ and Cl- transport by isolated rabbit ileum. *Am. J. Physiol.*, 228:1808–1814.
62. Okada, Y. (1979): Solute transport processes in intestinal epithelial cells. *Membr. Biochem.*, 2:2339–2365.
63. Patterson, J. Y. F., Sepulveda, F. V., and Smith, M. W. (1979): Two carrier influx of neutral amino acids into rabbit ileal mucosa. *J. Physiol.* (Lond.), 292:339–350.
64. Preston, R. L., Schaeffer, J. F., and Curran, P. F. (1974): Structure - affinity relationships of substrate for the neutral amino acid transport system in rabbit ilium. *J. Gen. Physiol.*, 64:443–467.
65. Quigley, J. P., and Gotterer, G. S. (1972): A comparison of the (Na+ - K) - ATP - ase activities found in isolated brush-border and plasma membrane of the rat intestinal mucosa. *Biochim. Biophys. Acta*, 255:107–113.
66. Reiser, S., and Christiansen, P. A. (1971): Stimulation of basic amino acid uptake by certain neutral amino acids in isolated intestinal epithelial cells. *Biochem. Biophys. Acta*, 241:102–113.
67. Reiser, S., and Christiansen, P. A. (1973): The properties of Na+ - dependent and Na+ - independent lysine uptake by isolated intestinal epithelial cells. *Biochim. Biophys. Acta*, 307:212–222.
68. Rivier, D. (1973): Kinetics and Na+ - dependence of riboflavin absorption by intestine *in vivo*. *Experimentia*, 29:1443–1446.
69. Robinson, J. W. L. (1968): Interaction between neutral and dibasic amino acids for uptake by the rat intestine. *Eur. J. Biochem.*, 7:78–89.
70. Robinson, J. W. L., and Alvarado, R. (1977): Comparative aspects of the interaction between sugar and amino acid transport systems. In: *Intestinal Permeation*, edited by M. Kramer and F. Lauterbach, Vol. 4, pp. 145–163. Excerpta Medica, Amsterdam.
71. Nose, R. C., Nahrwald, D. L., and Koch, M. J. (1977): Electrical potential profile in rabbit ileum: role of rheogenic Na+ transport. *Am. J. Physiol.*, 232:E5–E12.

72. Rouse, D. J., and Lack, L. (1979): Ionic requirements for taurochloate uptake by ileal brush border membrane vesicles. *Life Sci.*, 25:45–52.
73. Sacktor, B. (1981): L - glutamate transport in renal plasma membrane vesicles. *Mol. Cell. Biochem.*, 39:239–251.
74. Schneider, E. G., Hammerman, M. R., and Sacktor, B. (1980): Sodium gradient-dependent L - glutamate transport in renal brush border vesicles. *J. Biol. Chem.*, 255:7650–7656.
75. Schultz, S. G. (1981): Salt and water absorption by mammalian small intestine. In: *Physiology of the Gastrointestinal Tract. Vol. 2*, edited by L. R. Johnson, pp. 983–989. Raven Press, New York.
76. Schultz, S. G., Yu-tu, L., Alvarez, O. O., and Curran, P. F. (1970): Dicarboxylic amino acid influx across the brush border of rabbit ileum. *J. Gen. Physiol.*, 56:621–639.
77. Semenza, G. (1967): Sucrose and sugar transport in the small intestine. *Protides Biol. Fluids*, 15:210.
78. Siliprandi, L., Vanni, P., Kessler, M., and Semenza, G. (1979): Na⁺ - dependent, electroneutral L - ascorbate transport across brush border membrane vesicles from guinea pig small intestine. *Biochim. Biophys. Acta*, 552:129–142.
79. Stevenson, N. (1974): Active transport of L - ascorbic acid in the human ileum. *Gastroenterology*, 67:952–956.
80. Stevenson, N., and Brush, M. (1969): Existence and characteristics of Na⁺ - dependent active transport of ascorbic acid in guinea pig. *Am. J. Clin. Nutr.*, 22:318–326.
81. Toggenburger, G. M., Kessler, M., and Semenza, G. (1982): Phlorizin as a probe of the small intestinal Na⁺, D - glucose cotransporter. A model. *Biochim. Biophys. Acta*, 688:557–571.
82. Turnburg, L. A., Bieberdorf, F. A., Maranski, S. G., and Fordtran, J. S. (1970): Interrelationship of chloride, bicarbonate, sodium and hydrogen transport in the human ileum. *J. Clin. Invest.*, 49:557–567.
83. Turnberg, L. A., Fordtran, J. S., Carter, N. W., and Rector, F. C. (1970): Mechanism of bicarbonate absorption and its relationship to sodium transport in the human jejenum. *J. Clin. Invest.*, 49:548–556.
84. Wingrove, T. G., and Kimmich, G. A. (1983): Isolated intestinal cells as a model system for the study of glutamate and aspartate transport. *The Toxicologist*, 3:41.
85. Wright, E. M., Gunther, R. D., Kaunitz, J. D., Stevens, B. R., Harms, V., Ross, H. J., and Schell, R. E. (1983): Mechanisms of Na⁺ transport across brush border and basolateral membranes. In: *Intestinal Transport — Fundamental and Comparative Aspects*, edited by M. Gilles-Baillien and R. Gilles, pp. 122–132. Springer-Verlag, New York.

Intestinal Toxicology, edited by C. M. Schiller.
Raven Press, New York © 1984.

Alteration of Intestinal Function by Chemical Exposure: Animal Models

Carol M. Schiller, Chon R. Shoaf, and Dennis E. Chapman

Laboratory of Pharmacology, National Institute of Environmental Health Sciences, National Institutes of Health, Research Triangle Park, North Carolina 27709

Literally thousands of chemicals are mined, manufactured, and used in modern industry. In the process of using these chemicals, some escape and become environmental contaminants while others are deliberately applied in the environment. The amount of chemicals escaping or being applied is estimated to be in the range of millions of pounds per year (34). Although some of these chemicals are very short-lived in the environment by virtue of their physiochemical properties, others may persist for considerable time. Through a variety of processes these chemicals may be transported from the point of release to a site where they become an exposure hazard. Chemicals may contaminate the factory or plant in which they are produced and may result in widespread exposure to humans either directly or in their food and water. In some instances, chemicals become incorporated into the food chain with resultant magnification of concentrations and even higher levels of exposure. The full impact of chemically contaminated water and food chain on human health is yet to be understood.

The gastrointestinal tract shares with the skin and lung the distinction of being a major route of exposure for environmental chemicals as well as being a target for their action. Food- and water-borne chemicals enter the body via the gastrointestinal tract, whereas occupational exposure to chemicals occurs primarily through the skin and lungs. When injury occurs to the gastrointestinal tract by ingested chemicals, these chemicals alter their portal of entry directly, which in turn may enhance their deleterious effects on the whole organism. In addition, damage to the gastrointestinal barrier may enhance or suppress absorption of other substances. Since an intact gastrointestinal tract is necessary for the maintenance of the nutritional status, a chemically injured intestinal mucosa may alter the normal digestive and absorptive functions as reflected by poor nutritional status as well as by altered responsiveness to the chemical insult. The response of the gastrointestinal tract to viral agents or microorganisms may cause a self-limited diarrheal disease. The limited course of such disease tends to remove chemicals via the diarrheal secretions and increased motility. Intestinal toxins that result from interactions of chemicals, nutrients, and microorganisms add another dimension to the possible alterations of intestinal function by chemical exposure. The possible interactions of chemicals, nutrients, and microorganisms have not been explored completely (33).

NATURE OF CHEMICAL EXPOSURE

The number and amounts of potentially damaging chemicals entering the environment have increased steadily since the beginning of the Industrial Revolution. Their effects went unnoticed or were of little concern initially; however, gradual awareness has developed as to the risk posed to human health by chemically contaminated food and water (2). Although the rate of increase in chemical pollution has slowed, thousands of chemicals are still being emitted into the air, dumped into rivers and lakes, and buried in the land (51). It appears that large-scale degradation of surface waters has been stopped; however, water quality data indicate that surface water pollution from conventional and toxic pollutants is still widespread. Ground water has always been considered a pristine resource, but recent information reveals that in many locations ground water is contaminated. This contamination comes from many different sources and includes a variety of materials, e.g., synthetic organic chemicals and inorganic chemicals. The concentrations of these synthetic organic chemicals in the ground water are often orders of magnitude higher than those concentrations found in raw or surface water supplies. A third of all public supplies and 95% of all rural domestic supplies depend on ground water resources (9). Based on total use (withdrawal) fresh ground water is used predominantly for agricultural purposes (Table 1). The indentity of potential pollutants is largely unkown and uncharacterized at present. Of the more than 300 organic chemicals that have been identified in drinking water, less than 5% have been adequately tested for carcinogenicity in mammalian systems (10). The presence of volatile chlorinated solvents in raw and finished ground water from municipal sources indicates that trichloroethylene is frequently present and that *cis*-dichloroethylene is present at the greatest concentration (Table 2). From the standpoint of health, it is the total intake of pollutants that is important and there are many unknowns. The need for awareness of specific chemical species involved must be emphasized. For example, the inorganic arsenic that occurs in water is far

TABLE 1. *Fresh ground water use, 1950–1975*

| Use | Percentage of total | | | |
---	1950	1960	1970	1975
Public supplies	12	13	14	13
Rural supplies	8	6	5	5
Irrigation	62	68	66	69
Industry	18	13	15	14
Total withdrawals[a] (trillion gallons per year)	12.4	18.3	24.8	29.9

[a]Totals may not equal 100 because of rounding (11).

TABLE 2. *Concentrations of selected synthetic organic compounds in raw and finished ground water obtained from 39 cities*

Compound	No. of cities sampled		Percentage with chemical present		Concentration ($\mu g/L$ = parts per billion)					
					Mean		Range			
	Raw	Fin.	Raw	Fin.	Raw	Fin.	Raw		Fin.	
Trichloroethylene	13	25	38.5	36.0	29.72	6.76	0.2–125.0		0.11–53.0	
Carbon tetrachloride	27	39	7.4	28.2	11.5	3.8	3.0–20.0		0.2–13.0	
Tetrachloroethylene	27	36	18.5	22.0	0.98	2.08	0.1–2.0		0.2–3.1	
1,1,1-Trichloroethane	13	23	23.1	21.7	4.8	2.13	0.3–13.0		1.3–3.0	
1,1-Dichloroethane	13	13	23.1	23.1	0.7	0.3	0.4–0.9		0.2–0.5	
1,2-Dichloroethane	13	25	7.7	4.0	0.2	0.2	0.2–NA		0.2–NA	
Trans-dichloroethylene	13	13	15.4	15.4	1.75	1.05	0.2–3.3		0.2–1.9	
Cis-dichloroethylene	13	13	38.5	30.8	13.56	9.35	0.1–69.0		0.1–37.0	
1,1-Dichloroethylene	13	13	15.4	7.7	0.5	0.2	0.5–0.5		0.2–NA	
Methylene chloride	27	38	3.7	2.6	4.0	7.0	4.0–NA		7.0–NA	
Vinyl chloride	13	25	15.4	4.0	5.8	9.4	2.2–9.4		9.4–NA	

NA = not applicable (12).

more accessible to the the organism and its biologic processes than the organically bound arsenic in foods such as shellfish.

Comprehensive surveys reveal a vast array of chemical entities encompassed by the compounds added to foods by man. These entities include food additives and residues as well as those occurring as natural toxicants and contaminants. The food additives and residues are added in the course of food manufacture or preparation or arise as residues from seed, soil, or crop treatments, residues of drugs or other additives fed to animals, or residues from migration of packaging materials to food. Estimates of the number of compounds included in the food additive and residue category vary, but the figure of 10,000 is probably conservative. Since 95% of the food reaching the consumer has been processed in some way, the intentional food additives consumed have been estimated as 1.5 kg/yr/capita (34). As a toxicological consideration, the extensiveness of this consumption makes it difficult to draw attention to individual substances or groups of related compounds.

Special mention is made of agricultural chemicals as these may inadvertently or deliberately be allowed to escape in the environment. Such is the case with pesticides and fertilizers. Although agricultural chemicals such as pesticides are selected based on their biological activity, and in some instances from substantial information about their acute effects, long-term effects over several generations are frequently not known. The toxic water pollution problem of the south central states is largely caused by pesticides (51). Evidence exists that nutritional status may modify the biological effects of many chemicals. Efforts have been made to measure levels of residue in foodstuffs as a route of ingestion of pesticides. Since less is known about residue levels in water, few studies have attempted to quantify the total amount of residues retained by organisms as a consequence of food and water intake. The gastrointestinal tract, as a major portal of entry and a primary site of injury for water and food contaminants, is an appropriate organ system for investigation.

NATURE OF INTESTINAL FUNCTION

The principal function of the gastrointestinal tract is to modify ingested food so that the nutrients can be absorbed by the intestines, passed into the bloodstream/lymph, and transported throughout the organism. This function involves the processes of secretion, digestion, absorption, metabolism, and motility all working together (Table 3). In addition, the intestine serves as a selective barrier to foreign molecules, some of which provoke an antigenic response. Food- and water-borne

TABLE 3. *Major gastrointestinal functions*

Secretion:	Release of ions, substances, and enzymes
Digestion:	Intraluminal breakdown of ingested substances
Absorption:	Uptake of molecules across mucosal surface
Metabolism:	Intracellular synthesis and degradation
Motility:	Movement of intraluminal contents along tract

chemicals entering the gastrointestinal tract can injure the tract and alter these normal functions as well as modulate their own effects. Interactions of these chemicals within the gastrointestinal tract reflect the properties of the tract per se, the chemicals and the organisms. Examination of the roles of the gastrointestinal tract in this interaction requires an understanding of the luminal milieu (bacterial and biochemical components) as well as of dietary factors, the brush border, and the intracellular processes (metabolism of nutrients and chemicals). The ingested chemicals may vary in solubility, size, and reactivity, all of which affect their digestion, absorption, and interaction with the mucosal surface. Specific organism factors, such as age, genetic defects, and disease state, also influence the interactions of chemicals with the gastrointestinal tract. The major diseases of the gastrointestinal tract are at least, in part, environmentally determined (40).

Examination of the effects of ingested environmental chemicals on the gastrointestinal tract as a target organ system may focus on the time-course of damage, recovery, repair, and adaptation within this system. To better understand the impact of these chemicals, model systems are designed to evaluate these effects. This effort develops and exploits animal analogs of the disease processes. A number of approaches have been developed to examine various aspects of gastrointestinal tract function (see C. T. Walsh, *this volume*). The choice of approach reflects the focus of the project, which may include enzymes, isolated cells, intestinal sacs, or whole animals. Recent work examines intraluminal metabolism as well as intracellular metabolism.

APPROACHES TO STUDY CHEMICAL ALTERATION OF INTESTINAL FUNCTION

There is a rapidly growing body of knowledge concerning the effects of ingested chemicals on gastrointestinal function. The approaches utilized in the examination of chemically altered gastrointestinal function include *in vivo* exposure and *in vivo*, *in situ*, or *in vitro* evaluation, or *in vitro* exposure and *in vitro* evaluation (41). The various methodolgies for evaluating gastrointestinal function were reviewed previously. Specific examples of these approaches taken from the current literature are given in Table 4.

REVIEW OF GASTROINTESTINAL FUNCTIONS AFFECTED BY CHEMICAL EXPOSURE

Ingested food is processed by the gastrointestinal tract by mixing with a number of secretions produced primarily by the salivary glands, stomach, pancreas, liver, and intestines. These secretions consist of ions, water, enzymes, and bile. In some instances, the degradation processes are assisted by the intestinal flora. Although the salivary glands and their secretions are not essential to life, the secreted electrolytes, K^+ and HCO_3^-, and enzymes, α-amylase, lysozyme, and kallikrein, enhance the digestive process. The stomach elaborates electrolytes, intrinsic factor, pepsinogen, and mucus, which convert the ingested food into semiliquid form.

TABLE 4. *Evaluation of altered gastrointestinal function*

Method of exposure/ method of monitoring	Function studied	Environmental agent	Ref.
In vivo/in vivo	Digestion, flora Barrier	Methyl mercury Cadmium	47,48 25
In vivo/in situ	Absorption Absorption	Organochlorine compounds Cadmium	54 55
In vivo/in vitro	Absorption Motility Absorption	Dieldrin Hexachlorobenzene Lindane; DDT	28 37 29,32
In vitro/in vitro	Metabolism Absorption Motility	Salicylate Aluminum; DDT and DDE Amitraz (pesticide)	53 15,20 35

More specific enzymes enter the intestinal lumen from the pancreas, e.g., trypsin, chymotrypsin, carboxypeptidase, and pancreatic lipase. The liver secretes bile, up to a liter per day in man, which contains bile salts, mucin, hemoglobin breakdown products, phospholipids, cholesterol, and electrolytes. The bile salts are essential for the emulsification of the oil and water portions of the semidigested food and for the formation of micelles. The intestinal secretions play an important role as a lubricant, e.g., mucus.

Examination of the effects of known food and water contaminants and food additives on gastrointestinal secretion/digestion of food is in its infancy. As would be expected, agents that are identified as liver, pancreatic, stomach, or colon carcinogens would be anticipated to affect these normal functions. Also, agents that are destructive of the mucosal surfaces on contact would be expected to disrupt the secretory and digestive functions. Examples of such agents include gastric juices, aspirin (21), alcohol (27), and T-2 toxin (23).

The gastrointestinal tract contains a bacterial system within the lumen, particularly in the colon. These microorganisms contain enzymes that hydrolyze undigested food as well as chemicals. A well-known role of the gastrointestinal flora is the hydrolysis of glucuronide conjugates. Studies have shown that a variety of compounds secreted in the bile as glucuronide conjugates are hydrolyzed by the bacterial β-glucuronidase, which allows for reabsorption of the compounds. Facilitation of enterohepatic circulation by rat intestinal bacteria has been reported for phenytoin (8), phenacetin (50), diethylstilbesterol (16), digitoxin (56), and warfarin (36). More recently, these microorganisms have been demonstrated to convert methyl mercury to inorganic mercury (47,48). There are many recent examples of the effect of microorganisms on the concentration of ingested substances in the feces (Table 5).

The monitoring of substances in the feces is one approach to measuring the relative absorption of agents such as aliphatic hydrocarbons (1). The effects of a dioxin on lipid absorption has been examined in detail with the rat (42). Prior oral

TABLE 5. *Excretion of several chemicals in feces of conventional (control), germ-free, or antibiotic-treated animals*

Chemical	Conventional	Germ-free (% of dose)	Antibiotic-treated	Ref.
Warfarin	24	31	33	36
Inorganic mercury	9.3	—	1.8	48
Diphenylhydantoin	78	—	95	8

TABLE 6. *Altered absorption of nutrients by chemicals*

Chemical	Species	Method	Effect	Mechanism (suggested)	Ref.
DDT	Rats	Everted sacs	Inhibition of active transport of glucose and tyrosine	Inhibition of sodium pump	20
Dieldrin	Monkeys	Everted sacs	Augment glucose and depressed leucine uptake	Increased disaccharidase activity	28
Malathion	Rats	Tissue accumulation	Reduced glucose and glycine absorption	Depressed brush-border enzyme activities	3
TCDD	Rats	Everted sacs	No physiologically significant changes in glucose or leucine active transport	Monosaccharide and amino acid active transport unaffected	44

exposure to low doses of 2,3,7,8-tetrachlorodibenzo-*p*-dioxin markedly augments the appearance of lipid in the serum after a dose of corn oil (46). Several agents have been used to limit the absorption of lipophilic toxins, e.g., cholestryramine (14) and paraffin (37). Monitoring radiolabeled carbon dioxide production from radiolabeled nutrients has been utilized to examine malabsorption induced by chemical exposure. In this instance, careful selection of dose and time of monitoring would be essential to detect altered nutrient absorption and subsequent metabolism. Several investigators have used the everted sacs technique for examining alterations in intestinal absorptions of nutrients, e.g., simple sugars and amino acids (Table 6).

One aspect of the target organ approach that has changed in emphasis is the recognition that metabolism by an organ is not necessarily synonymous with detoxification. The role of intestinal metabolism of foreign substances by laboratory animals and humans is discussed fully in later chapters. The intestinal mucosa is an extremely active metabolic tissue. The proliferative nature of the crypt cells and differentiation to well-defined absorptive villous tip cells require marked synthesis of macromolecules. For instance, it has been estimated that 50 g of protein is sloughed per day (31). The active transport and synthetic components of intestinal

TABLE 7. *Estimated number of water supply systems in violation of Federal drinking water standards[a]*

Systems	Quality monitored		
	Turbidity	Bacteria	Inorganic
Very small (39,000)	200	3,400	3,600
All others larger (20,000)	500	1,800	1,800
Total (59,000)	700	5,200	5,400

[a]Based on 1979 data (13).

metabolism entail the production of large amounts of metabolic energy. Intestinal absorptive cells contain increased numbers of apical mitochondria. Isolated mucosal cells have been utilized to monitor the unique energy requirements, e.g., glucose and glutamine, for this tissue (45,49). Salicylate alters oxidative phosphorylation monitored in isolated gastric mucosal cells (53). It has been demonstrated that arsenate inhibits mitochondrial oxidative phosphorylation that is pyruvate-mediated (18). Intestinal pyruvate dehydrogenase has been implicated in that inhibitory process (43). The full impact of foreign substances on gastrointestinal metabolism is largely unknown.

Control of intestinal motility is complex and involves both cholinergic and adrenergic nervous system components (30). In general, cholinergic stimulation increases intestinal motility and adrenergic stimulation inhibits motility. Somnolence and constipation are side effects of many antihistamines (6). A formamidine pesticide, amitraz, is widely used to control ticks but with some toxicity to horses (38). The effects of amitraz on drug-induced contractions of guinea pig ileum *in vitro* indicates inhibition of the histamine H_1 agonists stimulated contractions (35). This action may be relevant to the intestinal stasis observed in horses. Recent approaches to monitor motility rely on marker substances other than polyethylene glycol, chromium sesquioxide, and barium sulfate. Of particular value as marker substances are the polystryene particles, which are available in varying sizes (50–100 μ and 800–1,000 μ) and are of low specific gravity (22). Phenol red alone and complexed with a high molecular weight anion exchange resin have also been confirmed as appropriate markers for gastrointestinal transit time in mammals (26) and poultry (19).

CONCLUSIONS

There is a growing appreciation of the gastrointestinal tract as a target organ system for ingested substances. This appreciation is reflected in the increasing interest in the gastrointestinal tract as a metabolic organ contributing to the homeostasis of the entire organism. There are several areas of gastrointestinal research that are at the forefront. These include the role of the bacterial ecosystem in the metabolism of nutrients and foreign substances (17,39), the role of enterohepatic circulation in affecting the absorption of substances from the lumen (4,7), the role of fibers in digestion, absorption, and protection of the intestines (52,57), and response of the local gastrointestinal immune system to toxic substances (5,24). Adaptation normally occurs in the gastrointestinal tract in response to increasing age, enteral feeding of nutrients, and after surgical removal of a section of intestines (42). The ability of the gastrointestinal tract to adapt after toxic insults is being explored. Because of the high metabolic and cell turnover rates of the intestinal mucosa, it is likely that this tissue is particularly susceptible to injury.

The trend of increased reliance on ground water for agricultural and drinking purposes and the discovery of increasing numbers of synthetic chemicals in these sources imply a need for concern about continued contamination of our water and food. The establishment of Federal standards for the various forms of contamination are not sufficient (Table 7). Awareness and understanding of potential health effects resulting from such contamination are essential. The use of animal models to explore these potential gastrointestinal effects from ingested chemicals offers an opportunity to establish such an understanding.

REFERENCES

1. Albro, P. W., and Fishbein, L. (1970): Absorption of aliphatic hydrocarbons by rats. *Biochim. Biophys. Acta*, 219:437–446.
2. Carson, R. (1962): *Silent Spring*. Houghton Mifflin Company, Boston.
3. Chowdhury, J. S., Dudeja, P. K., Mehta, S. K., and Makomood, A. (1980): Effect of a single oral dose of malathion on D-glucose and glycine uptake and on brush border enzymes in rat intestine. *Toxicol. Lett.*, 6:411–415.
4. Colburn, W. A. (1982): Pharmacokinetic and biopharmaceutic parameters during enterohepatic circulation of drugs. *J. Pharm. Sci.*, 71(1):131–133.
5. Dobbins, W. D. (1982): Gut immunophysiology: A gastroenterolgists's view with emphasis on pathophysiology. *Am. J. Physiol.*, 242(1):G1–8.
6. Douglas, W. W. (1980): Histamine and 5-hydroxytryptamine (serotonin) and their antagonists. In: *The Pharmacological Basis of Therapeutics*, edited by A. F. Gilman, L. S. Goodman and A. Gilman, pp. 609–646. MacMillan, New York.
7. Duggan, D. E., Hooke, K. F., Noll, R. M., and Kwan, K. C. (1975): Enterohepatic circulation of indomethacin and its role in intestinal irritation. *Biochem. Pharmacol.*, 25:1749–1754.
8. El-Hawari, A. M., and Plaa, G. L. (1978): Role of the enterohepatic circulation in the elimination of phenytoin in the rat. *Drug Metab. Dispos.*, 6:59–69.
9. Environmental Protection Agency (1975): *National Safety Drinking Water Strategy: One Step at a Time*. Draft Report. U.S. Environmental Protection Agency, Washington, D.C.
10. Environmental Protection Agency (1976): *Organic Compounds Identified in Drinking Water in the United States*, Health Effects Research Laboratory. U.S. Environmental Protection Agency, Cincinnati.
11. Environmental Protection Agency (1980): *Planning Workshops to Develop Recommendations for a Ground Water Protection Strategy*, Office of Drinking Water. U.S. Environmental Protection Agency, Government Printing Office, Washington, D.C.
12. Environmental Protection Agency (1980): *The Occurrence of Volatile Organics in Drinking Water*, Office of Drinking Water. U.S. Environmental Protection Agency, briefing paper.
13. Environmental Protection Agency (1980): *Community Water Systems: Financial Aspects of Compliance with Interium Primary Drinking Water Regulations*. U.S. Environmental Protection Agency, draft.
14. Ershoff, B. A. (1976): Protective effects of cholestyramine in rats fed low fiber diets containing toxic doses of sodium cyclamate and amaranth. *Proc. Soc. Exp. Biol. Med.*, 152:253–256.

15. Feinroth, M., Feinroth, M. V., and Berlyne, G. M. (1982): Aluminum absorption in the rat everted gut sac. *Miner. Electrolyte Metab.*, 8(1):29–35.
16. Fischer, L. J., Kent, T. H., and Weissinger, J. L. (1973): Absorption of diethylstilbesterol and its glucuronide conjugate from the intestines of five-and twenty-five-day-old rats. *J. Pharmacol. Exp. Ther.*, 185:163–170.
17. Flock, M. H., and Hentges, D. J. (1974): Intestinal microecology. *Am. J. Clin. Nutr.*, 27:1261–1355.
18. Fowler, B. A., Woods, J. S., and Schiller, C. M. (1979): Studies of hepatic mitochondrial structure and function: I. Morphometric and biochemical evaluation of *in vivo* perturbation by arsenate. *Lab. Invest.*, 41:313–320.
19. Goñalons, E., Rial, R., and Tur, J. A. (1982): Phenol red as indicator of the digestive tract motility in chickens. *Poult. Sci.*, 61(3):581–583.
20. Iturri, S. J., and Wolff, D. (1982): Inhibition of the active transport of D-glucose and L-tyrosine by DDT and DDE in the rat small intestine. *Comp. Biochem. Biophys.*, 71C(1):131–134.
21. Jacobson, E. D. (1978): The gastrointestinal system. In: *Essentials in Human Physiology*, edited by G. Ross, pp. 370–443. Year Book Medical Publishers, Chicago.
22. Jilge, B. (1982): Rate of movement of marker substances in the digestive tract of the rabbit. *Lab. Anim.*, 16(1):7–11.
23. Joffe, A. Z. (1971): Alimentary toxic aleukia. In: *Microbial Toxins, Vol. 7*, edited by S. Kadis, A. Ciegler and S. J. Ajl, pp. 139–189. Academic Press, New York.
24. Katz, A. J., Falchuk, Z. M., Strober, W., and Shwachman, H. (1976): Gluten - sensitive enteropathy: Inhibition by cortisol of the effect of gluten protein *in vitro*. *N Engl. J. Med.*, 295:131–135.
25. Keino, H., and Aoki, E. (1981): Scanning electron microscopic and enzyme histochemical observations on the cadmium-affected gastrointestinal villi of mice. *J. Toxicol. Sci.*, 6(3):191–202.
26. Kunihara, M., and Meshi, T. (1981): Measurement of gastrointestinal transit of solid food using a colestipol-phenol red complex as a marker. *J. Pharmacobiodyn*, 4(12):916–921.
27. Langman, M. J., and Bell, G. D. (1982): Alcohol and the gastrointestinal tract. *Br. Med. Bull.*, 38(1):71–75.
28. Mahmood, A., Agarwal, N., Sanyal, S., Dudeja, P. K., and Subrahmanyam, D. (1981): Acute dieldrin toxicity: Effect on the uptake of glucose and leucine and on brush border enzymes in monkey intestine. *Chem. Biol. Interact.*, 37(1-2):165–170.
29. Mahmood, A., Agarwal, N., Sanyal, S., and Subrahmanyam, D. (1978): Effects of DDT (chlorophenotane) administration on glucose uptake and brush border enzymes in monkey intestine. *Acta Pharmacol. Toxicol.*, 43(2):99–102.
30. Mayer, S. E. (1980): Neurohumoral transmission and the autonomic nervous system. In: *The Pharmacological Basis of Therapeutics*, edited by A. F. Gilman, L. S. Goodman and A. Gilman, pp. 56–90. Macmillan, New York.
31. Munro, H. N. (1966): Protein secretion into the gastrointestinal tract. In: *Postgraduate Gastro-Enterology*, edited by T. J. Thompson and I. E. Gillespie, pp. 58–67. Bailliere, Tindall and Cassell, London.
32. Nedkova-Bratanova, N., Ivanov, E., Savov, G., Mickaiolva, Z., Krusteva, A., and Petrova, S. (1979): Effect of the pesticides phosalone and lindane on the activity of some dipeptidases and disaccharidases in rat intestinal mucosa. *Enzymes*, 24(5):281–284.
33. Nelson, N., Chair (1976): *Human Health and the Environment — Some Research Needs*, U.S. Government Printing Office, Washington, D.C.
34. Nelson, N., Chair (1970): *Man's Health and the Environment — Some Research Needs*, U.S. Government Printing Office, Washington, D.C.
35. Pass, M. A., and Seawright, A. A. (1982): Effect of amitraz on contractions of the guinea pig ileum *in vitro*. *Comp. Biochem. Physiol.*, 73C(2):419–422.
36. Remmel, R. P., Pohl, L. R., and Elmer, G. W. (1981): Influence of the intestinal microflora on the elimination of warfarin in the rat. *Drug Metab. Dispos.*, 9(5):410–414.
37. Richter, E., and Schafer, S. G. (1981): Intestinal excretion of hexachlorobenzene. *Arch. Toxicol.*, 47(3):233–239.
38. Roberts, M. C., and Seawright, A. A. (1979): Armitraz induced large intestinal impaction in the mouse. *Aust. Vet. J.*, 55:553–554.
39. Savage, D. C. (1981): The microbial flora in the gastrointestinal tract. *Prog. Clin. Biol. Res.*, 77:893–908.

40. Schedl, H. P. (1977): Environmental factors and the development of disease and injury to the alimentary tract. *Environ. Health Perspect.*, 20:39–54.
41. Schiller, C. M. (1979): Chemical exposure and intestinal function. *Environ. Health Perspect.*, 33:91–100.
42. Schiller, C. M. (1982): Effects of toxins on gastrointestinal function: Developing systems. *Banbury Report*, 11:43–51.
43. Schiller, C. M., Fowler, B. A., and Woods, J. S. (1978): Pyruvate metabolism after *in vivo* exposure to oral arsenic. *Chem. Biol. Interact.*, 22:25–33.
44. Schiller, C. M., Shoaf, C. R., Chapman, D. E., and Walden, R. (1983): Alterations in lipid assimilation induced by 2,3,7,8-tetrachlorodibenzo-*p*-dioxin (TCDD) in male Fischer rats. *Fed. Proc.*, 42(3):355.
45. Schiller, C. M., Southern, J. S., and Walden, R. (1981): Glutamine and glutamate utilization by the hamster small intestine. *J. Appl. Biochem.*, 3:147–156.
46. Schiller, C. M., Walden, R., and Shoaf, C. R. (1982): Studies on the mechanism of 2,3,7,8 - tetrachlorodibenzo - *p* - dioxin toxicity: Nutrient assimilation. *Fed. Proc.*, 41(4):1426.
47. Seko, Y., Miura, T., and Takahashi, M. (1982): Reduced decomposition and fecal excretion of methyl mercury in cecum-resected mice. *Acta Pharmacol. Toxicol.*, 50(2):117–120.
48. Seko, Y., Miura, T., Takahashi, M., and Kayama, T. (1981): Methyl mercury decomposition in mice treated with antibiotics. *Acta Pharmacol. Toxicol.*, 49(4):259–265.
49. Shirkey, R. J., and Schiller, C. M. (1980): Preparation and properties of epithelial cell suspensions from rat small intestine. *J. Appl. Biochem.*, 2:196–207.
50. Smith, G. E., and Griffiths, L. A. (1976): Metabolism of a biliary metabolite of phenacetin and the acetanilides by the intestinal microflora. *Experientia*, 32(12):1556–1557.
51. Speth, G., Chair (1980): Environmental Quality — 1980. U.S. Printing Office, Washington, D.C.
52. Story, J. A. (1981): The role of dietary fiber in lipid metabolism. *Adv. Lip. Res.*, 18:229–246.
53. Tanaka, K., and Fromm, D. (1983): Effects of bile acid and salicylate on isolated surface and glandular cells of rabbit stomach. *Surgery*, 93(5):660–663.
54. Turner, J. C., and Shanks, V. (1980): Absorption of some organochlorine compounds by the rat small intestine — *in vivo*. *Bull. Environ. Contam. Toxicol.*, 24(5):652–655.
55. Valberg, L. S., Haist, J., Cherian, M. G., Delaquerriere-Richardson, L., and Goyer, R. (1977): Cadmium-induced enteropathy: Comparative toxicity of cadmium chloride and cadmium-thionein. *J. Toxicol. Environ. Health*, 2(4):963–975.
56. Volp, R. F., and Lage, G. L. (1978): The fate of a major biliary metabolite of digitoxin in the rat intestine. *Drug Metab. Dispos.*, 6:418–424.
57. Wise, A., Mullett, A. K., and Rowland, I. R. (1982): Dietary fiber, bacterial metabolism and toxicity of nitrate in rat. *Xenobiotica*, 12(2):111–118.

Intestinal Toxicology, edited by C. M. Schiller.
Raven Press, New York © 1984.

Intestinal Absorption and Metabolism of Xenobiotics in Laboratory Animals

Rajendra S. Chhabra and William C. Eastin, Jr.

Carcinogenesis and Toxicology Evaluation Branch, Toxicology Research and Testing Program, National Institute of Environmental Health Sciences, Research Triangle Park, North Carolina 27709

The chemicals foreign to biologic systems are referred to as xenobiotics. Epstein (16) has classified xenobiotics into four broad categories: (a) natural chemicals in excess such as nitrates, (b) natural fungal or plant toxins such as aflatoxins and cycasins, (c) air and water pollutants consisting of complex inorganic and organic chemical mixtures, and, the largest category of xenobiotics, and (d) drugs, agricultural chemicals such as pesticides and fertilizers, food additives, heavy metals, plasticizers, and industrial and household chemicals including solvents. The number of chemicals in everyday use is approximately 50 to 63,000 (39). There are more than 500 chemicals added intentionally to food in addition to unintentional contamination of food by a variety of other chemicals (46). The human population is exposed to xenobiotics through inhalation, ingestion, and dermal absorption. Oral exposure occurs by ingestion of therapeutic agents and environmental contaminants present in food and water as well as by swallowing part of inhaled pollutants. After intestinal absorption, the xenobiotics may be distributed in the bloodstream as well as in interstitial cellular and transcellular fluids. The physiochemical characteristics of xenobiotics—cardiac output and regional blood circulation—are the major determining factors that influence the rate, extent, and pattern of initial distribution. The lipid-soluble chemicals are readily distributed to all fluid compartments and in highly perfused tissues but move less into muscles and even more slowly into fats. After distribution, the xenobiotics can accumulate in tissues, which may serve as reservoirs and prolong the toxicity of chemicals or the therapeutic effect of chemicals when taken as medication. A large number of xenobiotics are lipid soluble, weak organic acids or bases that are not readily eliminated from the body. They must be transformed into more polar metabolites before they can be excreted from the body. After biotransformation, the end products of xenobiotics are usually less lipid soluble, more ionized at physiological pH, less bound to plasma and tissue protein, and less stored in fat.

This chapter presents an overview of xenobiotic absorption and metabolism by intestine; for in-depth information on this subject, the reader is referred to reviews on absorption (4,24,26,28,42,50) and metabolism of chemicals (9,19,38).

145

INTESTINAL ABSORPTION OF XENOBIOTICS

To be absorbed into the body, ingested chemicals must pass through the gastrointestinal mucosa, the major site of absorption being the small intestine. The movement of xenobiotics across the intestinal mucosa and into the blood or lymph system occurs by the same processes that are responsible for the absorption of nutrients. The effect of age-related changes on gastrointestinal physiology and absorption in the young and the elderly has been reviewed elsewhere and will not be discussed in detail here (4,35,47,48,64). Although some examples are given for purpose of illustration, the following is an overview of processes known to play a role in intestinal absorption of xenobiotics.

Active Transport

Active transport involves specialized cellular systems that require an expenditure of energy, can transport chemicals against an electrochemical gradient, and are substrate specific. These systems are responsible for the transport of substances important to normal intestinal function, e.g., absorption of specific amino acids, sugars, and electrolytes, and for the recovery of bile acids. Toxicants structurally similar to naturally occurring substrates can apparently compete for binding sites on the same transport mechanism and thus be actively absorbed. For example, the antitumor agents 5-fluorouracil and 5-bromouracil are actively transported across the rat intestinal epithelium by the same mechanism responsible for pyrimidines, uracil, and thymine absorption (42). Similarly, cobalt and manganese compete for the iron transport system (26,41,51,52). However, because of substrate specificity, these specialized transport systems are not considered major mechanisms for absorption of xenobiotics.

Pinocytosis

In pinocytosis, the intestinal absorptive cell membrane forms invaginations that finally close to form vesicles (phagosomes) containing extracellular milieu. These phagosomes migrate into the cytoplasm and coalesce with lysosomes, exposing the absorbed material to intracellular digestive processes. Undigested macromolecules may be released into the intercellular spaces by exocytosis. In the immature intestine of neonates and suckling animals, excessive quantities of antigens may be transported during the time when host defenses are developing. As the intestinal epithelial cell membrane matures, there is a decreased capacity of absorptive cells to transport macromolecules. Nevertheless, reports describing the pinocytosis of macromolecules in adult mammals, e.g., ferritin, virus particles (63), horseradish perioxidase (57), and azo dyes (2), suggest that this transport mechanism provides the potential for intestinal transport of xenobiotics. The role of pinocytosis in absorption of macromolecules and particulate matter has been reviewed by LeFevre and Joel (29), M. E. LeFevre and D. D. Joel, *this volume*, and Walker (56).

Filtration

Both lipophilic and hydrophilic compounds may pass through "pores" or aqueous channels in the cell membrane. The driving force for this type of transport is a hydrostatic or osmotic pressure gradient that produces a bulk flow of water. Solutes, depending on size and charge, may move with water through these channels. Xenobiotics with molecular weights around 100 may be absorbed through this process.

Absorption Via the Lymphatics

Dietary short-chained fatty acids and monoglycerides enter the absorptive cells by diffusion. Absorbed and resynthesized triglycerides are discharged as chylomicrons, most likely by exocytosis, into the extracellular space. These chylomicrons then enter the lymphatics and empty into the systemic venous blood, completely bypassing the liver (12,53). Few systematic studies on xenobiotic absorption through intestinal lymphatics are known. DeMarco and Levine (13) studied the absorption of some drugs through this process and showed that compounds such as *p*-amino-salicylic acid and tetracycline are absorbed to some extent through the lymphatic system, but the proportion of the dose absorbed is too low to be of any therapeutic significance. However, the absorption of environmental toxic chemicals through intestinal lymphatics may be important, since these chemicals can be distributed throughout the body without being transformed by the liver. Some environmental toxic chemicals are known to be partly absorbed through lymphatics. Sieber (44,45) studied the absorption of ^{14}C-labeled compounds structurally related to *p,p'*-DDT in thoracic cannulated rats and identified the parent DDT compounds and their metabolites in the lymph collected during the experiment. The DDT compounds varied in their lipid solubility and in the extent of their lymphatic absorption, but a strict correlation between lipid solubility and lymphatic absorption was not established, possibly because of other factors such as differences in rate and routes of excretion of each compound. The carcinogens, benzo[*a*]pyrene, 3-methylchol-anthrene (3-MC), and *cis*-dimethylaminostilbene have also been reported to be absorbed through intestinal lymphatics (25,40). (See A. Kuksis, *this volume.*)

In addition to lipid solubility, the absorption of xenobiotics through intestinal lymphatics is apparently influenced by the lymph flow rate. For example, the absorption of *p*-aminosalicylic acid and tetracycline was doubled when intestinal lymph flow was increased by the administration of tripalmitin (31).

Passive Diffusion

Most xenobiotics cross intestinal membranes by simple diffusion. Simple diffusion is dependent on physicochemical criteria, e.g., is not saturable and the transfer is directly proportional to the concentration gradient and to the lipid-water partition coefficient of the xenobiotic. The greater the concentration gradient and the higher the partition coefficient, the faster the rate of diffusion. As an illustration of this phenomenon, the rate of intestinal absorption of the industrial antioxidant 4,4′-thiobis-(6-t-butyl-*m*-cresol) was proportional to the administered dose over three orders of magnitude (5). When the concentrations become the same on both sides of the membrane, net passive movement of xenobiotics across the membrane stops. Absorption of structurally related chemicals occurs independently; coabsorption does not alter absorption rate of either chemical. In addition to lipid solubility, the rate of passive absorption of xenobiotics is influenced by the degree of ionization (42). For example, many weak acids and bases are readily absorbed whereas stronger, more highly ionized acids and bases are less readily transported, and completely ionized compounds are very slowly absorbed. The effect of degree of ionization on absorption can be illustrated by a study in which raising the pH in rat intestine increased the absorption of bases such as quinine and aminopyrine and decreased the absorption of acids, such as benzoate and salicylates (42). In addition to degree of ionization, the charge on the ion may affect absorption. For example, Eastin et al. (14) found that the rate of intestinal absorption of chromium was greater when the dissociated chromium complex carried a negative charge.

FACTORS AFFECTING INTESTINAL ABSORPTION OF XENOBIOTICS

The effect of normal physiological processes involved in digestion and the nutritional status of the animal can affect the intestinal absorption of xenobiotics. A study to examine the effect of food in the intestines on absorption indicated that serum levels of phenobarbital, when administered orally, were higher in fasted animals than in the animals that were fed ad libitum (27). The exact mechanism for increased serum phenobarbital levels in fasted animals is not clear. One reason for the difficulty in explaining mechanisms is that there are many physiological responses to the arrival of food and other substances into the digestive tract that may affect absorption. For example, bile is secreted into the small intestine to aid in the digestion and absorption of fats. The presence of bile in the intestine has also been shown to affect the absorption of some metals. Cikrt and Tichy (10) found that the absorption of ^{203}Pb administered into the duodenum of rats as ^{203}PbCl$_2$ was decreased by about 18% when normal bile flow to the intestine was interrupted by bile duct cannulation. In another study, a milk diet resulted in a markedly higher body retention of ^{109}CdCl$_2$ in mice compared with other groups receiving a laboratory chow diet (15). The authors suggest that the fatty substances in milk may have affected Cd absorption. Intestinal intracellular digestion, i.e., mucosal metabolism, has been shown to moderate the flux of some xenobiotics across the intestine. For example, White et al. (61) reported that intracellular hydrolysis of di-*n*-butyl phthalate (DBP) to mono-*n*-butyl phthalate (MBP) appeared to control the rate of entry of DBP to the serosal side in rat everted sac preparations. The flux of native MBP was unaffected by inhibition of this pathway.

After food and chemicals in the intestine are digested they move out of the intestinal cells and enter the circulation. The relationship between intestinal flow and absorption was the topic of a recent review (62). Based on experimental data, the author concluded that intestinal blood flow becomes rate-limiting as the absorbability of the xenobiotic increases.

Other factors that may influence the intestinal absorption of xenobiotics include changes in motility of intestinal tract, interaction with gastrointestinal microorganisms, changes in the rate of gastric emptying, and dissolution rate of xenobiotics. Further details on this topic are available in the literature (28,30,31).

METABOLISM OF XENOBIOTICS

The chemical reactions involved in metabolism of xenobiotics are classified as phase 1 and phase 2 reactions. The phase 1 or nonsynthetic reactions are oxidation, reduction, or hydrolysis. The phase 1 reactions of xenobiotic metabolism may result in activation, change in activity, or inactivation of the parent chemical. The phase 2 or synthetic reactions are concerned with formation of a complex between the parent chemical or its metabolite and an endogenous substrate, which usually results in inactivation of the parent compound. Liver is the major organ where phase 1 and phase 2 reactions, also known as biotransformation or toxication-detoxication reactions of xenobiotics, take place. In the liver, endoplasmic reticulum contains a group of nonspecific enzymes that catalyzes these metabolic reactions. These enzymes are also responsible for metabolism of natural substrates such as fatty acids and steroids. These enzyme systems require dihydronicotinamide adenine dinucleotide phosphate (NADPH), molecular oxygen, and an electron transport system consisting of NADPH cytochrome c reductase, lipid, and a carbon monoxide binding pigment, generally known as cytochrome P-450. The reaction products generated by these enzyme systems are usually less lipid soluble and are readily excreted as such or after conjugation. The hepatic metabolism of foreign chemicals has been extensively studied and reviewed (17,18).

For the last several years our laboratory has been studying the comparative aspects of biochemical properties of intestinal and hepatic xenobiotic metabolizing enzymes (9). All of these studies were conducted *in vitro* by using microsomal fractions prepared from intestinal and hepatic homogenates. The *in vitro* metabolism of model drug substrates was studied by standard analytical methods. The details of methodology for preparation of microsomal fractions and estimation of drug metabolizing enzymes are well documented (33). We describe the major characteristics of intestinal xenobiotic metabolism enzymes studied in our laboratory and others.

Localization, Distribution, and Some Biochemical Properties of Intestinal Xenobiotic Metabolizing Enzymes

The intestinal xenobiotic metabolizing enzymes are localized in the endoplasmic reticulum of epithelial cells. The distribution studies of these enzymes along the entire length of small intestine show that the activity of these enzymes is highest in the proximal part of the intestine and progressively declines toward the distal end. Chhabra and Fouts (7) studied the distribution of ethylmorphine-*N*-demethylase, aniline hydroxylase, and aryl hydrocarbon hydroxylase activities (AHH), and cytochrome P-450 content in the proximal 150 cm of rabbit intestine. The activities of xenobiotic metabolizing enzymes were highest in the first 76 cm of the intestine. However, the cytochrome P-450 contents were similar along the entire length of rabbit intestine used in this study. The rat and mice xenobiotic metabolizing enzymes also have a similar pattern of distribution in intestines (20,60). A study on distribution of xenobiotic metabolizing enzymes among mucosal cell populations showed that mature tip cells contained 6 to 10 times more cytochrome P-450 and xenobiotic metabolizing enzyme activity per milligram of microsomal protein than the crypt epithelial cells (22,23). A recent study showed (43) that crypt and tip cells differ in their response to the inductive actions of 2,3,7,8-tetrachlorodibenzo-p-dioxin (TCDD).

A comparison of rabbit intestinal versus hepatic metabolism of a number of drug substrates showed activities generally lower in the intestine. The activities of intestinal drug-metabolizing enzymes were 15 to 50% of those observed in hepatic microsomes. The study on biochemical properties of both hepatic and intestinal enzyme systems showed that both systems require NADPH and O_2 for maximum activity and are inhibited by cytochrome c, SKF-525A, and CO. The *in vitro* addition of drug substrates to microsomal fractions of both tissues produced typical type I and type II binding spectra (7), again suggesting similarities in both enzyme systems.

Perinatal Development of Intestinal Xenobiotic Metabolizing Enzymes

The postnatal development of aminopyrine N-demethylase, arylhydrocarbon hydroxylase (AHH), biphenyl 4-hydroxylase, 7-ethoxycoumarin O-deethylase, NADPH-cytochrome c reductase activities, and cytochrome P-450 content were compared in microsomes obtained from the rabbit liver and small intestines (54). The common developmental pattern observed was characterized by enzyme activities that were low or undetectable in the first week after birth and increased slowly during the first 25 days of life. Subsequently, the enzyme activities exhibited a rapid two- to fivefold increase in magnitude. By 30 to 40 days of age, values reached or exceeded adult levels (75 days). At 50 days there was a transient fall in enzyme activities below the adult level, but activities were regained to adult level by 75 days postpartum. A similar pattern of hepatic enzyme development was noticed except that maximum activities were usually observed later than those for the corresponding parameter in the small intestine. Also, no subsequent decline below adult values was observed for any of the hepatic enzyme activities studied during later development.

Lucier et al. (32) studied the developmental patterns of uridine diphosphate glucuronyl transferase (UDPGT) activities in guinea pig and rabbit intestine during the perinatal period. The guinea pig intestinal UDPGT activities were not detectable until birth and developed to adult levels by 3 weeks after birth. However, the rabbit intestinal UDPGT activities were detectable 10 days before birth, declined during the first week after birth, and attained adult levels by 4 weeks of age.

Rhythmic Variations in Intestinal Xenobiotic Metabolizing Enzymes

Changes in the susceptibility of the laboratory animals to therapeutic or toxic effects of chemicals may be influenced by the time of day at which they are exposed. Some aspects of circadian rhythms on rates of extrahepatic drug-metabolizing enzymes has been reported by our laboratory (55). The circadian variations in various microsomal drug-metabolizing enzymes from rabbit intestine are shown in Table 1. All enzyme activities showed a peak in activity around 0600 hr with a trough around 1200 to 1500 hr. The microsomal cytochromic P-450 content appeared less rhythmic than the enzymic activities measured.

Nutrition as Modifier of Intestinal Xenobiotic Metabolizing Enzymes

The importance of dietary components as potential effectors of intestinal drug-metabolizing enzymes has been extensively studied by Wattenberg and his colleagues (58–60). Most of their studies concentrated on the AHH enzyme system in the rat. In their studies on the effect of various diets on AHH activities in rat intestine and lung, it was shown that rats on semipurified diet lost all AHH activities in these tissues. From these experiments, it was suggested that intestinal enzyme activities observed in rats on normal laboratory chow was due to the exogenous factors present in the diet which induce enzymes present at very low levels. This hypothesis was confirmed by their findings that the addition of various vegetables to a semipurified diet caused increases in intestinal AHH activity in the rat (37,38). Table 2 shows our studies, where the rabbit was used as an experimental animal, and the effect of semipurified diet on some of the drug-metabolizing enzymes was compared with the enzymes in animals on regular laboratory rabbit chow. Unlike rats, as shown by Wattenberg (58), the intestinal enzymic activities in rabbits fed semipurified diets were not altered. The reason for this apparent species difference is not immediately obvious, but may be of considerable importance should a regulatory role be envisioned for diet in the control of enzyme activities in the small intestine of all animals, including man. The effect of dietary factors on intestinal xenobiotic metabolizing enzymes has recently been reviewed (6).

Differences in Intestinal Xenobiotic Metabolizing Enzymes and Their Alteration by Foreign Chemicals in Various Species

Table 3 shows that intestinal activities of various drug-metabolizing enzymes as a percentage of that of liver enzyme activity in various animal species. In the intestines from mice, rat, guinea pigs, and hamsters, some of the enzymic activities were either absent or required very sensitive methods of detection. The rabbit emerged as the species with the highest activities of drug-metabolizing enzymes. The interspecies difference noticed in intestinal drug-metabolizing enzymes could be due to genetic factors or to the induction of these enzymes by environmental chemicals present in the diet of these animals (8). Hoensch et al. (21) have reported the presence of xenobiotic metabolizing activities in surgical specimens of the human small intestine and in jejunal biopsy material obtained from patients.

TABLE 1. *Circadian variations in rabbit intestinal microsomal enzyme activities*

Enzyme activity	Time (hr)							
	0000	0300	0600	0900	1200	1500	1800	2100
AHH[a]	54 ± 8	58 ± 7	67 ± 6	61 ± 6	51 ± 2	61 ± 10	58 ± 11	53 ± 4
Benzphetamine N-demethylase[b]	0.51 ± 0.08	0.57 ± 0.06	0.64 ± 0.08	0.54 ± 0.04	0.48 ± 0.06	0.47 ± 0.10	0.59 ± 0.11	0.60 ± 0.04
NADPH-cytochrome c reductase[c]	86 ± 13	97 ± 7	104 ± 12	84 ± 8	81 ± 7	89 ± 16	89 ± 10	94 ± 11
Cytochrome P-450[d]	0.43 ± 0.03	0.44 ± 0.04	0.50 ± 0.05	0.45 ± 0.02	0.51 ± 0.02	0.49 ± 0.03	0.49 ± 0.06	0.48 ± 0.01

Animals were killed at the times shown and microsomal fractions were immediately prepared and stored. Enzyme activities were determined within 1 week of sacrifice. Each value is the mean ± SEM of four separate determinations.
[a]Activities are presented as nmol 3-hydroxybenzpyrene produced/mg microsomal protein·min.
[b]Activities are nmol formaldehyde produced/mg microsomal protein·min.
[c]Activities are nmol cytochrome c reduced/mg microsomal protein·min.
[d]Cytochrome P-450 contents are nmol/mg microsomal protein.
Data from Tredger et al. (54).

TABLE 2. *Effect of purified diet in intestinal drug-metabolizing enzymes in rabbit*

	Enzyme activity (% of controls)[a]			
Treatment	Ethylmorphine demethylase	Aniline hydroxylase	AHH	7-Ethoxycoumarin deethylase
Purified diet vs pair-fed controls	82	95	77	110
Purified diet vs ad lib controls	99	104	87	125

[a]Controls were fed a natural ingredient rabbit diet, either pair-fed to the purified group or fed ad lib.

TABLE 3. *Species differences in intestinal microsomal drug-metabolizing enzymes and cytochrome P-450 content*

	Enzyme activity in intestine as percentage of that in liver					
Species	Ethylmorphine N-demethylase	Biphenyl hydroxylase	Aniline hydroxylase	AHH	Cytochrome c reductase	Cytochrome P-450
Rabbit	18.6	14.1	20.4	30.0	75.7	34.6
Guinea pig	23.3	16.4	19.8	37.4	78.7	12.4
Rat	ND[a]	9.3	ND	4.6	42.0	ND
Mouse	ND	9.0	ND	6.0	79.6	4.0
Hamster	ND	6.8	ND	5.7	60.7	13.0

[a]Not detectable.
Data compiled from Chhabra et al. (8).

A number of foreign chemicals have been shown to increase the hepatic drug-metabolizing enzyme activities. These chemicals are classified into two major categories (11). The chemicals in Class I are those that increase the metabolism of a large number of drug substrates accompanied by an increase in cytochrome P-450, whereas the chemicals in Class II are more specific and induce the enzymic metabolism of a few drug substrates accompanied by the increase and shift of reduced cytochrome P450-CO absorption spectra from 450 nm to 448 nm. Class I is exemplified by phenobarbital, a commonly used inducer of drug-metabolizing enzymes. Class II chemicals are exemplified by 3-MC, one of the carcinogenic polycyclic hydrocarbons. Recent reports have shown that there are other categories of chemicals that induce different forms of cytochrome P-450 (36).

The effect of phenobarbital (PB) (Table 4) and 3-MC (Table 5) on some of the xenobiotic metabolizing enzymes in intestines of various species was studied in our laboratory. The effect of these inducers on cytochrome P-450 content is given in Table 6. Results from this study showed that rabbit intestinal xenobiotic metabolizing enzymes and cytochrome P-450 are not stimulated by either of the inducers used, whereas the induction of xenobiotic metabolizing enzymes in other species

TABLE 4. Activities of ethylmorphine demethylase, aniline hydroxylase, AHH, and 7-ethoxycoumarin deethylase in the small intestine of various animal species treated with PB[a]

Species	Ethylmorphine demethylase		Aniline hydroxylase		AHH		7-Ethoxycoumarin deethylase	
	Control	PB	Control	PB	Control	PB	Control	PB
Rat	Trace	Trace	Trace	Trace	33 ± 9	21 ± 5	0.049 ± 0.008	0.123 ± 0.019[b]
Mouse	Trace	Trace	Trace	Trace	32 ± 9	153 ± 23[b]	0.064 ± 0.012	0.260 ± 0.023[b]
Guinea pig	1.58 ± 0.15	1.79 ± 0.14	0.35 ± 0.03	0.23 ± 0.03	1472 ± 100	1257 ± 99	0.092 ± 0.010	0.150 ± 0.030
Rabbit	0.39 ± 0.06	0.44 ± 0.09	0.33 ± 0.05	0.27 ± 0.01	457 ± 120	410 ± 34	0.059 ± 0.020	0.041 ± 0.007

[a]Mean microsomal enzyme activity ± SE ($N = 4$). In some instances, tissues were pooled from a number of animals. N represents data from individual animals or different pooled samples.

[b]$p < 0.05$.

Data compiled from Miranda and Chhabra (34).

TABLE 5. Activities of aniline hydroxylase, AHH, and 7-ethoxycoumarin deethylase in the small intestine of various animal species treated with 3-MC[a]

Species	Aniline hydroxylase		AHH		7-Ethoxycoumarin deethylase	
	Control	3-MC	Control	3-MC	Control	3-MC
Rat	Trace	Trace	40 ± 13	646 ± 137[b]	0.026 ± 0.010	0.320 ± 0.050[b]
Mouse	Trace	Trace	50 ± 14	258 ± 64[b]	0.040 ± 0.008	0.010 ± 0.005[b]
Guinea pig	0.27 ± 0.02	0.26 ± 0.02	408 ± 43	980 ± 207[b]	0.102 ± 0.013	0.059 ± 0.017[b]
Rabbit	0.47 ± 0.15	0.32 ± 0.06	383 ± 95	316 ± 66	0.046 ± 0.009	0.044 ± 0.003

[a]Mean microsomal enzyme activity ± SE ($N = 4$). In some instances, tissues were pooled from a number of animals. N represents data from individual animals or different pooled samples.
[b]$p < 0.05$.
Data compiled from Miranda and Chhabra (34).

156   XENOBIOTIC ABSORPTION AND METABOLISM

TABLE 6. *Cytochrome P-450 content of microsomes from small intestine of various animal species treated with PB or 3-MC[a]*

| | Small intestine | | | |
Species	Control	PB	Control	3-MC
Rat	ND[b]	ND[b]	ND[b]	ND[b]
Mouse	ND[b]	ND[b]	ND[b]	ND[b]
Guinea pig	0.222 ± 0.02	0.231 ± 0.03	0.26 ± 0.014	0.26 ± 0.004
Rabbit	0.41 ± 0.06	0.40 ± 0.04	0.54 ± 0.12	0.34 ± 0.03

[a]Values are expressed in nmol of cytochrome P-450/mg of microsomal protein ± SE.
[b]Not determined.
Data compiled from Miranda and Chhabra (34).

TABLE 7. *Effect of purified diet and inducers on intestinal drug-metabolizing enzymes in rabbit enzyme activity (% of controls)[a]*

Treatment	Ethylmorphine demethylase	Aniline hydroxylase	AHH	7-Ethoxycoumarin deethylase
Purified diet plus PB (IP)	101	82	107	145
Purified diet plus 3-MC (IP)	—	59	101	68

[a]Controls were fed purified diet and injected with physiological saline (for PB) or corn oil alone (for 3-MC).

depended on the type of drug substrate selected. The lack of induction of xenobiotic metabolizing enzymes in the rabbit small intestine could be due to the maximum induced status of these enzymes caused by the chemical contaminant in the rabbit feed. To test this hypothesis, rabbits were fed semipurified diet for 6 to 7 weeks and then treated with PB or 3-MC for 3 days. Table 7 shows that the 3-MC or PB did not induce any of the enzymes studied and indicated the inability of the rabbit enzyme system to respond to chemical treatment. The resistance to induction of rabbit intestinal enzymes by foreign chemicals seems to be due to genetic factors rather than to dietary ones. Recently, Stohs and Wu (49) studied the effect of various xenobiotics and steroids on AHH activities of intestinal and hepatic microsomes from male rats. In general, hepatic AHH was more sensitive than intestinal AHH to inhibition by a wide variety of xenobiotics. Al-Turk et al. (1) have shown that AHH activity in the rat intestine when compared with activity in liver is less subject to regulation by androgen, estrogen, and the pituitary. These studies provide further support that hepatic and intestinal xenobiotic metabolizing enzyme systems differ in their responses to administration of foreign compounds to laboratory animals.

SUMMARY

There are five possible processes of intestinal absorption of xenobiotics. These are active transport, passive diffusion, pinocytosis, filtration through "pores," and lymphatic absorption. Passive diffusion is the major process for transport of foreign chemicals across the intestine. Though the lymphatic absorption of drugs is not of any major therapeutic significance, the uptake of toxic chemicals such as 3-MC, benzpyrene, and DDT through lymphatics may enhance their toxicity, since they are distributed to other organ systems in the body without being metabolized by the liver. A number of factors such as diet, motility of intestine, interference with gastrointestinal contents of microorganisms, changes in the rate of gastric emptying, age of the animal, and dissolution rate of xenobiotics can alter the rate of absorption of chemicals.

Liver is the major site of metabolism of xenobiotics, but the contribution of intestinal metabolism of xenobiotics can influence the overall bioavailability of chemicals. The xenobiotic metabolizing enzymes located in the endoplasmic reticulum of intestine possess biochemical characteristics similar to that of liver. In general, the rate of metabolism of xenobiotics by intestinal microsomal preparation is lower than that observed with similar hepatic microsomal preparations. The *in vitro* intestinal metabolism of xenobiotics is affected by several factors, including age, sex, diurnal variations, species, and nutritional status of the animal.

The intestinal xenobiotic metabolizing enzymes are stimulated by pretreatment of animals with foreign chemicals, but this depends on the drug substrate and the animal species used. Rabbit intestinal drug-metabolizing enzymes seem to be resistant to induction by foreign chemicals.

REFERENCES

1. Al-Turk, W. A., Stohs, S. J., and Roche, E. B. (1981): Effect of hypophysectomy and castration on hepatic, pulmonary and intestinal aryl hydrocarbon hydroxylase activities in the rat. *J. Pharmacol. Exp. Ther.*, 216:492–495.
2. Barrnett, R. J. (1959): The demonstration with the electron microscope of the end-products of histochemical reactions in relation to the fine structure of cells. *Exp. Cell Res.*, [Suppl.] 7:65–89.
3. Bender, A. D. (1968): Effect of age on intestinal absorption: Implications for drug absorption in the elderly. *J. Amer. Geriatr. Soc.*, 16:1331–1339.
4. Binns, T. B. (1971): The absorption of drugs from the alimentary tract, lung and skin. *Br. J. Hosp. Med.*, 6:133–142.
5. Birnbaum, L. S., Eastin, W. C., Jr., Johnson, L., and Matthews, H. B. (1983): Disposition of 4,4'-Thio-bis-(6-t-butyl-m-cresol) in rats. *Drug Metab. Dispos.*, 11:537–543.
6. Chhabra, R. S. (1981): Effect of dietary factors and environmental chemicals on intestinal drug metabolizing enzymes. *Toxicol. Environ. Chem.*, 3:173–199.
7. Chhabra, R. S., and Fouts, J. R. (1976): Biochemical properties of some microsomal xenobiotic-metabolizing enzymes in rabbit small intestine. *Drug Metab. Dispos.*, 4:208–214.
8. Chhabra, R. S., Pohl, R. J., and Fouts, J. R. (1974): A comparative study of xenobiotic-metabolizing enzymes in liver and intestine of various animal species. *Drug Metab. Dispos.*, 2:443–447.
9. Chhabra, R. S., and Tredger, J. M. (1978): Interactions of drugs and intestinal mucosal endoplasmic reticulum. In: *Nutrition and Drug Interrelations*, edited by J. N. Hathcock and J. Coon, pp. 253–274. Academic Press, New York.

10. Cikrt, M., and Tichy, M. (1975): Role of bile in intestinal absorption of [203]Pb in rats. *Experientia*, 31:1320–1321.
11. Conney, A. H. (1967): Pharmacological implications of microsomal enzyme induction. *Pharmacol. Rev.*, 18:317–366.
12. Davenport, H. W. (1982): *Physiology of the Digestive Tract.* pp. 211–225. Year Book Medical Publishers, Inc., Chicago.
13. De Marco, T. J., and Levine, R. R. (1969): Role of the lymphatics in the intestinal absorption and distribution of drugs. *J. Pharmacol. Exp. Ther.*, 169:142–151.
14. Eastin, W. C., Jr., Haseltine, S. D., and Murray, H. C. (1980): Intestinal absorption of 5 chromium compounds in young black ducks (Anas rubripes). *Toxicol. Lett.*, 6:193–197.
15. Engström, B., and Nordberg, G. (1976): Effects of milk diet on gastrointestinal absorption of cadmium in adult mice. *Toxicology*, 9:195–203.
16. Epstein S. S. (1972): Environmental pathology. *Am. J. Pathol.*, 66:352–371.
17. Gillette, J. R. (1966): Biochemistry of drug oxidation and reduction by enzymes in hepatic endoplasmic reticulum. *Adv. Pharmacol.*, 4:219–261.
18. Gillette, J. R., Davis, D. W., and Sasame, H. A. (1972): Cytochrome P-450 and its role in drug metabolism. *Ann. Rev. Pharmacol.*, 12:57–84.
19. Hartiala, K. (1973): Metabolism of hormones, drugs and other substances by the gut. *Physiol. Rev.*, 53:496–534.
20. Hietanen, E., and Vainio, H. (1973): Interspecies variations in small intestinal and hepatic drug hydroxylation and glucuronidation. *Acta Pharmacol. Toxicol.*, 33:57–64.
21. Hoensch, H. P., Hutt, R., and Hartmann, F. (1979): Biotransformation of xenobiotics in human intestinal mucosa. *Environ. Health Perspect.*, 33:71–78.
22. Hoensch, H., Woo, C. H., Raffin, S. B., and Schmid, R. (1976): Oxidative metabolism of foreign compounds in rat small intestine: Cellular localization and dependence on dietary iron. *Gastroenterology*, 70:1063–1070.
23. Hoensch, H., Woo, C. H., and Schmid, R. (1975): Cytochrome P-450 and drug metabolism in intestinal villous and crypt cells of rats: Effect of dietary iron. *Biochem. Biophys. Res. Commun.*, 65:399–406.
24. Jollow, D. J., and Brodie, B. B. (1972): Mechanisms of drug absorption and of drug solution. *Pharmacology*, 8:21–32.
25. Kamp, J. D., and Neumann, H.-G. (1975): Absorption of carcinogens into the thoracic duct lymph of the rat: Aminostilbene derivatives and 3-methylcholanthrene. *Xenobiotica*, 5:717–727.
26. Klaassen, C. D. (1980): Absorption, distribution and excretion of toxicants. In: *Casarett and Doull's Toxicology. The Basic Science of Poisons*, 2nd edition, edited by J. Doull, C. D. Klaassen and M. O. Amdur, pp. 28–55. Macmillan, New York.
27. Kojima, S., Smith, R. B., and Dolyisio, J. T. (1971): Drug absorption: Influence of food on oral absorption of phenobarbital in rats. *J. Pharmac. Sci.*, 60:1639–1641.
28. Kurz, H. (1975): Principles of drug absorption. In: *International Encyclopedia of Pharmacology and Therapeutics, Section 39B, Vol. 1*, edited by W. Forth and W. Rummel. Pergamon Press, New York.
29. Lefevre, M. E., and Joel, D. D. (1977): Intestinal absorption of particulate matter. *Life Sci.*, 21:1403–1408.
30. Levine, R. R. (1961): The influence of the intraluminal intestinal milieu on absorption of an organic cation and anionic agent. *J. Pharmacol. Exp. Ther.*, 131:328–333.
31. Levine, R. R. (1970): Factors affecting gastrointestinal absorption. *Am. J. Dig. Dis.*, 15:171–188.
32. Lucier, G. W., Sonawane, B. R., and Medancel, O. S. (1977): Glucuronidation and deglucuronidation reactions in hepatic and extrahepatic tissues during perinatal development. *Drug Metab. Dispos.*, 5:279–287.
33. Mazel, P. (1971): Experiments illustrating drug metabolism *in vitro*. In: *Fundamentals of Drug Metabolism and Drug Disposition*, edited by B. N. LaDu, H. G. Mandel and E. L. Way, pp. 551–578. Williams and Wilkins, Baltimore.
34. Miranda, C. L., and Chhabra, R. S. (1980): Species differences in stimulation of intestinal and hepatic microsomal mixed-function oxidase enzymes. *Biochem. Pharmacol.*, 29:1161–1165.
35. Morselli, P. L. (1976): Clinical pharmacokinetics in neonates. *Clin. Pharmacokinet.*, 1:81–98.
36. Nebert, D. W., and Negishi, M. (1982): Multiple forms of cytochrome P-450 and the importance of molecular biology and evolution. *Biochem. Pharmacol.*, 31:2311–2317.
37. Pantuck, E. J., Hsiao, J.-C., Loub, W. D., Wattenberg, L. W., Kuntzman, R., and Conney, A. H.

(1976): Stimulatory effect of vegetables on intestinal drug metabolism in the rat. *J. Pharmacol. Exp. Therap.*, 198:278–283.

38. Pantuck, E. J., Kuntzman, R., and Conney, A. H. (1976): Intestinal drug metabolism and bioavailability of drugs. In: *New Concepts in Safety Evaluation*, edited by M. A. Mehlman, R. E. Shapiro, and H. Blumenthal, pp. 345–367. Hemisphere Publishing Corporation, Washington, D.C.

39. Pienta, R. J. (1979): A hamster embryo cell model system for identifying carcinogens. In: *Carcinogens: Identification and Mechanism of Action*, edited by A. C. Griffin and C. R. Shaw, pp. 123–147. Raven Press, New York.

40. Rees, E. D., Mandelstam, P., Lowry, J. Q., and Lipscomb, H. (1971): A study of the mechanism of intestinal absorption of benzo(a)pyrene. *Biochim. Biophys. Acta*, 225:96–107.

41. Schade, S. G., Felsher, B. F., Glades, B. E., and Conrad, M. E. (1970): Effect of cobalt upon iron absorption. *Soc. Exp. Biol. Med.*, 134:741–743.

42. Schanker, L. S. (1971): Drug absorption. In: *Fundamentals of Drug Metabolism and Drug Disposition*, edited by B. N. LaDu, H. G. Mandel, and E. L. Way, pp. 22–40. Williams and Wilkins, Baltimore.

43. Schiller, C. M., and Lucier, G. W. (1978): The differential response of isolated intestinal crypt and tip cells to the inductive actions of 2,3,7,8-tetrachlorodibenzo-p-dioxin. *Chem. Biol. Interact.*, 22:199–209.

44. Sieber, S. M. (1974): The entry of foreign compounds into the thoracic duct lymph of the rat. *Xenobiotica*, 4:265–284.

45. Sieber, S. M. (1976): The lymphatic absorption of p,p'-DDT and some structurally-related compounds in the rat. *Pharmacology*, 14:443–454.

46. Siu, R. G. H., Borzelleca, J. F., Carr, C. J., Day, H. G., Fomon, S. J., Irving, G. W., Jr., LaDu, B. N., Jr., McCoy, J. R., Miller, S. A., Plaa, G. L., Shimkin, M. B., and Wood, J. L. (1977): Evaluation of health aspects of GRAS food ingredients: Lessons learned and questions unanswered. *Fed. Proc.*, 36:2527–2562.

47. Stevenson, I. H., Salem, S. A. M., O'Malley, K., Cusak, B., and Kelly, J. G. (1981): Age and drug absorption. In: *Drug Absorption*, The proceedings of the international conference on drug absorption. Edinburgh, September, 1979. ADIS Press Australia.

48. Stevenson, I. H., Salem, S. A. M., and Shepherd, A. M. M. (1979): Studies on drug absorption and metabolism in the elderly. In: *Drugs and the Elderly*, edited by J. Crooks and I. H. Stevenson, pp. 51–63. Macmillan, New York.

49. Stohs, S. J., and Wu, C. L. J. (1982): Effect of various xenobiotics and steroids on aryl hydrocarbon hydroxylase activity of intestinal and hepatic microsomes from male rats. *Pharmacology*, 25:237–249.

50. Ther, L., and Winne, D. (1971): Drug absorption. *Annu. Rev. Pharmacol.*, 11:57–70.

51. Thomson, A. B. R., Olatunbosun, D., and Valberg, L. S. (1971a): Interrelation of intestinal transport system for manganese and iron. *J. Lab. Clin. Med.*, 78:642–655.

52. Thomson, A. B. R., Valberg, L. S., and Sinclair, D. G. (1971b): Competitive nature of the intestinal transport mechanism for cobalt and iron in the rat. *J. Clin. Invest.*, 50:2384–2394.

53. Thomson, A. B. R., and Dietschy, J. M. (1981): Intestinal lipid absorption: major extracellular and intracellular events. In: *Physiology of the Gastrointestinal Tract*, edited by L. R. Johnson, pp. 1147–1220. Raven Press, New York.

54. Tredger, J. M., Chhabra, R. S., and Fouts, J. R. (1976): Postnatal development of mixed-function oxidation as measured in microsomes from the small intestine and liver of rabbit. *Drug Metab. Dispos.*, 4:17–23.

55. Tredger, J. M., and Chhabra, R. S. (1977): Circadian variations in microsomal drug metabolizing enzyme activities in rat and rabbit tissues. *Xenobiotica*, 7:481–489.

56. Walker, W. A. (1981): Intestinal transport of macromolecules. In: *Physiology of the Gastrointestinal Tract*, edited by L. R. Johnson, pp. 1271–1289. Raven Press, New York.

57. Warshaw, A. L., Walker, W. A., Cornell, R., and Isselbacher, K. J. (1971): Small intestinal permeability to macromolecules: Transmission of horseradish peroxidase into mesenteric lymph and portal blood. *Lab. Invest.*, 25:675–684.

58. Wattenberg, L. W. (1971): Enzymatic reactions and carcinogenesis. *Coll. Pop. Annu. Symp. Foundan. Cancer Res.*, 24:241–254.

59. Wattenberg, L. W. (1971): Studies of polycyclic hydrocarbon hydroxylases of the intestine possibly related to cancer. *Cancer*, 28:99–102.

60. Wattenberg, L. W., Leong, J. L., and Strand, P. J. (1962): Benzpyrene hydroxylase activity in the gastrointestinal tract. *Cancer Res.*, 22:1120–1125.
61. White, R. D., Carter, D. E., Earnest, D., and Mueller, J. (1980): Absorption and metabolism of three phthalate diesters by the rat small intestine. *Fed. Cosmet. Toxicol.*, 18:383–386.
62. Winne, D. (1980): Influence of blood flow on intestinal absorption of xenobiotics. *Pharmacology*, 21:1–15.
63. Worthington, B. S., and Syrotuck, J. (1976): Intestinal permeability to large particles in normal and protein-deficient adult rats. *J. Nutr.*, 106:20–32.
64. Yaffe, S. J., and Danish, M. (1978): Problems of drug administration in the pediatric patient. *Drug Metab. Rev.*, 8:303–318.

Intestinal Toxicology, edited by C. M. Schiller.
Raven Press, New York © 1984.

Normal and Abnormal Intestinal Absorption by Humans

William D. Heizer

University of North Carolina, School of Medicine, Chapel Hill, North Carolina 27514

Absorption of nutrients is the major function of the gastrointestinal system. Although the most prevalent gastrointestinal diseases such as peptic ulcer, cancers, and gallstones seldom cause clinically detectable changes in absorption, there are more than 30 less common human diseases that do cause malabsorption of one or more nutrients (1,2). These diseases and the clinical methods used to evaluate intestinal absorption are reviewed.

The approximate amounts of various nutrients ingested by normal adult Americans are shown in Table 1 (3). In addition, endogenous secretions must be digested and absorbed, and they contribute about 6,500 ml of water, 35 to 100 g protein, and possibly 20 to 30 g fat each day.

Table 2 summarizes the steps in digestion and in absorption of fats, carbohydrates, and proteins. For the sake of brevity, important gastric functions are not shown. Pancreatic lipase assisted by colipse, a low molecular weight protein that is also secreted by the pancreas, hydrolyzes ingested triglyceride predominantly to free fatty acids and β-monoglyceride (4). This mixture is solubilized to a clear micellar solution by the action of bile acids (5,6). The fatty acids and β-monoglyceride diffuse from the micelles into the intestinal mucosa while bile acids remain in the lumen and are absorbed by an active process in the terminal ileum (7). Within the mucosal cell, triglyceride is resynthesized and packaged with cholesterol, cholesterol esters, and specific proteins to form chylomicrons which leave the basolateral

TABLE 1. *Typical daily intake (2,600 calories)*

Food	Amount	Form
Fat	100 g	95% triglycerides 5% other
Carbohydrates	350 g	50% starch 35% disaccharides 5% fiber
Protein	75 g	Mixed proteins
Other	Few g	Vitamins, minerals
Water	2,300 ml	

161

TABLE 2. *Summary of intestinal absorption*

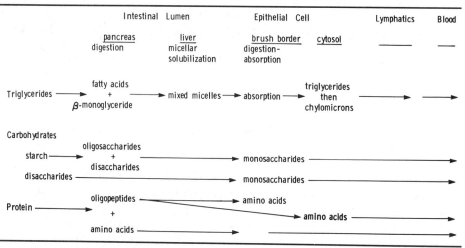

membrane of the cell, enter lymphatics, and eventually join the blood via the thoracic duct (8,9). The digestion and absorption of carbohydrates and proteins is less complex (8). Pancreatic amylase hydrolyzes starch only to maltose and small oligosaccharides (10). These products plus ingested dissacharides, primarily lactose and sucrose, are further cleaved to monosaccharides by disaccharidases in the brush border membrane of the epithelial cells. In contrast, approximately one-third to one-half the ingested protein is hydrolyzed completely to free amino acids by pancreatic enzymes. The peptides that remain, averaging two to six amino acids in length, are cleaved by peptide hydrolases while being transported through the epithelial cells. Peptide hydrolases are present not only in the brush border membrane but also in the cytosol. Peptides composed of three to six amino acids are hydrolyzed predominantly by brush border enzymes. Dipeptides may be either transported intact and hydrolyzed inside the cell or cleaved by surface enzymes (11). One or more proteases in the brush border are also capable of digesting whole protein.

The quantities of nutrients ingested (Table 1) are less than the absorptive capacity of the intestine. Although fecal fat does increase slightly as the amount of fat ingested is increased, normal subjects are capable of absorbing more than 350 g of fat daily (12). The reserve capacity for carbohydrate and protein is even greater than for fat. Reserve capacity is in part due to excess function including 9- to 10-fold more pancreatic enzyme activity (13), 2- to 3-fold higher bile salt concentration (2,7), and severalfold more surface area, at least for carbohydrate (14), than the minimum required for normal absorption. Adaptation also contributes to the reserve capacity of the intestine. Thus, following resection or bypass of part of the small intestine, the remaining segment undergoes changes in enzyme activity and morphology and an increase in absorbing capacity per centimeter of length (15,16). Also, resection or disease of the terminal ileum, which results in excessive fecal losses of bile acids, induces an increase in bile acid synthesis by the liver of up to 10-fold the normal rate (7). The digestive system can also partially compensate for total loss of pancreatic secretions (17,18). Although this reserve absorptive capacity is of obvious benefit, it often precludes early detection of conditions that cause malabsorption or detection of slight damage.

The malabsorption syndrome, i.e., steatorrhea and weight loss, is caused by many diseases which can be conveniently divided into groups based on the major deficiency leading to the absorptive defect (Table 3) (1,2). Most of these diseases cause malabsorption of many or all nutrients. There are other diseases that cause malabsorption of only one or a few related nutrients and that do not produce the malabsorption syndrome. The most important of these are categorized in Table 4 (19).

Although a great many tests have been proposed for detecting and diagnosing the cause of malabsorption, many of them are only different methods of gathering the same information. Therefore, a rational approach to investigation of suspected malabsorption need not involve a large number of tests. By history, most patients with malabsorption have diarrhea and weight loss, but occasionally the patient will complain predominantly of one or more other symptoms including weakness, bleeding tendency, sore tongue, tetany, bone pain, edema, amenorrhea, or peripheral neuritis. The physical exam is often unremarkable but may show signs of malnutrition or of specific vitamin deficiencies.

Since most patients who present with these symptoms and signs will not have malabsorption, appropriate tests must be done to rule out other more common

TABLE 3. *Conditions that cause malabsorption syndrome*

Insufficient pancreatic enzyme activity	Multiple defects
Chronic pancreatitis	Gastrin-secreting tumor
Pancreatic carcinoma	Scleroderma
Pancreatic resection	Ileal dysfunction—resection, disease
Cystic fibrosis	Steatorrhea following gastric surgery
Enterokinase deficiency	Radiation enteritis
Isolated lipase deficiency	Mechanism unknown
Insufficient bile acid	Mast cell disease
Extrahepatic biliary obstruction	Immune deficiencies
Intrahepatic biliary obstruction	Carcinoid
Intestinal stasis syndromes	Diabetes mellitus
Disease of the small intestinal wall	Hyperthyroidism
Celiac sprue	Adrenal innsufficiency
Tropical sprue	Parasitic infections—giardiasis,
Whipple's disease	strongyloidiasis
Infiltrative disease—amyloid,	Drugs
lymphoma	Colchicine
Small bowel ischemia—atherosclerosis	Cholestyramine
vasculitis	p-aminosalicylate
Jejunal resection	Cathartics
Intestinal lymphangiectasia	Neomycin
a-β-lipoproteinemia	Alcohol
	Clofibrate
	Phenindione

TABLE 4. *Conditions that cause malabsorption of specific nutrients*

Primary disaccharidase deficiency	Vitamin B_{12} malabsorption
Acquired lactase deficiency	Pernicious anemia
Congenital lactase deficiency	Congenital B_{12} malabsorption
Congenital sucrase-isomaltase deficiency	Alcohol
Monosaccharide malabsorption	Folic acid malabsorption
Glucose malabsorption	Oral contraceptives
Fructose malabsorption	Dilantin
Amino acid malabsorption	Alcohol
Cystinuria	
Hartnup's disease	
Methionine malabsorption	
Proline malabsorption	
Probably others	

conditions, including intestinal cancers, inflammatory bowel disease, and infectious diarrheas.

Initial procedures to investigate malabsorption generally include visual inspection of the stool, examination of the stool for meat fibers (20), and semiquantitative determination of fecal fat by counting microscopic lipid droplets after treatment of a stool specimen with a fat stain such as Sudan (20,21). Initial blood determinations include carotenoids and folic acid. Since these compounds are not synthesized by humans in appreciable quantities, the blood levels fall when absorption decreases if intake remains constant. Low folate and carotenoid levels are frequently the result of decreased intake rather than malabsorption, but carotenoid levels less than 20 µg/100 ml usually indicate malabsorption. Prothrombin time or serum alkaline phosphatase activity may be abnormal when vitamin K or vitamin D and calcium absorption, respectively, have been decreased for a long period of time. Blood levels of calcium, magnesium, phosphorus, cholesterol, and vitamin B_{12} may also be obtained, but the results are often normal or only slightly decreased even when malabsorption is clinically obvious. Plain radiographs of the abdomen and barium contrast studies of the upper gastrointestinal tract and small bowel are performed to look for evidence of pancreatic and small bowel disease.

Quantitative analysis of stool fat in a 72-hr collection is the most definitive test for malabsorption. The patient must be ingesting a known quantity of fat, greater than 50 g/day and preferably close to 100 g/day, beginning at least 48 hr before starting the collection. Accuracy of the test depends on (a) careful stool collection and estimation of fat intake; (b) avoidance of drugs that alter intestinal motility, avoidance of barium or other agents that interfere with the assay, and avoidance of cathartics or other suppositories that add fat to the stool; and (c) a properly performed assay.

Recently, a promising new test for fat malabsorption has been developed, the ^{14}C-triolein breath test (22). Triolein labeled with ^{14}C in the carboxyl group is given orally, and the percentage of administered label expired as $^{14}CO_2$ over the next 6 hr is determined. Constant collection of the expired CO_2 is possible, but impractical. Instead, a known quantity of the CO_2 is collected in hyamine at intervals, and its specific activity is determined by scintillation counting. The total label expired in 6 hr is then calculated by assuming a constant CO_2 production of 9 mmol/kg/hr for the patient at rest. The initial report (22), which indicates that this test is as sensitive and specific for fat malabsorption as the 72-hr fecal fat assay, requires confirmation. The breath test can also be done using ^{13}C-triolein, avoiding a radioactive label (23).

The D-xylose test is frequently used in evaluating intestinal absorption (24,25). D-Xylose is a 5-carbon sugar that is absorbed by the intestinal mucosa and that requires no intraluminal digestion. It is metabolized slowly in the body, and the amount excreted intact in the urine is a measure of the amount absorbed. After an oral dose, urine is collected for 5 hr and assayed colorimetrically D-xylose. Normally, 20% or more of the ingested dose is present in this urine specimen. Determination of blood levels of D-xylose 30 to 60 min following the dose may add significantly to the accuracy of the test. Low levels suggest a decrease in effective mucosal surface area or intestinal stasis in which bacteria metabolize the D-xylose before it can be absorbed. There are many causes of falsely low test results, and occasionally patients with documented mucosal disease have normal test results. For these reasons, use of the test may be decreasing in favor of proceeding directly to peroral intestinal biopsy for evaluating the intestinal mucosa (26).

Peroral biopsy of the intestinal mucosa is a safe, relatively simple procedure (27). Depending on the instrument used, one to four pieces of tissue can be obtained with a total weight of up to approximately 35 mg. A hydraulic instrument is available for research purposes which will permit biopsies of the same patient at multiple levels of the small intestine without having to repeatedly remove and reinsert the instrument (28). Biopsy specimens are used for many types of study, including light and electron microscopic examination, chemical and enzymatic assays, tissue culture, and uptake of various radio-labeled compounds.

There are a few other useful tests of intestinal function. Pancreatic secretory tests are used in which a tube is passed by mouth into the duodenum whereby secretions from the pancreas can be aspirated. The pancreas is then stimulated to secrete either by injecting the hormone secretin or by giving a standard meal. The volume, composition, and enzyme activity of the secreted pancreatic fluid is then measured and compared with established normal values (29). The Schilling test determines B_{12} absorption by measuring of radio-labeled B_{12} excreted in the urine for 24 hr following an oral dose (30). A large dose of nonlabeled vitamin is given parenterally to saturate tissue-binding sites. Intrinsic factor normally secreted by the stomach is necessary for B_{12} absorption; therefore, if the initial (first stage) test is abnormal, the test must be repeated, this time giving intrinsic factor with the oral B_{12} (second stage). A combined first- and second-stage test can be performed by use of B_{12} labeled with different isotopes of cobalt, one labeled product bound to intrinsic factor, and one free. An abnormal second-stage test indicates either dysfunction of the terminal ileum, where B_{12} is actively absorbed, or intestinal stasis, as the bacteria in this condition may bind B_{12} before it can be absorbed.

Excessive loss of whole protein from the intestine can be measured by giving ^{51}Cr albumin intravenously and measuring fecal radioactivity for several days. Chromium is practically nonabsorbable; therefore, any that leaks out into the intestinal lumen attached to albumin will remain and be passed in the stool, even though the protein is digested and absorbed (31).

Breath tests similar to the triolein test already described have been reported for detecting malabsorption or metabolism of other compounds labeled with ^{13}C or ^{14}C, including bile acid, D-xylose, and aminopyrine (32–34). When the bile acid, cholylglycine, labeled with ^{14}C in the glycine moiety is given orally to normal subjects, most of the compound is absorbed intact in the terminal ileum and enters the enterohepatic circulation so relatively little is metabolized. If the bile acid comes in contact with a large population of anerobic bacteria, deconjugation may occur, and the released glycine is metabolized to ^{14}CO$_2$, which is absorbed by the intestine and expired in the breath. Thus, either ileal dysfunction, which causes the bile acid to escape into the colon in excess quantities, or intestinal stasis, in which bacteria overgrow in the upper intestine, will cause excessive quantities of ^{14}CO$_2$ to be expired following administration of the labeled bile acid. The two conditions can be distinguished by measuring fecal radioactivity, which is elevated in the case of ileal dysfunction but not in intestinal stasis.

Finally, several new, apparently useful tests for malabsorption of various carbohydrates measure hydrogen in the breath following ingestion of the test carbohydrate (35,36). Bacteria, but not mammalian cells, produce hydrogen during metabolism of sugars. Hydrogen produced in the intestinal lumen by bacteria is readily absorbed from the intestinal tract and expired in the breath. Therefore, the presence of significant amounts of hydrogen in the breath following ingestion of any carbohydrate indicates that bacteria are coming in contact with the compound. Normally, ordinary doses of compounds such as lactose, sucrose, and glucose are 100% absorbed. Therefore, increased breath hydrogen following their ingestion indicates malabsorption or bacterial overgrowth in the upper intestine. On the other hand, lactulose is a sugar that is not absorbed by humans so that the time of appearance of hydrogen in the breath following its ingestion is used to measure intestinal transit time as well as bacterial overgrowth. A small percentage of normal individuals do not expire hydrogen even when given a nonabsorbed sugar, presumably because they do not harbor hydrogen-producing bacteria.

In summary, although absorption is the main function of the intestine, the system has a large reserve capacity so that most of the tests currently used are not likely to detect very early or mild changes. Measurements done on peroral intestinal biopsies and possibly some of the developing breath tests offer more sensitive methods for detecting intestinal dysfunction.

REFERENCES

1. Beck, I. T. (1973): The role of pancreatic enzymes in digestion. *Am. J. Clin. Nutr.*, 26:311–325.
2. Benson, J. A., Culver, P. J., Ragland, S., Jones, C. M., Drummey, G. D. and Bougas, E. (1957): The D-xylose absorption test in malabsorption syndromes. *N. Engl. J. Med.*, 2567:335–339.

3. Bond, J. H. (Jr.), Levitt, M. D., and Prentiss, R. (1975): Investigation of small bowel transit time in man utilizing pulmonary hydrogen (H_2) measurements. *J. Lab. Clin. Med.*, 85:546–555.
4. Borgstrom, B. (1975): On the interactions between pancreatic lipase and colipase and the substrate, and the importance of bile salts. *J. Lipid Res.*, 16:411–417.
5. Brindley, D. N. (1974): The intracellular phase of fat absorption. In: *Intestinal Absorption*, edited by S. H. Smythe, pp. 621–671. Plenum Press, New York.
6. Castle, W. B. (1968): Gastric intrinsic factor and vitamin B_{12} absorption. In: *Handbook of Physiology*, edited by C. F. Code, pp. 1529–1552, Washington, D.C.
7. Corring, T., and Borudon, D. (1977): Exclusion of pancreatic exocrine secretion from intestine in the pig: Existence of a digestive compensation. *J. Nutr.*, 107:1216–1221.
8. Curtis, K. J., Gaines, H. D., and Kim, Y. S. (1978): Protein digestion and absorption in rats with pancreatic duct occlusion. *Gastroenterology*, 74:1271–1276.
9. DiMagno, E. P., and Go, V. L. W. (1976): The clinical application of exocrine pancreatic function tests. *Disease-A-Month*, 22(12):September.
10. DiMagno, E. P., Go, V. L. W., and Summerskill, W. H. J. (1973): Relations between pancreatic enzyme outputs and malabsorption in severe pancreatic insufficiency. *N. Engl. J. Med.*, 288:813–815.
11. Drummey, G. D., Benson, J. A. Jr., and Jones, C. M. (1961): Microscopical examination of the stool for steatorrhea. *N. Engl. J. Med.*, 264:85–87.
12. Finlay, J. M., Hogarth, J., and Wightman, K. J. R. (1964): A clinical evaluation of the D-xylose absorption test. *Ann. Intern. Med.*, 61:411–422.
13. Flick, A., Quinton, W., and Rubin, C. (1961): A peroral hydraulic biopsy tube for multiple sampling at any level of the gastrointestinal tract. *Gastroenterology*, 40:120–126.
14. Goodhart, R. S., and Shils, M. E., editors (1973): *Modern Nutrition in Health and Disease.* Lea and Febiger, Philadelphia.
15. Gray, G. M. (1978): Mechanisms of digestion and absorption of food. In: *Gastrointestinal Disease*, edited by M. H. Sleisenger and J. S. Fordtran, pp. 241–250. W. B. Saunders, Philadelphia.
16. Gray, G. M. (1978): Maldigestion and malabsorption: clinical manifestations and specific diagnosis. In: *Gastrointestinal Disease*, edited by M. H. Sleisenger and J. S. Fordtran, pp. 272–294. W. B. Saunders, Philadelphia.
17. Hofmann, A. F. (1977): Fat absorption and malabsorption: physiology, diagnosis, and treatment. *Viewpoints on Dig. Dis.*, 9(4):September.
18. Hofmann, A. F. (1978): The enterohepatic circulation of bile acids. In: *Gastrointestinal Disease*, edited by M. H. Sleisenger and J. S. Fordtran, pp. 92–107. W. B. Saunders, Philadelphia.
19. Hofmann, A. F., and Lauterburg, B. H. (1977): Breath test with isotopes of carbon: progress and potential. *J. Lab. Clin. Med.*, 90:405–411.
20. Krawitt, E. L., and Beeken, W. L. (1975): Limitations of the usefulness of the D-xylose absorption test. *Am. J. Clin. Path.*, 63:261–263.
21. Lauterburg, B. H., Newcomer, A. D., and Hofmann, A. F. (1978): Clinical value of the bile acid breath test. Evaluation of the Mayo Clinic experience. *Mayo Clin. Proc.*, 53:227–233.
22. Matthews, D. M. (1975): Intestinal absorption of peptides. *Physiol. Rev.*, 55:537–608.
23. Milne, M. D. (1974): Hereditary disorders of intestinal transport. In: *Intestinal Absorption*, edited by D. H. Smythe, pp. 961–1013. Plenum Press, New York.
24. Moore, J. G., Englert, E., Jr., Bigler, A. H., and Clark, R. W. (1971): Simple fecal tests of absorption. A prospective study and critique. *Dig. Dis.*, 16:97.
25. Newcomer, A. D., Hofmann, A. F., DiMagno, E. P., Thomas, P. J., and Carlson, G. L. (1979): Triolein breath test: a sensitive and specific test for fat malabsorption. *Gastroenterology*, 76:6–13.
26. Newcomer, A. D., McGill, D. B., Thomas, P. J., and Hofmann, A. F. (1975): Prospective comparison of indirect methods for detecting lactase deficiency. *N. Engl. J. Med.*, 293:1232–1236.
27. Perera, D. R., Weinstein, W. M., and Rubin, C. E. (1975): Small intestinal biopsy. *Human Path.*, 6:157–217.
28. Rommel, K., Goebell, H., and Bohmer, editors (1976): *Lipid Absorption: Biochemical and Clinical Aspects.* MTP Press, Lancaster.
29. Schoeller, D. A., Schneider, J. F., Solomons, N. W., Watkins, J. B., and Slein, P. D. (1977): Clinical diagnosis with the stable isotope ^{13}C in CO_2 breath tests: methodology and fundamental considerations. *J. Lab. Clin. Med.*, 90:412–421.

30. Sleisenger, M. H., and Brandborg, L. L. (1977): Malabsorption. In: *Major Problems in Internal Medicine*, edited by L. H. Smith, Jr. W. B. Saunders, Philadelphia.
31. Trier, J. S. (1968): Morphology of the epithelium of the small intestine. In: *Handbook of Physiology*, edited by C. F. Code, pp. 1125–1275. American Physiological Society, Washington, D.C.
32. Waldmann, T. A. (1966): Protein-losing enteropathy. *Gastroenterology*, 50:422–443.
33. Watkins, J. B., Schoeller, D. A., Klein, P. D., Ott, D. G., Newcomer, A. D., Hofmann, A. F. (1977): ^{13}C-trioctanoin: a nonradioactive breath test to detect fat malabsorption. *J. Lab. Clin. Med.*, 90:422–430.
34. Weser, E. (1978): Intestinal adaptation after small bowel resection. *Viewpoints Dig. Dis.*, 10(2):March.
35. Williamson, R. C. N., and Chir, M. (1978): Intestinal adaptation: structural, functional, and cytokinetic changes. *N. Engl. J. Med.*, 298:1393–1402.
36. Wollaeger, E. E. (1973): Role of the ileum in fat absorption. *Mayo Clin. Proc.*, 48:836–843.

Intestinal Toxicology, edited by C. M. Schiller.
Raven Press, New York © 1984.

Intestinal Absorption and Metabolism of Xenobiotics in Humans

*Harald P. Hoensch and **Michael Schwenk

*Universitätsklinikum der GH-Essen, Med. Klinik und Poliklinik, Allgem. Innere Abteilung, D-4300 Essen 1, Germany; and **Institut für Toxikologie, Universität Tübingen, D-7400 Tübingen, Germany*

The food we eat contains not only nutrients, which serve as energy sources, but xenobiotics, which are chemical compounds foreign to the human body without a nutritional or physiological role and potentially toxic. These xenobiotics originate from many different sources: pharmaceutical drugs, plant ingredients (flavonoids), food additives (preservatives, coloring, flavoring), side products of food technology (nitrosamines), microbial metabolites (aflatoxin), and environmental contaminants (chlorinated hydrocarbons, heavy metals). Some xenobiotics are structurally related to nutrients, and others are not. In this chapter special emphasis is given to the biological fate of drugs entering the body by the oral route.

Xenobiotics are delivered with the food into the gastrointestinal tract. Although nutrients are degraded by digestive enzymes, xenobiotics are usually not chemically altered in the lumen of the upper intestine. However, they must be solubilized before they can get into contact with the intestinal mucosa.

The mucosa is a sheet of metabolically highly active cells (enterocytes) that are tightly connected to each other, forming a barrier between the "outside" and the "inside" of the organism.

A compound is considered absorbed when it has crossed the mucosal barrier and reached the intercellular space of the lamina propria, from where it may enter the blood capillaries or the lymphatics. If a compound is rapidly absorbed, the intestine's "permeability" for this molecule is high.

Most nutrients are efficiently and actively absorbed, whereas xenobiotics are absorbed to varying degrees. The pharmacologist aims at developing drugs with rapid absorption; the toxicologist worries about absorption of potentially hazardous xenobiotics. The factors determining the extent of absorption include physiochemical features of xenobiotics, events in the lumen, features of the mucosa, events in the submucosa, and pathophysiological conditions.

PRESYSTEMIC FATE OF XENOBIOTICS

Xenobiotics in the gastrointestinal lumen encounter a wide variety of different conditions on their way to the central circulatory system of the body. Presystemic or first-pass effect means irreversible extraction and/or biotransformation of xenobiotics on their passage through the intestinal wall and the liver. Under the influence of these tissue-specific factors, the physiochemical properties of the chemical compounds may change, and their fate within the body will be modified by the microenvironment to which they are exposed. Figure 1 depicts the various situations that determine the fate of drugs and other xenobiotics when they interact with the various tissues and organs of the organism.

Alterations by Gut Flora, Gastric, and Intestinal Secretions

Usually the stomach, the duodenum, and the jejunum of the human gut are relatively germ-free. If drugs pass into the lower small intestinal segments or into the colon, the intestinal flora can play a role in drug metabolism and degradation (102). Furthermore, when under pathological conditions such as intestinal blind loops and diminished propulsive motility or when achlorhydric gastric juices are present, drugs may be broken down by the ascending gut flora. Bacteria can break hydrolytic bonds (β-glucuronidases, ref. 105; glycoside hydrolysis, ref. 106) and carry out reduction and dehydrogenation reactions (30). Moreover, some drugs are unstable at acidic or neutral pH values, leading to unsoluble precipitates that are eliminated through the feces.

Intestinal and Hepatic First Pass

If a drug is soluble and is lipophilic to some degree, it passively permeates into the epithelial cell layer of the small intestine. Most drugs are absorbed at the level of the upper small intestine (duodenum, jejunum) owing to the huge surface area and the neutral pH value at this site. Intestinal first-pass effect of xenobiotics represents the irreversible extraction and/or biotransformation of xenobiotics while

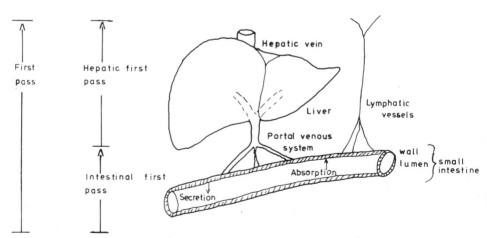

FIG. 1. Presystemic blood circulation. Presystemic fate of drugs and other xenobiotics on oral administration.

passing through the gut wall. The portal venous blood that drains the intestinal wall contains the unchanged drug as well as metabolic products of the intestinal biotransformation. However, some xenobiotics are channeled into the lymphatics or secreted back into the lumen (66) by the action of the epithelial cells. Highly lipophilic drugs (griseofulvin) can be incorporated into chylomicrons and leave the gut by the lymphatic vessels, thus bypassing the liver (115). Conjugated water-soluble compounds may be formed by intestinal metabolism and secreted into the lumen, thus being disposed of by the action of the intestinal tissue itself. Further-more, some compounds could stay within the epithelial cells of the mucosa, being sloughed into the lumen at the end of the life-span of these cells.

Intestinal biotransformation reactions of xenobiotics can be measured kinetically in the portal venous blood. In contrast to the liver, first-order drug kinetics do not apply because the enzymatic activity of the mucosa is saturated owing to the relatively high-tissue concentrations of xenobiotics. Therefore Michaelis-Menten kinetics are to be expected, since intestinal metabolism is capacity-limited (82). Salicylamide is completely conjugated at low doses and therefore therapeutically not effective (8). At higher doses the enzymatic activity is saturated, and the unmetabolized drug appears in the portal venous blood. The intestinal first-pass effect is responsible for the reduced bioavailability of drugs undergoing intestinal biotransformation (29). The systemic bioavailability, however, is largely dependent on the hepatic first-pass effect, which similarly means irreversible extraction and/or biotransformation on passage through the liver. Usually the hepatic first-pass effect of the liver is much greater than that of the intestine, since the liver contains the highest metabolic biotransformation capacity of the human body. The effect of the hepatic first pass can be measured directly when a catheter is placed into the hepatic vein and drug concentrations are monitored at that side. Recently, computer-aided methods using classical data of drug kinetics were used to determine and differ-entiate the first-pass effect of liver and gut (9,74). Thus, drugs entering the body by the oral route can be subject to a wide variety of modifications caused by the functional and morphological characteristics of the gut and liver.

PRINCIPLES OF XENOBIOTIC ABSORPTION

This chapter describes factors that are potentially rate-limiting in the absorption of xenobiotics. It also evaluates findings on the secretory function of the intestine for xenobiotics. For additional literature, the reader is referred to extensive mono-graphs on intestinal absorption in man (73) and on principles of drug absorption (51,63).

Mucosal Absorption of Xenobiotics

We will first assume that an ingested xenobiotic is well dissolved and gets in touch with the brush border membrane. There are two major possibilities for its mucosal absorption: There is the transcellular route where it is taken up by the brush border membrane, travels through the enterocyte, and is transferred to the intercellular space via the basal/lateral membrane. And there is the paracellular route where it migrates across the junctions between cells. The various mechanisms of transfer are depicted are Fig. 2 and are briefly discussed in the following sections.

Transcellular Diffusion

Diffusion via the transcellular route is the mechanism by which small hydrophilic (dimethylnitrosamine) or lipophilic (benzpyrene) xenobiotics can rapidly be absorbed (81,86). Small hydrophilic molecules presumably move through hydrophilic gaps at the protein-lipid interphases of the brush border membrane into the intracellular space and then through similar gaps of the basal/lateral membrane into the intercellular space. Lipophilic compounds may be integrated into the lipid layer of the brush border membrane and are then moved by lateral membrane flow to the basal/lateral membrane, where they are detached. Diffusion is neither saturable nor energy-dependent, and the substrates follow their electrochemical gradient. Based on the studies of Schanker and co-workers, it is believed that the majority of drugs are mainly absorbed by transcellular diffusion in the stomach (95), intestine (96), and colon (93).

Facilitated Diffusion

A more elaborate mode of absorption is "facilitated diffusion." Transport is facilitated by carrier proteins immersed into both the brush border membrane and the basal/lateral membrane. Absorption of short-chain fatty acids is catalyzed by

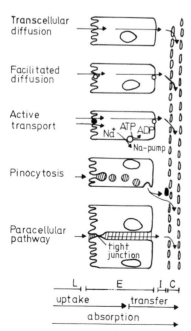

FIG. 2. Mucosal absorption of xenobiotics. *Open circles*, facilitated diffusion; *closed circles*, active transport. L, lumen; E, enterocyte; I, intercellular space; C, capillary. The basement membrane is not shown. ADP, adenosine diphosphate.

such mechanisms (65), and it appears possible that xenobiotics with carboxy groups might share similar routes (14). There are indications that heavy metal ions such as lead (5) or cadmium (26) in animals or zinc in humans (80) are absorbed by facilitated diffusion, and indirect evidence suggests that sulfate and glucuronide esters also follow this route, as outlined above. Since the involved carrier proteins are restricted in number, the transport capacity is limited. Carriers can transport their substrates in both directions; the net flux follows the downhill electrochemical gradient of the substrates.

Active Transport

This is an even more complex mechanism. A carrier, similar to that of facilitated diffusion, located in the brush border membrane, moves the substrate into the cell. The carrier's action, however, is coupled to a biological energy source, such as cellular adenosine triphosphate (ATP) or a transmembraneous Na^+ gradient. The substrate can therefore be taken up by enterocytes even against its electrochemical gradient. In the case of sugars, which have been best studied, the substrate is then transferred from the cells into the submucosa by facilitated diffusion (57).

Active transport is the mode of absorption of hydrophilic nutrients like sugars, amino acids, vitamins, and nucleosides. Therefore it is not surprising that therapeutically used antimetabolites such as 5-fluorouracil (94) or antibiotics with peptide-like structures (108) are also specifically absorbed. Active absorption of xenobiotics that are dissimilar to nutrients has also been reported (23,62).

It is not clear whether it is facilitated diffusion or active transport that is of general importance for those hydrophilic xenobiotics that are poor diffusers. Carrier-mediated transport can only be experimentally assessed on intact intestinal preparations in the absence of metabolism and with relevantly low substrate concentrations. These conditions were not always considered in the past. Further experiments involving the whole intestinal wall or preparations such as brush border membrane vesicles (89) and isolated intestinal cells (38) may help to resolve this question of carrier involvement.

Pinocytosis

It is clinically evident that some large xenobiotic molecules such as hemagglutinins or phalloidins are, to certain degrees, absorbed by the intestine, since they cause systemic intoxications. Even the absorption of particles has been observed and has been termed "persorption." By analogy to the absorption of immunoglobulins in the newborn, it has been assumed that large molecules and particles are taken up by pinocytosis (110): The brush border membrane invaginates, enclosing a vesicle with luminal content. The vesicle is delivered to the lateral aspect of the membrane and empties its contents into the intercellular space. This process can be visualized in electron microscopy studies (92). Interest in intestinal pinocytosis has decreased since it became clear that pinocytosis was not involved in fat absorption (91). To which extent it is involved in xenobiotic absorption is not clear at the moment. But as an alternative to pinocytosis, large molecules might be absorbed via the paracellular route.

Paracellular Pathway

The "tight junctions" connect neighboring enterocytes with bands of macromolecules just beneath the brush borders and thus assure the barrier function of the mucosa. Even intact junctions are not completely tight. They are, to a certain extent, permeable to water and inorganic cations, and it has been assumed that they are also permeable to xenobiotics (90). These molecules migrate along the paracellular pathway by diffusion. The quantitative importance of the paracellular pathway compared with the transcellular pathway is a matter of dispute. Since the tight junctions are leakier in the duodenum and jejunum than in the ileum (83), further comparative studies between absorption in jejunum and ileum are required to resolve this problem.

Luminal Factors

Ingested xenobiotics are delivered via the stomach into the upper small intestine, where they may be dissolved in the aqueous phase of the luminal content. Solubilized molecules are promoted and "stirred" by intestinal motility in the lumen; however, prior to reaching the mucosa, they have to diffuse through three different layers, the largest being the "unstirred layer." Physically it is a layer of immobile water, adjacent to the mucosa. It has a diameter of about 200 to 500 μ, and reduces the intestinal stirred surface by a factor of 100 compared with the mucosal surface (113). This unstirred layer decreases the rate of absorption, both of actively transported nutrients and passively transported drugs, but its barrier function is greatest for hydrophobic molecules. The second layer is a mucus layer, which protects the mucosa surface from injuries; it may restrict diffusion (12). The third layer is a proton-rich sheet called "acid microclimate," which affects the protonation of weak acids and bases (50). It is opposed by the fixed negative charges of the membrane surface. The acid microclimate layer influences the permeability of weak acids and weak bases. At the neutral pH of the intestinal lumen, weak acids diffuse through the unstirred layer and the mucus layer mainly in the anionic form, whereas weak bases diffuse in the protonized form. Weak acids may take up a proton at the acid microclimate layer, thus becoming lipophilic and then diffuse into the membrane. Weak bases will remain protonized and this may favor their approach to the negatively charged membrane surface.

Lipophilic molecules are contained in the fat fractions of food (75). Because of their poor aqueous solubility, their concentration in the diffusion layers would be very low if there was not a specific fat digestion process: When the gastric content is emptied into the duodenal lumen, the gallbladder contracts and releases bile into the duodenum. The biliary micelles solubilize not only fat and cholesterol, but also lipophilic xenobiotics to varying extents (48). Since the micelles are readily water soluble, they may diffuse to the brush border, carrying along the xenobiotics in high concentrations (Fig. 3). When the micelles are degraded by digestive enzymes, the xenobiotic molecules are released and may be absorbed into the lipid phase of the brush border membrane. Sometimes micelle formation has, however, an inhibitory effect. This may occur if a xenobiotic has, by itself, a reasonable water solubility. Its insertion in micelles may then decrease its free concentrations at the brush border surface and thus delay its absorption (2). Many experimental studies on uptake of lipophilic xenobiotics were either performed in the absence of micelles or they employed undigestible, unphysiological solubilizers. Therefore, our knowledge on the luminal events in the *in vivo* absorption of lipophilic xenobiotics is still very restricted.

Submucosal Factors

If a compound is absorbed and enters the submucosal space, its further fate depends on a variety of factors. One of them is the binding to macromolecules. Some xenobiotics such as DDT are partly incorporated into chylomicrons (101). These large aggregates do not fit through the fenestrae between the endothelial cells and are therefore delivered with the lymph. Other xenobiotics are incorporated into lipoproteins (72). But the majority is bound to serum albumin or blood cells and therefore readily enters the blood capillaries. In each instance, association with macromolecules acts like a sink, lowering the free concentration of the xenobiotic in the intercellular space and thus promoting its absorption. Xenobiotic absorption is also enhanced by a mechanism called "solvent-drag": Water that is actively absorbed pulls dissolved molecules into the submucosal space (77). Furthermore, the rate of absorption depends on blood flow (115). Blood delivers oxygen required for active transport processes, "stirres" the submucosa, and carries away absorbed xenobiotics. Finally, it has been proposed that a countercurrent distribution within the villus (114) may delay absorption. However, the exchange distance in the human villus is short so that the venous-arterial exchange is probably negligible.

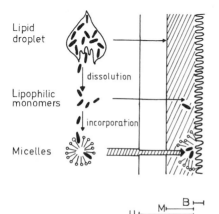

FIG. 3. Approach of lipids to the brush border. B, brush border; M, mucus; U, unstirred layer; L, lumen. The width of the *arrows* indicates the rates of diffusion.

Localization of Absorption Along the Gastrointestinal Tract

Some compounds are well absorbed from the buccal mucosa (mouth), and this route is utilized therapeutically for rapid treatment of angina pectoris with nitro compounds. The absorptive capacity of the esophagus has not been extensively studied. The stomach usually absorbs considerably less than 20% of ingested xenobiotics. The peculiarity of the stomach is its acidic luminal milieu. Weak organic acids are protonized and readily diffuse across the membrane (49), thus transporting protons into the cells. Consequently, the intracellular space is acidified, which may lead to cellular damage.

The duodenum and jejunum have a large inner surface and possess a higher paracellular permeability (83) than other parts of the gastrointestinal tract, thus providing better conditions for absorption. Some heavy metals are preferentially absorbed from the duodenum (25), whereas nutrients and most drugs are mainly absorbed in the jejunum. The transport systems for bile acids and cobalamine are exclusively localized in the ileum. The localization of postulated xenobiotic carriers has not been studied. The colon and rectum readily absorb a variety of drugs, as indicated by the therapeutic usefulness of enemas. Drugs absorbed via this route can bypass the liver on their way to the systemic circulation.

Intestinal Secretion of Xenobiotics

The intestine is not only the major organ of xenobiotic absorption, but also a secretory organ for xenobiotics. Hydrophilic organic compounds of differing chemical structure, such as cardiac glycosides, ammonium bases, and anionic dyes (66), are actively secreted into the intestinal lumen. Furthermore, heavy metal ions (39) and highly lipophilic xenobiotics (15,87) are also delivered into the gut lumen. Interestingly, fecal elimination of such lipophilic toxins can be augmented by oral administration of paraffin (87) or cholestyramine (33), and has been used in attempts to detoxify humans (33).

The mechanisms of secretion are still unknown; however, various possibilities are depicted in Fig. 4. Active secretion may be either mediated by the absorptive enterocytes or by cells specialized for excretion of mucus and enzymes. Passive

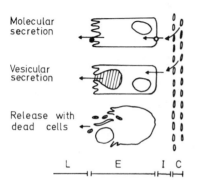

FIG. 4. Intestinal elimination of xenobiotics. L, lumen; E, enterocytes; I, intercellular space; C, capillary. *Open circle*, facilitated diffusion; *closed circle*, active transport.

elimination of xenobiotics may occur together with the release of dead cells; this may be the route for heavy metals and highly lipophilic chemicals.

HUMAN INTESTINAL ABSORPTION

Human intestinal absorption is governed by the principles of absorption laid out in the former chapter. However, a wide variety of pathophysiological conditions exist which alter the process of intestinal absorption. If a given gastrointestinal disease is diagnosed, it is important to identify the pathophysiological mechanism in order to predict the effects on absorption.

Methods

In man the absorption of drugs is usually measured by comparing the bioavailability after intravenous (i.v.) and oral administration (88). After oral administration if the bioavailability—as determined by the area under drug concentration versus time curve—is reduced when compared with i.v. administration, it could mean decreased absorption on the one hand or a high degree of first-pass elimination on the other hand. Therefore when using this method, it is essential to measure the metabolite concentrations as well as to determine the extent of absorption. To quantify the rate of absorption in humans, computer programs have been used (64).

The application of radiolabeled drugs to measure drug retention in the body (using the whole body, urinary, and fecal excretion of radioactivity) is a very reliable method for estimating absorption (11,79). Recently, a simultaneous i.v., and oral administration of differently labeled drugs (i.v. ^{3}H; orally, ^{14}C) was given to obtain a convenient estimate of drug absorption (56).

Simple intestinal perfusion studies with intubation of the upper small intestine yield information on the disappearance of drugs from the lumen (42). Disappearance could mean absorption, but it could also mean binding to the epithelial surface or uptake in the mucosal layer without transfer into circulation. If a drug is completely excreted into the urine then, of course, the amount of drug in the urine can be taken as the fraction of drug absorbed.

Therefore, when studying drug absorption, the biological and physiochemical properties of the compound determine the method to be used. Furthermore, methods applicable to measuring the intestinal first-pass effect of drugs can also be used to assess the absorption rates and is mentioned later.

Factors Affecting Gastrointestinal Absorption

The absorption rate of a drug is highest in the upper small intestine, since in this segment the greatest surface area is available for passive diffusion (60). For absorption all drugs have to be in a soluble form and should possess some lipophilic properties (51). Thus, absorption of particulate drug formulations depends on the dissolution rate of tablets, as has been shown for aspirin (69) and phenacetin (76).

Also, the intraluminal milieu, especially the pH value, fluid, and food content, influences the solubility and the water-fat coefficient of drugs. Mechanical factors, especially the "mixing gut motility," increase the disintegration and dissolution rates, and the intraluminal juices derived from bile, stomach, pancreas, and intestinal mucosa contribute to the composition of intestinal fluid and to the stability of the drug solution (76,100). Table 1 lists the factors known to modify human drug absorption.

The gastric emptying rate is reduced by a fatty meal and inhibition of gastric motility delays acetaminophen absorption (84). Food, in general, decreases drug absorption rates; however, some drugs (doxycycline, griseofulvin, nitrofurantoin) are absorbed faster probably by a bile-acid-mediated mechanism (107). Intestinal motility is accelerated in hyperthyroidism and in enteritis with diarrhea, leading to reduced drug absorption when the dissolution or absorption process of a drug is slow (76). The surface area is diminished in patients with gluten-sensitive enteropathy and after intestinal resection (short bowel syndrome). Enterohepatic circulation (intestinal reabsorption after biliary drug excretion) can lead to prolongation and a second peak of absorption (3,61), and this mechanism is interrupted by cholestyramine or colestipol. Using these anion-binding resins, digitoxin intoxication can be treated by interfering with its reabsorption. The permeability of the intestinal mucosa is increased in patients with gluten-sensitive enteropathy, thus allowing entry of large sugar molecules (cellobiose) into the bloodstream (34). Under these circumstances nonabsorbable toxic carbohydrates like acarbose, which is a new therapeutic agent for diabetes mellitus, could pass into the circulation. However, other investigators have shown that in treated patients with sprue-syndrome, low molecular weight polyethylene glycol less efficiently permeates through the small intestinal mucosa (17). Intestinal blood flow rarely limits drug absorption except when a general circulatory failure is present as in shock syndrome (51,76). Some drugs, when taken simultaneously on oral administration, form insoluble complexes that render them nonabsorbable. If iron salts and tetracyclines are administered together, a precipitating complex is formed which inhibits the absorption of either drug (76).

TABLE 1. *Factors affecting drug absorption*

Gastric emptying rate
Gastric pH
Intestinal motility
Food content
Surface area of small intestine
Intestinal blood flow
Enterohepatic circulation
Permeability of mucosa
Concomitant drug therapy

See also (4) and (32).

Clinical Consequences of Changes in Drug Absorption

If the aforementioned factors reduce drug absorption, some alterations of pharmacokinetics and pharmacodynamics are to be expected to have various clinical consequences. Reduced gastric emptying, food, and diminished mucosal surface area delay peak blood concentrations of drugs and lower maximum serum levels even though the total amount absorbed may be unchanged. When high blood levels are necessary to obtain the desired therapeutic effect (such as high bactericidal levels of antibiotics), delayed absorption rates may render a drug ineffective. On the other hand, when maintenance of a therapeutic level over a long time period is needed (such as for theophylline in asthmatics), slow extended absorption rates are an advantage, particularly since high theophylline concentrations can easily reach the toxic range. Thus, for drugs with a low therapeutic index (ratio between toxic and therapeutic drug levels) like theophylline, a sustained-release form is preferred whereas for drugs with a high index (penicillin), an accelerated absorption rate of short duration is acceptable or sometimes desirable. Therefore, changes in the absorption rate can significantly affect drug blood levels and bioavailability and consequently explain differences of drug action among individuals. Basically the same principles and factors can govern the absorption of xenobiotics. However, little data have been published in relation to absorption of environmentally important foreign compounds. Recently it was shown that the highly lipophilic chemical pollutant chlordecone is reabsorbed while undergoing extensive enterohepatic circulation and that its elimination can be increased by intraluminal binding to cholestyramine (33).

PRINCIPLES OF INTESTINAL DRUG METABOLISM

There are two different systems of intestinal xenobiotic metabolism. The first is located in the intestinal lumen and catalyzed by microorganisms. Its function has been reviewed elsewhere (97) and will not be considered here. The other is located in the intestinal mucosa and is catalyzed by enzymes of the enterocytes. It has been reviewed by Hartiala (75) and will be the subject of this chapter.

Like other epithelial cells (19), enterocytes are capable of performing phase 1 and phase 2 biotransformations of xenobiotics. Most phase 1 reactions involve cytochrome P-450, a drug-metabolizing enzyme system, immersed in the endoplasmatic reticulum, which catalyzes various oxidative and reductive reactions and often introduces free hydroxy groups into foreign molecules. These products usually undergo phase 2 reactions, in which they are conjugated with hydrophilic residues such as sulfate or glucuronic acid.

Though the intestinal cytochrome P-450 contents and the rates of most phase 1 reactions are about 10 times below the corresponding hepatic values, the intestine clearly contributes to the oxidation of various xenobiotics, such as benzo[a]pyrene (10) or perazine (13).

Some phase 2 reactions, such as glucuronidation and sulfation, proceed at almost the same velocity in intestinal cells as in liver cells. This might lead to an intestinal presystemic detoxication of plant phenols. Furthermore, intestinal conjugation reduces the bioavailability of phenolic drugs such as salicylamide (8), estrogens (99), isoprenaline (28), morphine (109), and others. The mucosa also contains hydrolases for the cleavage of conjugates, but in most cases studied, the equilibrium is on the side of conjugate formation.

Several peculiarities of mucosal drug metabolism are worth mentioning: First, the newly formed metabolites can leave the enterocytes not only via the basal/lateral membrane into the circulation, but also via brush border membrane back into the lumen. This has been documented for salicylamide (8) and estrogens (98,99). The disposition in the intestine thus becomes a complex kinetic event, including elimination and reabsorption (58) of conjugates (Fig. 5).

Second, the intestinal mucosa is exposed to higher concentrations of xenobiotics than other organs. Since some of these xenobiotics, e.g., benzopyrene or flavones, are powerful enzyme inducers of the drug-metabolizing system, the activity of these systems varies with the content of natural inducers in the chow of experimental animals. Finally, the drug-metabolizing enzymes are contained only in the mature tip cells but not in the proliferative crypt cells (47). This local separation of cell division from the hazardous reactive intermediates formed in phase 1 reactions may be a cause for the very low cancer incidence in the small intestine.

HUMAN INTESTINAL BIOTRANSFORMATION

Human Intestinal Biotransformation *In Vivo*

The biotransformation capacity of the small intestine and colon has been largely investigated in experimental animals, and a wide variety of metabolic reactions were found to be catalyzed by mucosal enzymes (18,24,35,40,47,103). The xenobiotic metabolizing activity of the gut was firmly established and thoroughly examined at the enzymatic or tissue level, and the results of these studies proved that the metabolic machinery exists in the intestinal mucosa. It is, however, difficult to

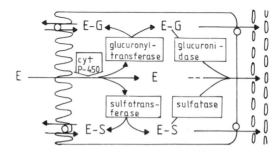

FIG. 5. Metabolic disposition of estrogens in intestinal mucosa cells (58,98,99). E, estrogen; E-G, estrogen glucuronide; E-S, estrogen sulfate. *Open circles*, membrane transport systems. Only a small fraction of estrogens are hydroxylated by cytochrome P-450. Large fractions are conjugated with sulfate and glucuronic acid. Part of the conjugate is transiently released into the lumen; the other part is transferred into blood, being partly deconjugated.

demonstrate whether or not the intestinal enzyme activity has a functional impact *in vivo*. Therefore, it is essential to show that drugs are biotransformed on their passage through the gut wall by studying the venous outflow of the parent compound and its metabolites in the blood draining the gut segment before the liver is reached (115). Other models for studying the intestinal biotransformation of animals *in vivo* include the everted gut segments (41), isolated intestinal epithelial cells (36), and perfusion experiments (42). In humans the *in vivo* significance of intestinal biotransformation of xenobiotics was investigated by several methods (Table 2).

Methods

The cannulation of the portal venous blood draining an isolated gut segment is the most valuable approach to determining the quantitative and qualitative aspects of biotransformation (Table 2). These procedures are used either during an abdominal operation or in patients with portal hypertension as part of their hemodynamic workup. However, under these circumstances a cautious interpretation of the data is necessary since the stress of the operation, the hemodynamic pertubation caused by the catheter or the portal hypertension have to be taken into account. Furthermore, there is a recirculation of blood coming from the liver into the portal venous system, which reaches the gut by the arterial blood supply. However, the portal cannulation is still the most direct approach to investigate intestinal biotransformation *in vivo*.

The intestinal biotransformation can also be evaluated indirectly by measuring the intestinal first-pass effect (29). If the area under concentration versus time curve after oral, intraperitoneal (i.p.), and i.v. drug administration is known, the intestinal contribution can be determined by subtracting the oral from the i.p. area (27,88). Recently computer-aided models have been described which use published data and conventional drug kinetics to calculate hepatic and intestinal presystemic elimination (9,74).

TABLE 2. *Human intestinal metabolism of xenobiotics* in vivo

Substrate	Type of metabolism	% of dose metabolized	Model	Refs.
Androstenedione	Hydroxylation (3α + β)	80	Isolated intestinal loop	59
Androstanolone	Sulfate conjugation (3α)	67	with intraluminal	
	Glucuronidation (3β)	12	application and	
Androstenolon-glucuronide	Hydrolysis	100	portal venous drainage	
Oestriol	Glucuronidation	n	Isolated intestinal loop	22
Oestron			(see above)	
Pivampicillin	Hydrolysis	99	Intraportal cannulation	70
Flurazepam	N-Dealkylation	90	Intraportal cannulation	71
	N-Hydroxylation			
Phenacetin	O-Dealkylation	10	Intraportal cannulation	52

n, Amount metabolized not reported ("considerable").

Metabolic Reactions In Vivo

There are only a few investigations that have directly established the extent and type of intestinal biotransformation *in vivo* (Table 2).

Steroid hormones can undergo hydroxylation reactions (phase 1 metabolism) and thereafter the polar product is conjugated with either glucuronic acid or sulfate (phase 2 metabolism). Glucuronidation reactions are very actively catalyzed by the intestinal mucosa, thus permitting a high degree of biotransformation of phenolic compounds. From the benzodiazepines, flurazepam is almost completely metabolized by monooxygenases in the small intestine at least in patients with liver cirrhosis and portal hypertension. The direct approach by portal cannulation can not be performed in subjects with normal liver function who might yield different data.

Insufficient liver function could be compensated for by metabolic adaptation of the intestinal mucosa. Originally it was assumed that the analgesic drug phenacetin could be mainly metabolized by the gut (20). The direct portal cannulation method however did not support this concept, since only less than 10% of the dose was biotransformed in the intestinal wall in man (52). Therefore, results of enzymatic studies have to be substantiated by *in vivo* experiments to validate the physiological significance of these observations.

Antibiotics such as pivampicillin are almost completely hydrolyzed by the intestinal mucosa. Hydrolysis of luminally absorbed glucuronides of steroid hormones was equally effective. Based on evidence from animal experiments, it is likely that a wide variety of other drugs are subject to intestinal biotransformation. Glucuronidation of morphine, for instance, takes place in the gut wall on oral administration of this compound leading to a pharmacologically inactive drug metabolite (54). Therefore, morphine is a more effective drug when given intravenously. Other drugs including nalorphine, naloxone, buprenorphine, salicylamide, terbutaline, isoprenaline, and isoproterenol, are conjugated by glucuronidation and sulfation, thus losing their pharmacodynamic effect despite their high degree of absorption (27,43,67,85). Glycosides like proscillaridin probably lose their cardiac activity by intestinal conjugation (3).

Intestinal Biotransformation *In Vitro*

Methods

Intestinal mucosa can be obtained by several types of biopsy tubes, which under fluoroscopic control are placed into the upper jejunum. Multiple biopsy particles of the mucosa are taken by a hydraulic mechanism of the instrument that delivers sufficient material for histological and biochemical investigations (45). The tissue can be incubated for cell culture studies (31) or homogenized to prepare the subcellular enzyme-containing fraction (45). Surgically obtained specimens of gut tissue can be used to isolate microsomes from the small intestinal mucosa (45). These specimens yield enough material to determine the content of cytochrome P-450 and to perform enzyme kinetics. Since the human small intestine is equipped with stationary Kerckring's folds which prevent a simple scraping of the mucosa, a special freezing and thawing technique was developed to sample human intestinal enterocytes (45).

Metabolic Reactions In Vitro

There are some drugs that are candidates of intestinal first-pass biotransformation, since their *in vitro* metabolism has been demonstrated in intestinal tissue samples or preparations (Table 3). The capability of the intestinal mucosa for sulfate conjugation and glucuronidation of steroid hormones was confirmed *in vitro*. Other synthetic enzymatic reactions include acetylation and methylation. Oxidative metabolism of xenobiotics can be mediated by the cytochrome P-450 dependent enzyme system of the smooth endoplasmic reticulum (microsomal fraction) of the enterocytes (45) and include the following reactions: hydroxylation of aromatic polycyclic hydrocarbons and dealkylation of side chains of model drugs (Table 3). Biologically active sympathomimetic amines of the food can be detoxified by intestinal monoamine oxidase which are cytosolic enzymes. Hydrolytic cleavage of esters and deacetylation might assume significance for the bioavailability of some clinically important drugs (Table 3). The intestinal first-pass biotransformation of the drugs mentioned in Table 3 needs to be established by appropriate *in vivo* studies.

Most of the *in vitro* studies have been performed in the small intestinal mucosa, which possesses a higher enzyme activity than the colonic mucosa (112). However, the human colon contains monooxygenases and conjugation enzymes (glucuronidation, sulfate, and glutathion conjugation) with a wide range of activities among individuals (6), which might play a role in colonic carcinogenesis. The conjugation of hydroxylated benzo[*a*]pyrenes in this tissue proceeds preferentially by sulfation and glutathion conjugation.

TABLE 3. *Types of xenobiotic metabolism of human intestinal mucosa* in vitro

Type of metabolism	Substrate	Model	Refs.
Sulfate conjugation	Ethinyl estradiol	Culture of jejunal biopsies	7
Glucuronidation	Testosterone	Microsomes of jejunal mucosa	21
Acetylation	INH, PAS, sulfonamides	Jejunal mucosa (autopsy)	55
Hydroxylation	Tetrahydrocannabinols	Culture of jejunal biopsy	31
Dealkylation	7-Ethoxycoumarin	Microsomal enzymes of jejunum	45
Monooxygenation	Benzo[*a*]pyrene	Culture of colonic biopsies	6
Monoamine oxidation	Tyramine	Homogenate of jejunal biopsies	68
Esterhydrolysis	Clofibrate, aspirin	Purified enzymes	53
Deacylation	Procaine, acetyl gitoxin	Intestinal mucosal homogenate	37

INH, Isoniazid; PAS, *p*-aminosalicylic acid.

Modification of Intestinal Biotransformation

In experimental animals it has been shown that the xenobiotic metabolizing monooxygenase activity of the small intestine can be affected by factors that either elevate or reduce its activity (43). Cytochrome P-450 mediated enzyme activity is inducible by lipophilic xenobiotics with a long half-life in the tissue. Therefore, increased activity was found when the intestine was exposed to aromatic hetero-cyclic hydrocarbons (cigarette smoke, charcoal-broiled meat) or flavones and in-doles (vegetable-enriched diet). The inducing effect of the aromatic hydrocarbons was much higher when the inducer (methylcholanthrene) was administered orally than parenterally (i.v. or i.p.) (1). Nutrients that are essential for the structural integrity of the microsomal membrane such as cholesterol and for the molecular structure of cytochrome P-450 such as iron have to be present in the food. Their deficiency causes a rapid reduction of enzyme activity, occurring within 24 hours for iron (47). Unique is the exclusive dependency of the intestinal enzymes on the luminal supply of these factors, which suggests a delicate adaptation of biotrans-formation activity on exogenous factors arising from dietary nutrition (43). In man the enzymatic biotransformation capacity of the small intestine is controlled by similar influences as mentioned earlier.

Diet

Jejunal biopsy samples of healthy subjects were shown to exhibit activities of dihydronicotinamide adenine dinucleotide phosphate (NADPH)-cytochrome *c* re-ductase—the electron supplying enzyme for monooxygenation—and of 7-ethoxy-coumarin O-deethylase (EOD)—the dealkylating cytochrome P-450 dependent monooxygenase (45). On a presumably inducer-free semisynthetic diet, the activity of the monooxygenase was half that found on a normal home diet (46), while the reductase was unchanged. The normal home diet contains natural-inducing com-pounds from vegetables (indoles, flavones) and from incomplete pyrolysis of organic material (polycyclic hydrocarbons) (111). Furthermore, by feeding charcoal-broiled meat, which is an efficient inducer of the intestinal monooxygenases (78), the metabolism of phenacetin was enhanced *in vivo*, as has been shown by pharma-cokinetic studies (20).

Sex

There was a clear-cut sex difference of monooxygenase activity in jejunal biopsy tissue (46). The intrinsic enzyme activity was lower in female subjects than in males on semisynthetic diet, and this difference was maintained while the subjects were consuming the inducing home diet (Fig. 6). In human liver biopsies this sex difference was not found (45).

Disease

The gluten-sensitive enteropathy (nontropical sprue-syndrome) leads to a destruc-tion of the villous structure of the small intestinal mucosa with diminution or loss

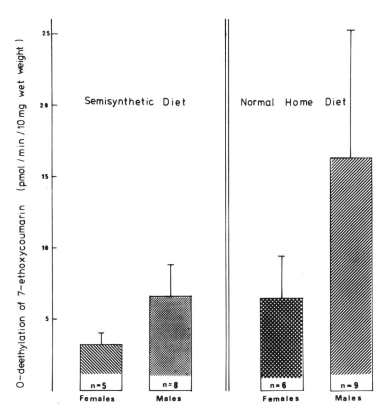

FIG. 6. Sex dependency of monooxygenase activity in jejunal mucosa of volunteers determined in 20,000 g supernatant of homogenate. The male subjects had significantly higher activities of 7-ethoxycoumarin O-deethylase than females on semisynthetic diets as well as on normal home diets. n = number of subjects per group.

of the villous height. In the jejunal mucosa of patients with this disease, the monooxygenase activity, and to a lesser degree the reductase activity, was clearly depressed or even absent (45). In patients with various forms of intestinal malassimilation, the monooxygenase activity was reduced despite maintenance of the villous structure (45). Therefore, the monooxygenase activity of the human small intestinal mucosa is mainly depleted by the loss of the villous morphology and less strikingly by undernutrition of the enterocytes.

Physiological Significance of Intestinal Biotransformation

Detoxification

The intestinal mucosa is exposed to a high concentration of a wide variety of xenobiotics contained in food. These foreign compounds include preservatives, colors, flavors, congeners, and industrial contaminations. No other organ of the body is challenged with such an amount and so high a concentration of potentially harmful chemicals as the intestinal mucosa.

Under these circumstances it is amazing that the gut mucosa is almost resistant to the development of functional and morphological damage by chemical injuries. The small intestinal mucosa particularly seems to deal effectively with toxic and carcinogenic compounds. Although these compounds rarely hurt the upper gut, the colonic mucosa is rather susceptible to damage by carcinogens like dimethylhydrazine and by laxatives like anthraquinone derivatives. The biological system for resistance to chemical injuries might reside in the microsomal enzyme system of the enterocytes which could protect the mucosal tissue from toxic damage by xenobiotics (43). Although the remainder of the body can be protected by the biotransformation capacity of the liver, the intestine itself as the portal of entry of xenobiotics has to rely on its own mechanisms of detoxification. That this metabolic system is highly effective was shown by the intestinal bioinactivation of phenol. On oral administration, this toxic compound is almost completely conjugated in the gut wall before it enters the bloodstream (16). Although the enzymatic biotransformation appears to explain the unique intestinal resistance to drugs, other properties e.g., the rapid shedding of epithelial cells and the local immune system, could contribute to this feature.

Some compounds could be cleared by the mucosal cells without ever reaching the blood circulation. Thus, it was shown that the mucosa contains intrinsic mechanisms that are responsible for uptake, conjugation, and luminal secretion of carcinogens like benzo[a]pyrene (41). This bioinactivation system may be capable of handling the relatively small amounts of dietary toxins (43).

The in vitro intestinal transfer of diphenolic laxatives is capacity-limited by the metabolic conjugation of these compounds (104). Transport to the serosal side of the gut wall is dependent on the degree of conjugation. The water-soluble conjugates travel to the mucosal side of the jejunum in contrast to the colon, where they are transported to the serosal side. These results suggest that the upper gastrointestinal tract may dispose of these potential toxins by enzymatic biotransformation and luminal secretion whereas the colonic mucosa lacks this disposal mechanism. The much higher incidence of cancer and inflammatory damage in the colon could be explained by its low biotransformation capacity; however, additional factors, e.g., bacterial flora, long exposure time of toxins, and longer turnover time of colonic cells, have to be considered.

Bioavailability

Despite their complete absorption, drugs that undergo extensive intestinal biotransformation might be pharmacologically inactive. This could be the reason why morphine and other strong analgesics are ineffective when administered orally. Animal experiments indicate that these compounds are conjugated and oxidatively metabolized by intestinal microsomes (85). For the analgesic drug salicylamide, there is a dose that is completely metabolized in the intestinal mucosa, thus saturating the microsomal enzymes. By increasing the dose, the capacity of glucuronidation and sulfation is overwhelmed, and the active, unmetabolized drug appears in the bloodstream (8). Therefore, to overcome the intestinal first-pass effect, a breakthrough dose is required.

However, in most instances the liver contributes more to the first-pass effect of drugs than the intestine, as was shown for propranolol, which is largely metabolized by hepatic enzymes.

CONCLUSION

Intestinal absorption and biotransformation of xenobiotics are processes that influence the biological fate of drugs and numerous other foreign compounds in man. The intestinal mucosa plays a decisive role in the interaction of drugs within the human body. This epithelial cell layer is positioned at the port of entry of orally taken xenobiotics. The properties of the mucosa plus the molecular structure of the chemical compound will determine whether the compound can travel into the organism. If absorption takes place, the biotransformation capacity of the mucosa can modify the character of the drug. Its profile of action can be changed by metabolic activation or inactivation and by controlling the transfer of the drug into the various body compartments.

Thus, the intestinal tissue is involved in the detoxification of xenobiotics and controls the bioavailability of certain drugs. Functional and morphological alterations of the gut mucosa affect the xenobiotic metabolizing enzyme activity of this tissue and could consequently influence the drug action in man. Therefore, intestinal factors have to be taken into account to explain the wide interindividual variability of the biological action of drugs and other xenobiotics.

REFERENCES

1. Aitio, A. (1974): Different elimination and effect on mixed function oxidase of 20-methylcholanthrene after intragastric and intraperitoneal administration. *Res. Comm. Chem. Pathol. Pharmacol.*, 9:701–709.
2. Amidon, G. E., Higuchi, W. I., and Ho, N. F. H. (1982): Theoretical and experimental studies of transport of micelle-solubilized solutes. *J. Pharm. Sci.*, 71:77–84.
3. Anderson, K. E., Bergdahl, B., Dencker, H., and Wettrell, G. (1977): Proscillaridin activity in portal and peripheral venous blood after oral administration to man. *Eur. J. Clin. Pharmacol.*, II:277–281.
4. Aslaksen, A., Aanderud, L. (1980): Drug absorption during physical exercise. *Br. J. Clin. Pharmacol.*, 10(4):383–385.
5. Aungst, B. J., and Fung, H. L. (1981): Kinetic characterization of in vitro lead transport across the rat small intestine. *Toxic. Appl. Pharmacol.*, 61:39–47.
6. Autrup, H. (1982): Carcinogen metabolism in human tissues and cell. *Drug Metabol. Rev.*, 13(4):603–646.
7. Back, D. J., Bates, M., Breckenridge, A. M., Ellis, A., Hall, J. M., Maciver, M., Orne, M. L'E., and Rowe, P. H. (1981): The in vitro metabolism of ethinyloestradiol, mestranol and levonorgestrel by human jejunal mucosa. *Br. J. Clin. Pharmacol.*, 11(3):275–278.
8. Barr, W. H., and Riegelmann, S. (1970): Intestinal drug absorption and metabolism II: Kinetic aspects of intestinal glucuronide conjugation. *J. Pharm. Sci.*, 59:164–168.
9. Bloch, R., Sweeney, G., Ahmed, K., Dickinson, C. J., and Ingram, D. (1980): "Mac Dope": a

simulation of drug disposition in the human body: applications in clinical pharmacokinetics. *Br. J. Clin. Pharmacol.*, 10(6):596–602.

10. Bock, K. W., Clausbruch von, U. C., and Winne, D. (1979): Absorption and metabolism of naphthalin and benzo(a)pyrene in the rat jejunum in situ. *Med. Biol.*, 57:262–264.

11. Bopp, B. A., Sonders, R. C., and Kesterson, J. W. (1982): Metabolic fate of selected selenium compounds in laboratory animals and man. *Drug Metab. Rev.*, 13(2):271–318.

12. Braybrooks, M. P., Barry, B. W., and Abbs, E. T. (1975): The effect of mucin on the bioavailability of tetracycline from the gastrointestinal tract; in vivo, in vitro correlations. *J. Pharm. Pharmacol.*, 27:508–515.

13. Breyer, U., and Winne, D. (1977): Absorption and metabolism of the phenothiazine drug perazine in the rat intestinal loop. *Biochem. Pharmacol.*, 26:1275–1280.

14. Bridges, J. W., Houston, J. B., Humphrey, M. J., Lindup, W. E., Parke, D. V., Shillingford, J. S., and Upshall, D. G. (1976): Gastrointestinal absorption of carbenoxolene in the rat determined in vitro and in situ: deviations from the Ph-partition hypothesis. *J. Pharm. Pharmacol.*, 28:117–126.

15. Bungay, P. M., Dedrick, R. L., and Matthews, H. B. (1981): Enteric transport of chlordecone (kepone) in the rat. *J. Pharmacokinet. Biopharm.*, 9:309–341.

16. Cassidy, M. K., and Houston, J. B. (1979): Protective role of intestinal and pulmonary enzymes against environmental phenols. *Proc. B.P.S.*, 316P.

17. Chadwick, V. S., Phillips, S. F., and Hofmann, A. F. (1977): Measurement of intestinal permeability using low molecular weight polyethylene glycols (PEG 400). II: Application to normal and abnormal permeability states in man and animals. *Gastroenterology*, 73:247–251.

18. Chhabra, R. S. (1979): Intestinal absorption and metabolism of xenobiotics. *Environ. Health Perspect.*, 33:61–69.

19. Connelly, J. C., and Bridges, J. W. (1980): The distribution and role of cytochrome P-450 in extrahepatic organs. In: *Progress in Drug Metabolism*, Vol. 5, edited by J. W. Bridges and L. F. Chasseaud, pp. 1–112. John Wiley & Sons, Chichester.

20. Conney, A. H., Pantuck, E. J., Hsiao, K.-C., Garland, W. A., Anderson, K. E., Alvares, A. P., and Kappas, A. (1976): Enhanced phenacetin metabolism in human subjects fed charcoal-broiled beef. *Clin. Pharmacol. Ther.*, 20:633–642.

21. Dahm, K., and Breuer, H. (1966): Characterisierung und Kinetik einer Mikrosomalen UDP-Glucuronat-Testeron-Glucuronyltransferase beim Menschen. *Hoppe-Seyler's 2. Physiol. Chem.*, 345:139–149.

22. Diczfalusy, E., Franksson, C., Lisboa, B. P., and Martinsen, B. (1962): Formation of oestrone glucosiduronate by lumen intestinal tract. *Acta Endocrinol.*, 40:537–551.

23. Dietschy, J. M., and Carter, N. W. (1965): Active transport of 5,5-dimethyl-2,4-oxazolidinedione. *Science*, 150:1294–1296.

24. Fang, W.-F., and Strobel, H. W. (1978): The drug and carcinogen metabolism system of rat colon microsomes. *Arch. Biochem. Biophys.*, 186:128–138.

25. Forth, W., and Rummel, W. (1975): Gastrointestinal absorption of heavy metals. In: *Pharmacology of Intestinal Absorption: Gastrointestinal Absorption of Drugs*, edited by W. Forth and W. Rummel, pp. 599–746. Pergamon Press, Oxford.

26. Foulkes, E. C. (1980): Some determinants of intestinal cadmium transport in the rat. *J. Environ. Pathol. Toxicol.*, 3:471–481.

27. George, C. F. (1981): Drug metabolism by the gastrointestinal mucosa. *Clin. Pharmacokinet.*, G:259–274.

28. George, C. F., Blackwell, F. W., and Davies, D. S. (1974): Metabolism of isoprenaline in the intestine. *J. Pharm. Pharmacol.*, 26:265–267.

29. Gibaldi, M., and Perrier, D. (1974): Route of administration and drug disposition. *Drug Metab. Rev.*, 3(2):185–199.

30. Goldmann, P. (1978): Biochemical pharmacology of the intestinal flora. *Annu. Rev. Pharmacol. Toxicol.*, 18:523–539.

31. Green, M. L., and Saunders, D. R. (1974): Metabolism of tetrahydrocannabinol by the small intestine. *Gastroenterology*, 66:365–372.

32. Greenblatt, D. J., Divoll, M., Abernethy, D. R., and Shader, R. J. (1982): Physiologic changes in old age: relation to altered drug disposition. *J. Am. Geriatr. Soc.*, 30(II):6–10.

33. Guzelian, P. S. (1982): Chlordecone poisoning: A case study in approaches for detoxification of humans exposed to environmental chemicals. *Drug Metab. Rev.*, 13:663–679.

34. Hamilton, I., Cobden, I., Rothwell, J., and Traxon, A. (1982): Intestinal permeability in coeliac disease: the response to gluten withdrawal and single dose gluten challenge. *Gut*, 23:202–210.
35. Hartiala, K. (1973): Metabolism of hormones, drug and other substances by the gut. *Physiol. Rev.*, 53:496–534.
36. Hartmann, F., Owen, R., and Bissell, M. D. (1982): Characterization of isolated epithelial cells from rat small intestine. *Am. J. Physiol.*, 242:G147–G155.
37. Haustein, K. O., Pachaly, C., Megges, R., and Franke, P. (1978): Investigation into the species-specific deacylation of pentaacetyl-gitoxin. *Eur. J. Clin. Pharmacol.*, 14(6):425–430.
38. Hegazy, E., Lopez del Pino, V., and Schwenk, M. (1983): Isolated enterocytes of high viability from guinea pig. *Eur. J. Cell. Biol.*, 30:132–136.
39. Henning, C. H., and Forth, W. (1982): The excretion of thallium (I)-ions into the gastrointestinal tract in situ of rats. *Arch. Toxicol.*, 49:149–158.
40. Hietanen, E. (1974): Effect of sex and castration on hepatic and intestinal activity of drug-metabolizing enzymes. *Pharmacology*, 12:84–89.
41. Hietanen, E. (1981): Oxidation and subsequent glucuronidation of 3,4-benzopyrene in everted intestinal sacs in control and 3-methyl-cholanthene-pretreated rats. *Pharmacology*, 21:233–243.
42. Ho, N. F. H., Park, J. Y., Amidon, G. E., Ni, F. P., and Higuchi, W. I. (1979): Methods for interrelating in vitro, animal and human absorption studies. In: *Gastrointestinal Absorption of Drugs*, edited by A. J. Aguiar. American Pharmaceutical Association, Academy of Pharmaceutical Sciences, Washington, D.C.
43. Hoensch, H. P., and Hartmann, F. (1981): The intestinal enzymatic biotransformation system: potential role in protection from colon cancer. *Hepatogastroenterology*, 28:221–228.
44. Hoensch, H., Hartmann, F., Schomerus, H., Bieck, P., and Doelle, W. (1979): Monooxygenase enzyme activity in alcoholics with varying degrees of liver damage. *Gut*, 20:666–672.
45. Hoensch, H. P., Hutt, R., and Hartmann, F. (1979): Biotransformation of xenobiotics in human intestinal mucosa. *Environ. Health Perspect.*, 33:71–78.
46. Hoensch, H., Steinhardt, H. J., Weiss, G., Haug, D., Maier, A., and Malchow, H. (1984): Effects of semisynthetic diets on xenobiotic metabolizing enzyme activity, disaccharidase activity and morphology of small intestinal mucosa in man. *Gastroenterology, (in press)*.
47. Hoensch, H. P., Woo, C. H., Raffin, S. B., and Schmid, R. (1976): Oxidative metabolism of foreign compounds in rat small intestine: cellular localization and dependence on dietary iron. *Gastroenterology*, 70:1063–1070.
48. Hofmann, A. F. (1976): Fat digestion: The interaction of lipid digestion products with micellar bile acid solutions. In: *Lipid Absorption: Biochemical and Clinical Aspects*, edited by K. Rommel and G. Goebell, pp. 3–22. MTP-press, Lancaster.
49. Hogben, C. A., Schanker, L. S., Tocco, D. J., and Brodie, B. B. (1957): Absorption of drugs from the stomach. II. The lumen. *J. Pharmacol. Exp. Ther.*, 120:540–545.
50. Hogben, C. A., Tocco, D. J., Brodie, B. B., and Schanker, L. S. (1959): On the mechanism of intestinal absorption of drugs. *J. Pharmacol. Exp. Ther.*, 125:275–282.
51. Houston, J. B., and Wood, S. G. (1980): Gastrointestinal absorption of drugs and other xenobiotics. In: *Progress in Drug Metabolism, Vol. 4*, edited by J. W. Bridges and L. F. Chasseaud, pp. 57–130. John Wiley & Sons, Chichester.
52. Inaba, T., Mahon, W. A., and Stone, R. M. (1979): Phenacetin concentrations in portal and hepatic venous blood in man. *Int. J. Clin. Pharmacol. Biopharmacy*, 17:371–374.
53. Inoue, M., Morikawa, M., Tsuboi, M., Ito, Y., and Sugiura, M. (1980): Comparative study of human intestinal and hepatic esterases as related to enzymatic properties and hydrolizing activity for ester-type drugs. *Jpn. J. Phmarmacol.*, 30(4):529–535.
54. Iwamoto, K., and Klaasen, C. D. (1977): First pass effect of nalorphin in rats. *J. Pharmacol. Exp. Ther.*, 203:365–376.
55. Jenne, J. W. (1963): Isoniazid acetylation by human liver and intestinal mucosa. *Fed. Proc.*, 22:540 (abstract).
56. Kenny, M. T., and Strates, B. (1981): Metabolism and Pharmacokinetics of the antibiotic rifampin. *Drug Metab. Rev.*, 12(1):159–218.
57. Kimmich, G. A. (1981): Gradient coupling in isolated intestinal cells. *Fed. Proc.*, 40:2474–2479.
58. Knapstein, P., Rindt, W., Treiber, L., and Oertel, G. W. (1966): Rekonjugation von (7-³H) androstenolon- (³⁵S)sulfat und (7-³H) androstenolon- (¹⁴C)-glucuronid in Dünndarm und Leber des Meerschweinchens. *Hoppe Seylers Z. Physiol. Chem.*, 346:192–197.
59. Knapstein, P., Treiber, L., Wendelberger, F., and Oertel, G. W. (1967): Metabolismus und Re-

konjugation von (7α-³H) Androstendion, (17α-³H) Androstenolon und (7α-³H) Androstenolon-sulfat in der menschlichen Darmwand in vivo. *Hoppe Seyler's Z. Physiol. Chem.*, 348:401–404.

60. Knoefel, P. K., Huang, K. C., Klingele, H. O., Le Fvre, P. G., Scharf, T. G., and Westphal, U. F. (1972): *Absorption, Distribution, Transformation and Excretion of Drugs*, pp. 39–55. C.C. Thomas, Springfield.

61. Kwan, K. C., Breault, G. O., Davis, R. L., Lei, B. -W., Czerwinski, A. W., Besselaar, G. H., and Duggan, D. E. (1978): Effects of concomitant aspirin administration on the pharmacokinetics of indomethacin in man. 3. *Pharmacokinet. Biopharm.*, 6(6):451–476.

62. Kunze, H. (1968): Aktiver Transport als Komronente der enteralen Phenolrotresorption. *Naunyn Schmiedebergs Arch. Pharmacol.*, 259:260–265.

63. Kurz, H. (1975): Principles of drug absorption. In: *Pharmacology of Intestinal Absorption: Gastrointestinal Absorption of Drugs, Vol. 1*, edited by W. Forth and W. Rummel, pp. 245–296. Pergamon Press, Oxford.

64. Lambert, C., and du Sonich, P. (1981): Drug absorption: a practical method to estimate the absorption rate constant. *Res. Commun. Chem. Pathol. Pharmacol.*, 34(2):217–229.

65. Lamers, J. M. J., and Hülsmann, W. C. (1974): The effects of fatty acids on oxidative decarbox-ylation of pyruvate in rat small intestine. *Biochem. Biophys. Acta*, 394:31–45.

66. Lauterbach, F. (1977): Intestinal secretion of organic ions and drugs. In: *Intestinal Permeation*, edited by M. Kramer and F. Lauterbach, pp. 173–195. Excerpta Medica, Amsterdam.

67. Leopold, G. (1977): First pass-effect. *Arzneim. Forschl. Drug Res.*, 27(I):241–249.

68. Levine, R. J., and Sjoerdsma, A. (1963): Estimation of monoamine oxidase activity in man: Techniques and applications. *Ann. NY Acad. Sci.*, 107:966–974.

69. Levy, G. (1978): Clinical pharmacokinetics of aspirin. *Pediatrics*, 62:867–872.

70. Lund, B., Kampmann, J. P., Lindahl, F., and Hansen, J. M. (1976): Pivampicillin and ampicillin in bile, portal and peripheral blood. *Clin. Pharmacol. Ther.*, 19:587–591.

71. Mahon, W. A., Inaba, T., and Stone, R. M. (1977): Metabolism of flurazepam by the small intestine. *Clin. Pharmacol. Ther.*, 22:228–233.

72. Maliwal, B. P., and Guthrie, F. E. (1982): In vitro uptake and transfer of chlorinated hydrocarbons among human lipoproteins. *J. Lipid Res.*, 23:474–479.

73. McColl, I., editor (1975): *Intestinal Absorption in Man*. Academic Press, London.

74. Minchin, R. E., and Ilett, K. F. (1982): Presystemic elimination of drugs: theoretical considerations for quantifying the relative contribution of gut and liver. *J. Pharm. Sci.*, 71(4):458–460.

75. Morgan, R. G. H., and Hofmann, A. F. (1970): Synthesis and metabolism of glyceryl ³H-triether a nonabsorbable oil phase marker for lipid absorption studies. *J. Lipid. Res.*, 11:223.

76. Nimmo, J. (1980): Drugs: absorption and action. In: *Scientific Foundation of Gastroenterology*, edited by W. Sircus and A. N. Smith, pp. 141–147. William Heinemann Medical Books, London.

77. Ochsenfahrt, H., and Winne, D. (1974): The contribution of solvent drag to the intestinal absorption of the basic drugs amidopyrine and antipyrine from the jejunum of the rat. *Arch. Pharmacol.*, 281:175–196.

78. Pantuck, E. J., Hsiao, K. C., Kuntzman, R., and Conney, A. H. (1975): Intestinal metabolism of phenacetin in the rat: effect of charcoal-broiled beef and rat chow. *Science*, 187:744–746.

79. Payton, K. B. (1982): Technique for determination of human zinc absorption from measurement of radioactivity in a fecal sample or the body. *Gastroenterology*, 83:1264–1270.

80. Payton, K. B., Flanagan, P. R., Stinson, E. A., Chpdirker, D. P., Chamberlain, M. J., and Valberg, L. S. (1982): Technique for determination of human zinc absorption from measurement of radio-activity in a fecal sample or the body. *Gastroenterology*, 83:1264–1270.

81. Pegg, A. E. (1980): Formation and subsequent repair of alkylation lesions in tissues of rodents treated with nitrosamines. *Arch. Toxicol. [Suppl.]*, 3:55–68.

82. Pieniaszek, H. J., and Bates, T. R. (1979): Capacity-limited gut wall metabolism of 5-aminosal-icylic acid, a therapeutically active metabolite of sulfasalazine, in rats. *J. Pharmacol. Sci.*, 68:1323–1325.

83. Powell, D. W. (1981): Barrier function of epithelia. *Am. J. Physiol.*, 241:6275–6288.

84. Prescott, L. F. (1980): Kinetics and metabolism of paracetamol and phenacetin. *Br. J. Clin. Pharmacol.*, 10(2):2915–2985.

85. Rance, M. J., and Shillingford, J. S. (1976): The role of the gut in the metabolism of strong analgesics. *Biochem. Pharmacol.*, 25:735–741.

86. Rees, E. D., Mandelstam, P., Lowry, J. Q., and Lipscomb, H. (1971): A study of the mechanism of intestinal absorption of benzo(a)pyrene. *Biochem. Biophys. Acta*, 225:96–107.

87. Richter, E., Fichtl, B., and Schäfer, S. G. (1982): Effects of dietary paraffin, squalane and sucrose polyester on residue disposition and elimination of hexachlorobenzene in rats. *Chem. Biol. Interact.*, 40:335–344.

88. Rowland, M., Riegelman, S., Harris, P. A., Sholkoff, S. D., and Eyring, E. J. (1967): Kinetics and acetylsalicylic acid disposition in man. *Nature*, 215:413–414.

89. Ruifrok, P. G. (1981): Uptake of quaternary ammonium compounds into rat intestinal brush border membrane vesicles. *Biochem. Pharmacol.*, 30:2637–2641.

90. Ruifrok, P. G., and Mol, W. E. M. (1983): Paracellular transport of inorganic and organic ions across the rat ileum. *Biochem. Pharmacol.*, 32:637–640.

91. Sabesin, S. S., and Frase, S. (1977): Electron microscopic studies of the assembly, intracellular transport and secretion of chylomicrons by rat intestine. *J. Lipid Res.*, 18:496–511.

92. Sanders, E., and Ashworth, C. (1961): A study of particulate absorption and hepatocellular uptake. *Exp. Cell Res.*, 22:137–145.

93. Schanker, L. S. (1959): Absorption of drugs from the rat colon. *J. Pharmacol. Exp. Ther.*, 126:283–290.

94. Schanker, L. S., and Jeffrey, J. J. (1961): Active transport of foreign pyrimidines across the intestinal epithelium. *Nature*, 190:727–728.

95. Schanker, L. S., Shore, P. A., Brodie, B. B., and Hogben, A. M. (1957): Absorption of drugs from the stomach I: The rat. *J. Pharmacol. Exp. Ther.*, 120:528–539.

96. Schanker, L. S., Tocco, D. J., Brodie, B. B., and Hogben, C. A. (1958): Absorption of drugs from the rat small intestine. *J. Pharmacol. Exp. Ther.*, 123:81–88.

97. Scheline, R. R. (1973): Metabolism of foreign compounds by gastrointestinal microorganisms. *Pharmacol. Rev.*, 25:452–523.

98. Schwenk, M., Frank, B., Bolt, H. M., and Winne, D. (1981): Intestinal first pass effect of estrone sulfate and estrone in the rat. *Drug Res.*, 31:1254–1257.

99. Schwenk, M., Schiemenz, C., Lopez del Pino, V., and Remmer, H. (1982): First pass biotransformation of ethinylestradiol in rat small intestine in situ. *Naunyn Schmiedebergs Arch. Pharmacol.*, 321:223–225.

100. Scott, A. K., and Hawsworth, G. M. (1981): Drug absorption. *Br. Med. J.*, 282:462–463.

101. Sieber, S. M., Cohn, V. H., and Wynn, W. T. (1974) The entry of foreign compounds into the thoracic duct lymph of the rat. *Xenobiotica*, 4:265–284.

102. Smith, R. V. (1978): Metabolism of drugs and other foreign compounds by intestinal microorganisms. *World Rev. Nutr. Diet*, 29:60–76.

103. Stohs, S. J., Grafström, R. C., Burke, M. D., and Orrenius, S. (1976): Xenobiotic metabolism and enzyme induction in isolated rat intestinal microsomes. *Drug Metab. Dispos.*, 4:517–521.

104. Sund, R. B., and Hillestad, B. (1982): Uptake, conjugation and transport of laxative diphenols by everted sacs of the rat jejunum and stripped colon. *Acta Pharmacol. Toxicol.*, 51(4):377–387.

105. Takada, H., Hirooka, T., Hiramatsu, Y., and Yamamoto, M. (1982): Effect of beta-glucuronidase inhibitor on azoxymethane-induced colonic carcinogenesis in rats. *Cancer Res.*, 42:331–334.

106. Tamura, G., Gold, C., Ferro-Luzzi, A., and Ames, B. N. (1980): Fecalase: a model for activation of dietary glycosides to mutagens by intestinal flora. *Proc. Natl. Acad. Sci. USA*, 77:4961–4965.

107. Toothaker, R. D., and Welling, P. G. (1980): The effect of food on drug bioavailability. *Annu. Rev. Pharmacol. Toxicol.*, 20:173–199.

108. Tsuji, A., Nakashima, E., Kagami, I., and Yamana, T. (1981): Intestinal absorption mechanism of amphoteric β-lactam antibiotics II: Michaelis-Menten kinetics of cyclacillin absorption and its pharmacokinetic analysis in rats. *J. Pharm. Sci.*, 70:772–777.

109. Villar del, E., Sanchez, E., and Tephly, T. R. (1974): Morphine metabolism II. Studies on morphine glucuronyltransferase activity in intestinal microsomes of rats. *Drug Metab. Dispos.*, 2:370–374.

110. Walker, W. A., and Isselbacher, K. J. (1974): Uptake and transport of macromolecules by the intestine. *Gastroenterology*, 67:531–550.

111. Wattenberg, L. W. (1972): Dietary modification of intestinal and pulmonary aryl hydrocarbon hydroxylase activity. *Toxicol. Appl. Pharmacol.*, 23:741–748.

112. Wattenberg, L. W., Leong, J. L., and Strand, P. J. (1962): Benzpyrene hydroxylase activity in the gastrointestinal tract. *Cancer Res.*, 22:1120–1125.

113. Wilson, F. A., and Dietschy, J. M. (1974): The intestinal unstirred layer: Its surface area and effect on active transport kinetics. *Biochim. Biophys. Acta*, 363:112–126.
114. Winne, D. (1975): The influence of villous countercurrent exchange on intestinal absorption. *J. Theor. Biol.*, 53:145–176.
115. Winne, D. (1980): Influence of blood flow on intestinal absorption of xenobiotics. *Pharmacology*, 21:1–15.

Intestinal Toxicology, edited by C. M. Schiller.
Raven Press, New York © 1984.

Environmental Contaminant Effects on Human Intestinal Function

John G. Banwell

*Division of Gastroenterology, University Hospitals of Cleveland, Case Western Reserve
University School of Medicine, Cleveland, Ohio 44106*

Environmental contaminants that have their major effect on the intestine are a disparate group of chemical agents that defy easy classification. Their study, in any effective manner, often requires the scientific disciplines of epidemiology together with those of pharmacology, toxicology, bacteriology, and biochemistry. They represent a challenge to a diversity of disciplines as well as to different investigational techniques attempting to provide the factual data with which to better the social environment. Information to determine whether these contaminants should be eliminated from the environment, monitored closely for possible deleterious effects, investigated for their role in disease causation, or whether to require the development of practical methods for reducing their deleterious effects on the gastrointestinal (GI) tract are the combined aims of these efforts.

Chemical agents affecting the intestine will be considered under three categories: (a) bacterial, viral, and parasitic agents; (b) food and plant substances; and (c) metabolic interactions of toxic substances, i.e., toxic agents in the diet and environment that are dependent for their effect on interaction with the intestinal bacterial flora, other physical agents in the intestine, and the nutritional status of the subject. Several experimental model systems have been applied to the study of toxic compounds of these types.

BACTERIAL, VIRAL, AND PARASITIC AGENTS

Bacteria-Associated Intestinal Disease

Bacterial, viral, and parasitic agents usually enter the GI tract in food and water. Acute infections of the intestinal tract are among the commonest forms of infection in the population (21). Acute infectious diarrheal disease is the world's leading cause of infant and child mortality and accounts for 8% of U.S. infant mortality (24). Among adults these agents are responsible for sporadic U.S. outbreaks abroad, epidemic diarrhea in developing countries, and are a predictable hazard for millions of travelers (39). Bacteria within our environment that injure/infect the intestine include *Salmonella*, *Shigella*, *Escherichia coli*, *Yersinia*, *Vibrio*, *Bacillus cerius*, *Campylobacter*, and many other organisms (25). They are known contaminants of our water supply, household pets, domestic and farm animals, and food (20). Over one-half of the outbreaks of gastroenteritis, for instance, are related to *Salmonella*-contaminated poultry products (5).

The mode of transmission, intestinal colonization, and pathogenesis of bacterial infections have received increased study in recent years. In general, such agents are either toxigenic organisms *(Vibrio, E. coli)*, elaborating enterotoxins but with minimal invasive potential, or invasive organisms causing direct damage to the mucosal surface of the bowel *(Shigella, Salmonella*, and viruses). Toxigenic organisms exert their effect through the toxin's influence on the intestinal mucosal surface, with the organism itself rarely gaining access to the host tissue. The enterotoxic injury is subtle, often occurring without significant morphological changes in the mucosal surface, although functional changes causing massive fluid and electrolyte secretion accompany the intoxication (7).

Invasive organisms enter the plasma membrane of the mucosal cell, cause cell death and necrosis with further spread of the inflammatory response in the underlying submucosa, causing ulceration and inflammation of the bowel wall (21). Initial entry of the organisms depends on their engulfment into phagosomes (48), their division within the mucosal cell with subsequent death of the enterocyte, and release of the organisms into the tissue. The inflammatory response is dependent on the presence of the living organisms (27). The pathogenetic role of any toxins generated by invasive bacteria in these forms of inflammatory reaction remains uncertain at this time (51).

Host-Defense Mechanisms

The intestinal mucosal surface of mammals is composed of epithelial cells, many of which are in direct continuity with the external environment (34,50). These tissues constitute a large surface area on which microbial pathogens and toxic agents to the host first make their contact (18,77). A variety of mechanisms has evolved to prevent damage and invasion by these agents. The mechanisms include both immune and nonimmune mechanisms. The major immune mechanism is the secretion of secretory IgA, whose potential functions include inhibition of bacterial adherence, toxin and virus neutralization, and prevention of antigenic uptake by epithelial cells (11). These aspects of resistance are discussed in detail in several recent review articles (11,46,56,64).

Mucous Biofilm

Mucus produced by goblet cells and glycoproteins, derived from desquamated cells and degradation of cell surface glycoproteins, serves to form a continuous "biofilm" over the surface of the cells of the intestinal epithelium. This surface is probably in continuous movement owing to peristaltic movement and to the regular synthetic rate for mucus discharged onto the surface. This coat of mucus is the preferred habitat of many bacteria. Only recently, with improved techniques for stabilization, has it been readily identified (16). It plays a physiological role in the diffusion barrier at the intestinal surface and in limiting access of pathogenic organisms to the epithelial surface. The intestinal surface of new born animals is exquisitely susceptible to colonization by pathogenic organisms (18). Similarly, loss of the autochthonous intestinal microflora may be of importance in the overgrowth of *Clostridium difficile*, which results in the development of antibiotic-associated colitis (25). A vigorous autochthonous bacterial flora in the mucous biofilm may provide a barrier to pathogenic colonization by spatial occlusion of potential adherence sites.

Bacterial Adherence

The normal commensal bacterial population of the intestine must retain its hold against the shear forces of fluid movement and peristalsis as well as against the continuous desquamation of the epithelial cell mucosa and its membrane surface structures (42,46). Little is known of the factors involved in this process. However, studies with scanning and electron microscopy have indicated that only a few of the many bacterial organisms actually present in the mucous biofilm actually adhere to the microvillous surface glycocalyx of the intestinal cell.

It has been demonstrated that for enterotoxigenic or pathogenic strains of *E. coli* to cause diarrhea in piglets, they must possess not only the ability to produce enterotoxin but also the ability to colonize the small intestine (16,18). Adherence is a necessary attribute for both proliferation and colonization. The mechanisms for adherence of pathogenic organisms depends on the presence of specific fine filamentous proteinacious structures or fimbriae (pili) on the surface of bacteria. These structures protrude from the bacterium and are involved in adherence by specific ligand-receptor binding to receptor sites on the intestinal cell (56).

Several varieties of fimbriae have been recognized with different antigenic features. Receptors for the fimbriae probably involve the oligosaccharide side chains of intestinal membrane glycoproteins or glycolipids. However, since most strains of enterotoxigenic *E. coli* are not inhibitable by simple sugars, other sites of binding may also be important. Also, other forces such as hydrophobic binding and van der Waal's forces may also be involved (64).

Evidence that supports the concept of fimbriae being associated with these adherence properties have been defined as follows: (a) Genetic control of fimbriae development results in loss or gain of the ability to adhere to the intestine; (b) enteric infections with entertoxigenic *E. coli* result in production of circulatory types specific antipilis antibody; (c) immunization of animals with purified pilus vaccines protect against challenge with the specific organism; and (d) diarrhea in humans is produced by bacteria with such pili but not by organisms lacking these structures.

Vibrio cholerae **Infections**

Much of our understanding of bacterial diarrheal disease is derived from studies of the severe, often epidemic, diarrheal disease, cholera (7,21). After ingestion of *V. cholerae* in food or water, the organism passes through the gastric environment, escaping destruction when gastric pH is buffered by food or is abnormally high because of prior illness and entering the small intestine. Organisms then adhere to the microvillus surface of the epithelium where they proliferate and elaborate an enterotoxin. The toxin binds and causes the subsequent cellular interactions that lead to secretion of large volumes of fluid and electrolyte which exceed the reabsorptive capacity of the colon, with diarrheal fluid production (5). All manifestations of the natural illness can be caused by the administration of cholera toxin (13,17,26).

Cholera Enterotoxin

Cholera toxin is a protein (approximate MW 84,000 daltons) comprised of two components called A and B (28). The B component, responsible for binding of the molecule to the cell receptor, is composed of five identical subunits (11,600 daltons). The A component, which activates adenylate cyclase in various cell preparations, consists of two fragments, A_1 (23,500 daltons) and A_2 (5,500 daltons), joined by a disulfide bond. The molecule consists of the five B subunits surrounding a single A subunit. This subunit structure is very similar to that of several other toxic peptides in which one component is a binding subunit and the other a toxic moiety (28,55) (Table 1). Cholera toxin binds to its receptor, the ganglioside known as GM_1. Gangliosides are common constituents of cell membranes, and cholera toxin binds via its B subunit. After conformational changes have occurred in the membrane, the A component, through hydrophobic interaction, enters the membrane where the A_1 fragment is released by reduction of the -SH bond between A_1 and A_2. The A_1 fraction activates adenylate cyclase, located in the lateral basal membrane of the intestinal cell, via a complex series of enzymatic events involving the release of nicotinamide adenine dinucleotide (NAD) from dihydronicotinamide

TABLE 1. *Protein toxins that act within the cell*

	Receptor	Whole molecule (MW, daltons)	Active fragment	Effect
Diphtheria	?	63,000	24,000	ADP-ribosylation
Cholera	Ganglioside GM_1	84,000	21,000	ADP-ribosylation
E. coli (LT)	Ganglioside GM_1	75,000	21,000	ADP-ribosylation
Ps. aeroginosa	Galactose	65,000	30–32,000	Protein inhibition
Abrin-ricin	?		27,000	ADP-ribosylation
Colicin 3	?		?	16S ribosome inhibition

adenine dinucleotide (NADH) and adenosine diphosphate (ADP)-ribosylation (28,76). These reactions, in a manner still poorly understood, change the epithelial transport process to cause fluid and electrolyte secretion. Cholera toxin causes fluid secretion by blocking the coupled influx (from blood to lumen) of sodium chloride while stimulating the secretion (cells to lumen) of chloride and water (25,28). Recent studies have produced evidence that the crypt cell epithelium may be the site of the fluid secretion.

E. coli

Our understanding of the importance of *E. coli* as a cause of diarrheal disease was facilitated by studies of cholera and cholera toxin. During the past 15 years intensive research into the cause of acute diarrhea has led to the recognition of several groups of *E. coli* as important diarrheal pathogens (23,24):

1. Enterotoxigenic *E. coli*, which produces enterotoxins, is an important cause of diarrhea in infants, young children, and adults in developing countries and also in travelers to these countries.

2. Enteropathogenic *E. coli*, which has been responsible for frequent outbreaks of infantile diarrhea, is known to have specific serotypes. Sporadic cases have also been identified with this group of bacteria.

3. Enteroinvasive *E. coli* is invasive and has a pathological behavior similar to *Shigella*.

Enterotoxigenic E. coli

Heat Labile Toxin

Enterotoxin-producing strains of *E. coli* may elaborate one or two distinct toxic products, although many strains produce both toxins. One such product is closely related to cholera toxin (49). It is the heat labile toxin (LT), which has a molecular weight of approximately 75,000 daltons. It has a B (binding) region of approximately 45,000 daltons and an enzymatically active A domain composed of subunits corresponding to A_1 and A_2 of cholera toxin. *E. coli* LT is much less active than cholera toxin. The reason for this is still uncertain, but it may be due to the difficulty of the A subunit passing through the cell membrane or to the fact that once inside the cell, it shows little enzymatic activity, perhaps because of the failure to release the A_1 fragment by proteolysis. LT exhibits ADP-ribosyl transferase activity in a way that is almost indistinguishable from that of cholera toxin. It is therefore also an activator of adenylate cyclase. LT and cholera toxin are also immunologically related, since antibodies that neutralize cholera toxin are also active against LT. The main difference between the two toxins relates to the genetic basis for their production. The gene for cholera toxin production is based on the chromosome but that for *E. coli* LT is found on extrachromosomal transferable genetic elements or plasmids. Genetic information for enterotoxin production can thus be transferred from one strain of *E. coli* to another as well as to other bacterial species.

Heat stable toxin

E. coli produces another enterotoxin, distinct from LT, which is remarkable for its unusual resistance to inactivation by heat, acid, and proteolysis (71). It is known as the heat stable toxin (ST) and is recognized to be a group of small molecular weight peptides (1,800–2,500 daltons), depending on the source of origin. It is a weak immunogen. ST causes activation of guanylate cyclase but has no activity against adenylate cyclase. In addition, ST exerts it metabolic activity only on the intestinal mucosa in an instantaneous manner in contrast to the effect of LT on intact cells when activation of adenylate cyclase may be delayed. Activation of guanylate cyclase is accompanied by elevation of levels of cyclic guanosine 3',5'-monophosphate (GMP) (17,24,26). This substance will inhibit NaCl cotransport across the mucosal cell membrane. Genetic information for ST, like LT, is transmissible by an extrachromosomal plasmid.

Enteropathogenic E. coli

In the 1940s it was recognized that certain varieties of *E. coli,* having specific serotypes such as 055, 0111, and 0127, caused outbreaks of infantile gastroenteritis and also was identified as producing such effects when fed to volunteers. Subsequently, some 15 serological strains have been recognized as causing diarrheal disease, although neither ST nor LT enterotoxins have been identified as factors in relation to the pathogenic mechanisms for them (23,24).

Recently it has been observed that several of these enteropathogenic *E. coli* (EPEC) organisms have a different pathogenetic mechanism. One mechanism results from colonization of the EPEC organisms on the microvillus surface of the intestine (23). Colonization results in destruction of the brush border and in pedestal formation of the intestinal epithelial cell plasma membranes (61). These features have been described in children with prolonged diarrhea as well as in animal infections with similar organisms.

An additional mechanism of some importance may result from observations by O'Brien and colleagues who have observed that EPEC produces a heat-stable *Shigella dysenteriae* organism type 1-like toxin (51). Both these features may contribute to the pathogenicity of EPEC organisms. However, other mechanisms may yet remain to be identified.

Mucosal Invasion by Pathogenic Enteric Bacteria

Pathogenic bacteria for the intestinal tract are pathogens by means of elaboration of enterotoxins; however, there are a wide variety of bacteria which invade the mucosal surface to a greater or lesser degree. Such organisms include *Salmonella, Shigella, Yersinia enterocolitica, Campylobacter* (15), and *V. parahaemolyticus* (27).

There are several general characteristics of these organisms which are different from those of toxogenic bacteria. The inoculum of invasive organisms necessary to cause infection in a susceptible subject is usually much lower (several hundred organisms of *Shigella* in contrast to $> 10^9$ organisms for enterotoxic *E. coli*) than that of the noninvasive organisms. Invasive organisms have a predilection to colonize and invade the ileum and colon instead of the small intestine, and the degree of invasion of the bowel wall varies from involvement of the epithelial cells alone to transmucosal spread and dissemination throughout the body by the lymphatic and vascular system (43). Focal or generalized ulceration of the colonic mucosa occurs with shigellosis causing an acute inflammatory response and the bloody diarrhea associated with this condition. In *Salmonella*, *Campylobacter*, and *Yersinia* the involvement is usually less generalized and more patchy in distribution (21,27).

In contrast to the information available with respect to the action of enterotoxins, details of the mechanisms for invasion of pathogenic bacteria are less well characterized. Bacterial organisms bind to the epithelial surface prior to invasion. Invasion involves a process resembling endocytosis or the uptake of material into intracytoplasmic vesicles (42). It is presumed, but poorly understood, that pathogenic organisms are "recognized" for binding by the enterocyte. Phagocytic uptake of nonencapsulated bacteria occurs when cells are coated with specific immunological ligands, immunoglobulins (IgG), and complement (C_3) (1). It is not known whether similar interactions are necessary prior to ingestion of bacterial pathogens or whether, through some form of mimicry, the pathogen induces phagocytosis. Uptake of *Shigella flexneri* by HeLa cells is similar to uptake to opsonized particles by macrophages. Fc receptors have been shown to be present in the intestinal villus (27,48). It can be readily understood that entry of a pathogen will require both viable organism and intestinal epithelial cells. Details of uptake of organisms into receptosomes and their subsequent transport into the cell remain poorly understood (72).

Invasive Organisms that Produce Exotoxins

Several other invasive organisms that produce inflammatory lesions of the intestinal tract after bacterial invasion also manufacture exotoxins, which can be identified in the supernate of broth cultures. Such toxins have been identified for *Salmonella*, *Shigella*, *Yersinia*, *Campylobacter*, *Pseudomonas*, and *Bacillus cereus*. Several are heat-stable and resemble the ST toxin of *E. coli* (27,56).

Mechanisms of fluid secretion in invasive diarrhea

Diarrheal fluid loss in invasive diarrheal disease may be dependent on both reduction of fluid absorption due to damage to the mucosal surface activation of cell secretory mechanisms. It has been proposed that secretory mechanisms are dependent on release of prostaglandins and their metabolic products, which may then cause secretion by action on nearby viable epithelial cells (59). Prostaglandin infusion will induce net fluid secretion in the dog intestine. An active inflammatory exudate is necessary for *Salmonella*-induced secretion. Indomethacin, a prostaglandin synthetase inhibitor, will inhibit these secretory responses. Similar features have been observed to occur in other inflammatory diseases of the bowel such as idiopathic ulcerative colitis (68).

Viruses

Viral gastroenteritis is the second leading cause of illness in the U.S. It can result in death in the elderly, in the malnourished, and in the debilitated patient. Fecal examination utilizing immune electron microscopy has defined two major virus groups as causative of this process (14,21).

Parvoviruses are 27 nm DNA viruses that produce an acute illness associated with myalgia, vomiting, and diarrhea in adults or older children. Attack rates exceed 50%, and immunity does not develop to attack by other similar virus agents.

Rheovirus or rotavirus infection is a major cause of acute diarrheal disease in children. The agent is a 70-nm particle readily identified in duodenal biopsies by electron microscopy with double-shelled capsids.

Both Parvovirus- and Rheovirus-like agents multiply in the intestines to reach concentrations of 10^8 organisms per gram feces. They cause an inflammatory disease of the villi of the small bowel, which is localized to this area of the intestine. No gastric or colonic involvement has been noted. Intestinal mucosal changes gradually return to normal after 2 to 3 weeks (66). Development of suitable vaccines for treatment of these agents has not been successful but nevertheless remains a possibility.

Many other viral agents may pass through the GI tract and even replicate in the intestinal mucosa (poliomyelitis), but they do not usually result in GI symptoms. However, several viral agents, including cytomegalovirus and herpesvirus, may cause symptoms and specific lesions in the esophagus, small intestine, and rectum in specific populations of patients who have either reduced immunosurveillance and increased susceptibility to viral infection or unusual modes of exposure (57).

Protozoa and other intestinal parasites

The intestine is also exposed to a myriad of other protozoal and parasitic organisms during ingestion of food and water. The propensity for infection of the host is dependent on a multitude of factors, including the size and frequency of the protozoa inoculum and host susceptibility and resistance. These features are well reviewed in several books and reviews of parasitology (20,21).

Human protozoal infections represent a range of involvement of the intestinal mucosal surface similar to that observed within enteric bacterial pathogens. *Giardia lamblia,* an environmental contaminant of water, mountain streams, and even the city water supply, may cause acute or chronic diarrheal disease (81). The trophozoite, after hatching from the ingested cyst, comes to reside in the upper 25% of the intestine, adhering to the microvilli of the columnar cells near the base of the villi wedged into furrows or lodged in the mucus layer (53). It produces no apparent ultrastructural damage although marks of the site of the adherence disc on the microvillus surface are visible after detachment. Other studies have defined specific adherence lectins as being present on these organisms. *Cryptosporidia*, a protozoa of importance in veterinary practice and recently recognized as a cause of both acute and chronic infections in man, invades the surface membrane of the epithelial surface but does not progress further through the bowel wall, and generalized spread of the organism does not occur (19,57,67,74).

In contrast, amebiasis, a protozoal infection of widespread world importance, causes ulceration, proliferation, and invasion in the colon and rectum (21). Development of trophozoites from cysts is dependent on specific features of the association with the other enteric microflora. The normal colonic milieu is normally inimical to the appearance of the free trophozoites. Invasion of amebae trophozoites may be dependent on a cell lectin for adherence and, on production of the humoral agent serotonin, for induction of intestinal fluid secretion (40,60). Other intestinal parasites, nematodes and trematodes, have life cycles that result in colonization of other animal vectors and cycles of progression out of the bowels into other tissues of the body. These biological contaminants are well described in several reviews (21).

NATURAL FOOD AND PLANT SUBSTANCES

In addition to the microbiological contaminants that enter food, as it were, by natural contamination, nature itself has introduced many more toxic substances into food than has man through his own processes (Table 2). Usually by trial and error, man has, in the past, discovered how to avoid, minimize, and eliminate these agents (70). We, perhaps, may even have become adapted to traces of such compounds (78). Many of the toxic compounds are present in plants and have recognized toxic effects after absorption by the GI tract. However, few of these agents after absorption have as their main target the GI tract. Likewise, direct carcinogens are

TABLE 2. *Toxic chemicals in food*

Origin	Type

Natural	Natural contaminants of natural food
	  Microbiological
	  Nonmicrobiological (mercury, selenium
	    consumed by mammals)
	  Normal components of natural foods

Human	Agricultural chemicals
	Food additives
	Chemicals from food packaging
	Chemicals from food processing (heat, etc.)
	  Food preparation
	  Contaminants of utensils
	  Environmental pollution
	  Contamination during storage or processing

recognized to occur in foodstuffs but have their major effect as primary liver carcinogens after absorption by the intestine, rather than on the bowel mucosa (36).

Animal nutritionists have been aware that extracts from plants contain properties of agglutinating red blood cells, features that led to the isolation and purification of many different phytohemagglutinins (PHA) or lectins in food (33,37). The antinutritional feature of these compounds in red kidney beans *(Phaseolus vulgaris)* and soybeans *(Glycine max)* has been recognized for a long time (20,45). Many other plant substances may have antinutritional effects, e.g., impairing weight gain, growth, protein and fat absorption, and inducing pancreatic hypertrophy. These antinutritional effects have largely been avoided by heat treatment or presoaking of the beans and seeds from which they are derived. Such measures remove most plant agglutinins (PHA), trypsin inhibitors, and other complex proteins that may have these effects. Certain lectins, such as ricin, from the castor oil bean *(Ricinus communis)* are poisonous even in minute quantities. However, the antinutritional influence of the other more widely used dietary agents cannot strictly be viewed as toxic. For instance, growth inhibition, pancreatic hypertrophy, and malabsorption are reversible with reinstitution of a normal diet after lectin feeding (30,32,58,75).

The significance of these other dietary "antinutritional factors" and their role in human nutrition has received little attention (44). Potent effects for some of these mitogenic compounds have been demonstrated in other organ systems, and the binding affinity of their carbohydrate end groups suggests that they may have potential importance in the GI tract as well. Pathogenesis of the malabsorptive processes that accompany the impaired nutritional state has recently been defined (8,9). This raises the possibility that transient or sustained dietary-induced malabsorption may accompany ingestion of other complex proteins in man as well as in animals.

It is noteworthy that a complex sulfated polysaccharide—carrageenan—will cause ulcerating lesions in the cecum of the guinea pig and rabbit but not in man (4,52). This effect is ameliorated by clindamycin and co-trimoxazole therapy, suggesting a synergistic effect of anaerobic organisms in this inflammatory process (25). A similar interrelationship between bacterial metabolism is present in the antinutritional effects of PHA in animal studies. The germ-free state or antibiotic administration restores growth rates to normal in PHA-fed animals (8).

Mycotoxins

Mycotoxins, the toxic agents of fungi, are toxic to the intestine only in the condition of alimentary toxic aleukia, which in the period of 1943–1947 was widely present in certain states of the USSR following the consumption of bread made from gain that had over-wintered in the snow (6,35). The disease is caused by eating adequate quantities of contaminated grain over a period of weeks. Contamination with *Fusarium* was identified, and the toxic materials were identified as tricothescenes or scerpenes. The cat has proved to be an acceptable animal model for this disease. These agents cause a burning sensation in the throat, esophagus, and stomach, causing vomiting, abdominal pain, and diarrhea before later features of depression of bone marrow, leucopenia, anemia, and the development of hemorrhagic phenomena on the body surfaces occur (35). Specific studies are not available to determine the effect of these agents on the alimentary tract prior to causing bone marrow depression. It would be of interest to define their mode of action on the intestinal mucosa.

Scombrotoxin

Intoxication by eating fish is named icthyosarcotoxin (47). Symptoms of scombroid, that form associated with ingestion of contaminated mackerel or tuna, are abdominal cramps, vomiting, diarrhea, flushing, and hypotension. These manifestations are thought to be due to the release of histamine by bacterial enzymatic breakdown of histidine, which is present in the flesh of these fish. Treatment with H_1 receptor antagonists moderates symptoms. Outbreaks of this problem have been recognized in this country in recent years (47).

ENVIRONMENTAL AND INDUSTRIAL PRODUCTS

The occurrence in food and water of chemical substances used as preservatives, of contaminants introduced in farming as insecticides, or in other ways, have been identified by routine surveillance in food sources for many years. The identity of those materials that are toxic to the intestines is often difficult to define (2,3,31). Epidemiological data indicate intestinal illness associated with gross contamination in occasional instances [Epping jaundice due to diaminodiphenylmethane contamination of flour (41)] but rarely in situations where an exposure to low concentrations of chemicals has occurred. At this time there is evidence that many hundreds of chemical substances—ranging from insecticides, pesticides, polychlorinated biphenyls to heavy metals, such as lead, cadmium, and mercury—contaminate the environment and enter the digestive tract from the mouth or even via the respiratory tract (70). Their target effects on the intestine are, if any, unknown. They are discussed above and in another chapter in this volume.

METABOLIC INTERACTIONS OF TOXIC SUBSTANCES IN THE INTESTINE

Metabolic effects related to the intestine per se may occur intraluminally by reaction with intraluminal bacteria at the brush-border membrane interface between mucosal cells and the lumen, and within the mucosal cell itself.

Intraluminal Metabolism by Bacteria

The metabolism of ingested compounds by GI organisms has received considerable attention in recent years, and many metabolic reactions are defined as occurring in this environment (2,20,65). Several examples of the pharmacological significance of these reactions with bacterial organisms are available. Sulfasalazine undergoes cleavage of the azo bond with release of 5-aminosalicylate and sulfapyr-idine (29). Sulfasalazine is relatively insoluble. Sulfapyridine appears to be well absorbed and is recovered in the urine either as the free drug or its metabolite. 5-Aminosalicylate, on the other hand, seems to remain in the colon and to be excreted in the feces, whereas its acetylated derivative can be recovered in both urine and feces. The disposition of sulfasalazine and its metabolites is, therefore, complex, and at this time the definition of the major therapeutic agent responsible for improvement of patients with ulcerative colitis remains uncertain (29). It is likely, however, that deconjugation is a prerequisite for its target effect on the bowel mucosa. Anthraquinone laxatives, likewise, require deconjugation and release of free anthraquinone from the glucuronide prior to exerting their cathartic effect on the colonic mucosa (12,69). In other instances, therapeutic compounds such as digoxin have been observed to be degraded by a single colonic organism: the anerobe *Eubacterium lentum* (63).

The importance of these bacterial metabolic pathways in toxicology is of intense interest in regard to (a) conversion of drugs, chemical substances, and additives in food to toxic products or carcinogens (79,80) and (b) the prolongation of action of environmental agents by deconjugation, resulting in reabsorption of an agent pri-marily secreted into the gut after prior conjugation in the liver. Several examples of these actions are known. The glycoside of cycasin, found in the cycad plants of Guam, is hydrolyzed to methylazoxymethanol, which is both hepatotoxic and carcinogenic. Nitrosamine formation may result from the conversion of nitrates to nitrites and secondary amines; such agents are thought to play a role in carcinoma of the stomach (62,73). The development of new short-term tests assaying for mutagenicity which can readily identify environmental mutagens and carcinogens will be of great use for early detection of hazardous dietary materials.

Intestinal Brush Border Enzymes

Reactions between dietary agents and the brush border membrane may be del-eterious to health. This is well illustrated in conditions of congenital or acquired enzyme deficiency associated with lactase or other disaccharidase deficiency. Under such conditions orally ingested disaccharides, such as lactose, may cause fluid accumulation in the bowel lumen and severe diarrhea due to the osmotic effects of the unabsorbed disaccharide and its breakdown products in the colon (10).

Intestinal Mucosal Cell Metabolism

The mucosal cell has many metabolic properties that, to date, are poorly defined. Estrogens are conjugated to glucuronides, cholesterol is synthesized, and striking interactions have been demonstrated between dietary agents and intestinal metab-olism of drugs. Chemicals that act as inducers of mucosal cell metabolic activity in animals and man include such agents as halogenated hydrocarbons, including polychlorinated biphenyls, metals, and cigarette smoke, as well as normal constit-uents in the diet (e.g., charcoal-broiled beef) (54). Such agents enhance metabolism and decrease absorption and bioavailability of a variety of drugs (54). The activity of the phenacetin metabolizing enzyme system in the mucosa of rats is increased by such agents. At the present time, the functional role of these intestinal enzymes and their relation to mucosal metabolism of ingested toxic agents require further definition (38).

Whereas at least several of the metabolic pathways in the intestinal mucosal cell are defined, interactions in other regions of the bowel wall are poorly defined, and often only by chance are local toxic effects noted. A recent example was the observation that practolol, a beta-adrenergic blocking agent used in Europe, caused the formation of dense peritoneal thickening and adhesions that resulted in small-bowel stasis and obstruction. Other beta-adrenergic blocking agents do not appear to have this effect, and no cause has yet been defined for such a localized action on the peritoneal surface (45).

Likewise, very little is known of factors that may alter proliferation of the crypt cells or of the underlying mesochymal elements that surround the crypt cells and that may have an important modulating role in their proliferation. Humoral (gastrin, beta-adrenergic agents, thyroxin, serotonin, growth hormone) as well as dietary products are known to enhance epithelial cell renewal in the mucosa. Chalones—substances that may inhibit mitotic activity—are well recognized in developmental processes, but little information is available as to their role in the adult intestine and as to whether environmental toxins might exert their effect on the small-bowel through chalones (22).

Our concepts of the metabolism of toxic agents in the intestine are rudimentary. Nevertheless, development of methods of organ and isolated cell culture as well as rapid methods to detect mitogenicity of fecal and food materials may lead to a quickening in the rate of understanding of this complex organ in its reaction to environmental substances and to those chemical substances that are usual constituents of the diet in different regions of the world.

ACKNOWLEDGMENT

This work was supported in part by Grant AM 31093 from the National Institutes of Health.

REFERENCES

1. Abrahamson, D. R., and Rodewald, R. (1981): Evidence for the sorting of endocytotic vesicle contents during the receptor-mediated transport of IgG across the newborn rat intestine. *J. Cell. Biol.*, 91:270.
2. Ames, B. (1983): Dietary carcinogens and anticarcinogens. *Science*, 221:1256–1263.
3. Ames, B. N. (1979): Identifying environmental chemicals causing mutations and cancer. *Science*, 204:587.
4. Anver, M. F., and Cohen, B. J. (1976): Animal model of human disease. Ulcerative colitis. Animal model: ulcerative colitis induced in guinea pigs with degraded Carrageenan. *Am. J. Pathol.*, 84:421.
5. Aserkoff, B., Schroeder, S. A., and Brachman, P. S. (1970): Salmonellosis in the United States. A five year review. *Am. J. Epidemiol.*, 92:13.
6. Austwick, P. K. C. (1976): Mycotoxins. *Br. Med. Bull.* 31:222.

7. Banwell, J. G., and Sherr, H. (1973): Effect of bacterial enterotoxins on the gastrointestinal tract. *Gastroenterology*, 65:467.
8. Banwell, J. G., Boldt, D. J., Meyers, J., and Weber, F. L. (1983): Phytohemagglutinin derived from red kidney bean *(Phaseolus vulgaris)*: A cause for intestinal malabsorption associated with bacterial overgrowth in the rat. *Gastroenterology*, 84:506–515.
9. Banwell, J. G., Abramowsky, C. R., Weber, F., and Howard, R. (1984): Phytohemagglutinin induced diarrheal disease. *Dig. Dis. Sci. (in press)*.
10. Bayless, T. M., and Christopher, N. L. (1969): Disaccharidase deficiency. *Am. J. Clin. Nutr.*, 22:181.
11. Bienenstock, J., and Befus, A. D. (1980): Mucosal immunology. *Immunology*, 41:249–270.
12. Binder, H. J., and Donowitz, M. (1975): A new look at laxative action. *Gastroenterology*, 69:1001.
13. Binder, H. J. (editor) (1979): *Mechanisms of Secretion*. Alan R. Liss, Inc., New York.
14. Blacklow, N. R., and Cukor, G. (1981): Viral gastroenteritis. *N. Engl. J. Med.*, 304:397–406.
15. Blaser, M. J., and Reller, L. B. (1981): Campylobacter enteritis. *N. Engl. J. Med.*, 305:1444–1452.
16. Cheng, K. J., Irvin, R. T., and Costerton, J. W. (1981): Autochthonous and pathogenic colonization of animal tissue by bacteria. *Can. J. Microbiol.*, 27:461–490.
17. Cuatrecasas, P., editor (1978): *The Specificity and Action of Animal, Bacterial and Plant Toxins (Receptors and Recognition, Series B, Vol. 1)*. Chapman and Hall, London.
18. Costerton, J. W., and Irvin, R. T. (1981): The bacterial glycoalyx in nature and disease. *Annu. Rev. Microbiol.*, 35:299–324.
19. Current, W. L., Reese, N. L., Ernest, J. V., Bailey, W. S., Heyman, M. B., and Weinstein, W. M. (1983): Human cryptosporidiosis in immunocompetent and immunodeficient persons. *N. Engl. J. Med.*, 308:1251–1258.
20. Drasar, B. S., and Hill, M. J. (1974): In: *Intestinal Flora*, pp.193–222. Academic Press, London.
21. DuPont, H. L., and Pickering, L. K. (1980): *Infections of the Gastrointestinal Tract*. Plenum Medical Books, New York.
22. Eastwood, G. L. (1977): Gastrointestinal epithelial renewal. *Gastroenterology*, 72:962.
23. Edelman, R., and Levine, M. M. (1983): Summary of a workshop on enteropathogenic *Escherichia coli*. *J. Inf. Dis.*, 147:1108–1118.
24. Elliott, K., and Knight, J., editors (1976): *Acute Diarrhea in Childhood. Ciba Foundation Symposium No. 42*, Elsevier Associated Scientific, New York.
25. Fekety, R. (1983): Recent advances in management of bacterial diarrhea. *Rev. Infect. Dis.*, 56:246–257.
26. Field, M. (1974): Intestinal secretion. *Gastroenterology*, 66:1063–1084.
27. Giannella, R. A. (1981): Pathogenesis of acute bacterial diarrheal disorders. *Annu. Rev. Med.*, 32:341–357.
28. Gill, D. M. (1977): Mechanism of action of cholera toxin. *Adv. Cyclic Nucleotide Res.*, 8:85.
29. Goldman, P. (1973): Therapeutic implications of the intestinal microflora. *N. Engl. J. Med.*, 289:623.
30. Hewitt, D., Coates, M. E., Kakade, M. L., and Liener, I. E. (1973): A comparison of fractions prepared from navy (haricot) beans *(Phaseolus vulgaris* L.) in diets for germ-free and conventional chicks. *Br. J. Nutr.*, 29:423.
31. Higginson, J., Jenson, O. M., and Muir, C. S. (1981): Environmental carcinogenesis: A global problem. *Curr. Probl. Cancer*, 5:1.
32. Honavar, P. M., Shih, C. V., and Liener, I. E. (1962): Inhibition of the growth of rats by purified hemagglutinin fractions isolated from *Phaseolus vulgaris*. *J. Nutr.*, 77:109.
33. Jaffe, W. G. (1980): Hemagglutinins (lectins). In: *Toxic Constituents of Plant Foodstuffs*, Chapter 3, 2nd Edition, edited by I. Liener, pp. 73–98. Academic Press, New York.
34. Jersild, R. A. (1982): Restricted mobility and endocytosis of anionic sites on newborn rat jejunal brush border membranes. *Anat. Rec.*, 202:61.
35. Joffe, A. Z. (1972): Alimentary toxic aleukia. In: *Microbial Toxins*, edited by S. J. Ajl, S. Kadis, and A. J. L. Cieglar. Academic Press, New York.
36. Jurland, L. T. (1964): Third Conference on the toxicity of cycads. *Fed. Proc.*, 23:1337.
37. Kakade, M. L., and Evans, R. J. (1965): Nutritive value of navy beans *(Phaseolus vulgaris)*. *Br. J. Nutr.*, 19:269.
38. Kaplowitz, N. (1977): Selected Summaries. Intestinal barbeque monooxygenase: Friend or Foe? *Gastroenterology*, 73:1455.

39. Kean, B. H., and Waters, S. (1958): The diarrhea of travellers. I. Incidence in travellers returning to the United States from Mexico. *Arch. Ind. Health*, 18:148–150.
40. Kobiler, D., and Mirelman, D. (1980): Lectin activity in *Entamoeba histolitica* trophozoites. *Infect. Immun.*, 29:221–225.
41. Kopelman, H., Robertson, M. H., Sanders, P. G., and Ash, I. (1966): The Epping Jaundice. *Br. Med. J.*, I:514.
42. Lamont, J. T., and Ventola, A. (1980): Synthesis and secretion of colonic glycoproteins: Evidence for shedding *in vivo* of low molecular weight membrane components. *Biochim. Biophys. Acta*, 629:553.
43. Levine, M. M., Dupont, H. L., Formal, S. B., Hornick, R. B., and Takeuchi, A. (1973): Pathogenesis of *Shigella dysenteriae* I (Shiga) dysentery. *J. Infect. Dis.*, 127:261.
44. Liener, I. E. (1974): Phytohemagglutinins: their nutritional significance. *J. Agr. Food Chem.*, 22:17.
45. Marshall, A. J., Baddeley, H., Barritt, D. W., Davies, J. D., Lee, R. E. J., Low-Beer, T. S., and Read, A. E. (1977): Practolol peritonitis. *Q. J. Med.*, 181:135.
46. McNabb, P. C. (1981): Host defense mechanisms at mucosal surfaces. *Annu. Rev. Microbiol.*, 35:477–498.
47. Merson, M. H., Baine, W. B., Gangarosa, E. J., and Swanson, R. C. (1974): Scombroid fish poisoning. Outbreak traced to commercially canned tuna fish. *JAMA*, 228:1268.
48. Michl, J. (1980): Receptor mediated endocytosis. *Am. J. Clin. Nutr.*, 33:2462–2471.
49. Moss, J., Osborne, J. C., Fishman, P. H., Nakaya, S., and Robertson, D. C.: *Escherichia coli* heat-labile enterotoxin. *J. Biol. Chem.*, 256:12861–12865.
50. Neutra, M. R., and Madara, J. L. (1982): Structural basis of intestinal iron transport. In: *Fluid and Electrolyte Transport In Exocrine Glands*, edited by P. M. Quinton, San Francisco Press.
51. O'Brien, A., LaVelk, G. D., Thompson, M. R., and Formal, S. B. (1982): Production of *Shigella dysenteriae* Type I—like cytotoxin by *Escherichia coli*. *J. Inf. Dis.*, 146:736–764.
52. Onderdonk, A. B., Hermos, J. A., and Barlett, J. G. (1977): The role of the intestinal microflora in experimental colitis. *Am. J. Clin. Nutr.*, 301:819.
53. Owens, R. L., Nemanic, P. C., and Stevens, D. P. (1979): Ultrastructural observations on giardiasis in a murine model. *Gastroenterology*, 76:757–769.
54. Pantuck, E. J., Hsiao, K. C., Kuntzman, R., and Conney, A. H. (1975): Intestinal metabolism of phenacetin in the rat: Effect of charcoal-broiled beef and raw chow. *Science*, 187:744.
55. Pappenheimer, A. M., Jr., and Gill, D. M. (1973): Diphtheria. Recent studies have clarified the molecular mechanisms involved in its pathogenesis. *Science*, 182:353.
56. Peterson, P. K., and Quie, P. G. (1981): Bacterial surface components and the pathogenesis of infectious diseases. *Annu. Rev. Med.*, 32:29–43.
57. Quinn, T. C., Stamm, W. E., Godell, S. E., Mkrtichian, E., Benedetti, J., Corey, L., Schuffler, M. D., and Holmes, K. K. (1983): The polymicrobial origin of intestinal infections in homosexual men. *N. Engl. J. Med.*, 309:576–582.
58. Rackis, J. J. (1974): Biological and physiological factors in soybeans. *J. Am. Oil Chemists Soc.*, 51:161A.
59. Rask-Madsen, J., and Buckhave, K. (1979): Prostaglandins and chronic diarrhea: Clinical aspects. *Scand. J. Gastroent.*, [14:Suppl.] 53:73–78.
60. Ravdin, J. I., and Guerrant, R. L. (1981): Role of adherence in cytopathogenic mechanisms of *Entamoeba Histolytica*. *J. Clin. Invest*, 68:1305–1313.
61. Rothbaum, R., McAdams, J., Giannella, R., and Partin, J. L. (1982): A clinicopathologic study of enterocyte-adherent *Escherichia coli*: A cause for protracted diarrhea in infants. *Gastroenterology*, 83:441–454.
62. Ruddell, W. S. G., Bone, E. S., Hill, M. J., Blendis, L. M., and Walter, C. L. (1976): Gastricjuice nitrite. A risk factor for cancer in the hypochlorhydric stomach. *Lancet*, II:1037.
63. Saha, J. R., Butler, V. P., Neu, H. L., and Lindenbaum, J. (1983): Digoxin inactivating bacteria: identification in human gut flora. *Science*, 220:325–328.
64. Savage, D. C. (1977): Microbial ecology of the gastrointestinal tract. *Annu. Rev. Microbiol.*, 31:107–133.
65. Scheline, R. R. (1973): Metabolism of foreign compounds by gastrointestinal microorganisms. *Pharmacol. Rev.*, 25:451.
66. Schreiber, D. S., Trier, J. S., and Blacklow, N. R. (1977): Recent advances in viral gastroenteritis. *Gastroenterology*, 73:174.

67. Schultz, M. G. (1983): Emerging Zoonoses. *N. Engl. J. Med.*, 308:1285–1286.
68. Sharon, P., Ligumsky, M., Rachmilewitz, D., and Zor, U. (1978): Role of prostaglandins in ulcerative colitis. *Gastroenterology*, 75:638–640.
69. Smith, B. (editor) (1972): *The Neuropathology of the Alimentary Tract.* Williams & Wilkins, Baltimore.
70. Spicèr, A. (1975): Toxicological assessment of new foods. In: *Chemicals in Food and Environment*, edited by M. Webb. *Br. Med. Bull.*, 31.
71. Staples, S. J., Asher, S. E., and Giannella, R. A. (1980): Purification and chemical characterisation of the heat-stable enterotoxin produced by a procine strain of *E. coli* pathogenic for man. *J. Biol. Chem.*, 255:4716–4721.
72. Takeuchi, A., Formal, S. B., and Sprinz, H. (1968): Experimental acute colitis in the rhesus monkey following peroral infection with *Shigella flexneri. Am. J. Pathol.*, 52:503.
73. Tannenbaum, S. R. (1983): N-Nitroso compounds: A perspective on human exposure. *Lancet*, i:629–631.
74. Trier, J. S., Moxey, P. C., Schimmel, E. M., and Robles, E. (1974): Chronic intestinal coccidiosis in man: intestinal morphology and response to treatment. *Gastroenterology*, 65:923–935.
75. Untawale, G. G., Pietraszek, A., and McGinnis, J. (1978): Effect of diet on adhesion and invasion of microflora in the intestinal mucosa of chicks. *Proc. Soc. Exp. Biol. Med.*, 159:276–280.
76. Vaughan, M., and Moss, J. (1981): Mono(ADP-ribosyl) transferases and their effects on cellular metabolism. *Curr. Top. Cell. Regul.*, 20:205.
77. Walker, W. A. (1975): Antigen absorption from the small intestine and gastrointestinal disease. *Pediatr. Clin. North Am.*, 22:731.
78. Webb, M. (1975): Chemicals and food and environment. *Br. Med. Bull.*, 32:220.
79. Weisburger, J. H., Spingarn, N. E., Yang, Y. Y., and Vuolo, L. L. (1981): Assessment of the role of mutagens and endogenous factors in large bowel cancer. *Cancer Bull.*, 33:124–128.
80. Wilkins, T. D., Lederman, M., Van Tassell, R. L., Kingston, D. G. I., and Henion, J. (1980): Characterisation of a mutagenic bacterial product in human feces. *Am. J. Clin. Nutr.*, 33:2513–2520.
81. Wolfe, M. S. (1978): Giardiasis. *N. Engl. J. Med.*, 298:319.

Intestinal Toxicology, edited by C. M. Schiller.
Raven Press, New York © 1984.

Environmental Agents and Intestinal Disease in Man

Harold P. Schedl

Department of Internal Medicine, The University of Iowa, College of Medicine, Iowa City, Iowa 52242

This chapter addresses the question of human diseases caused by environmental chemicals. These agents comprise the "natural" chemicals present in the human diet as well as the myriad of man-made chemicals introduced into the environment at an ever increasing rate. The potential scope of environmental disease is vast, ranging from the Chinese restaurant syndrome to cancer of the large intestine. In this chapter the alimentary tract is the organ system examined and the focus is on small and large intestine. To consider the role of environmental factors in causing disease or injury to the alimentary tract, it is essential to develop the setting in which these events occur. This requires relating the organ system and its normal function to the environmental factors and examining homeostasis within the system (54). The ultimate aim is to assess whether environmental factors are important determinants of diseases of the alimentary tract. If so, how can we identify, treat, and prevent the diseases (53)?

ALIMENTARY TRACT AS PORTAL OF ENTRY FOR ENVIRONMENTAL AGENTS

Chemical agents are integral to the home and work environment. Their potential for producing intestinal disease depends on their dosage, properties, how they enter and are distributed in the body, and how they are excreted. Chemicals must enter the body in order to cause intestinal disease, and effects depend, in part, on portal of entry. The dynamics of exposure to environmental agents are illustrated in Fig. 1. The alimentary tract is the major portal of entry of food- and water-borne chemicals. Secondary portals of entry for environmental agents are skin and lungs, and these organs share with the alimentary tract increased potential for damage, since they are also exposed to the entering concentration of environmental agents. The load of agent presented to the alimentary tract may be increased by pulmonary-to-alimentary tract exchange: inhaled substances dissolved in secretions and coughed into the pharynx may be swallowed. The distributive pathway (Fig. 1) of agents entering via skin and lung is potentially the entire body, since they pass through the circulatory system before reaching the liver. During circulation the gut is exposed to these agents from the blood, but their concentrations are greatly diluted by distribution in the body pool prior to uptake by the gut. Agents taken up from the circulation by the gut pass through the mucosa into the lumen and establish a steady state. The gut is also exposed to agents taken up from the circulation by the liver and excreted in bile into the duodenum.

THE LUMEN OF THE ALIMENTARY TRACT

General

Luminal contents of the alimentary tract consist of solid and liquid components. During and after meals, motor activity of the gastric antrum (a) reduces the size of the solid components by a grinding action and allows only fine particles to enter the duodenum; and (b) converts the liquid component to an aqueous phase and an emulsion composed of the lipid components of the diet. Since dietary lipids are chiefly triglycerides, which are liquid oils at body temperature, the lipid phase is essentially a fat emulsion. The emulsion is stabilized by the other dietary components. In the proximal small intestine, the emulsion is further mixed by peristalsis and stabilized by bile. The aqueous phase in the proximal small intestine is essentially an isotonic electrolyte solution containing digestion products of carbohydrate and protein. The fat emulsion is attacked at the oil-water interface by pancreatic lipase and colipase. This converts the water-insoluble triglyceride in the oil phase to free fatty acids and β-monoglyceride. These digestion products are virtually insoluble in water and are solubilized by interacting with bile acids to form mixed micelles. At intraluminal concentrations of bile acids above the critical micelle concentration, bile acids become oriented to form small spheres (5 μm in diameter, two orders

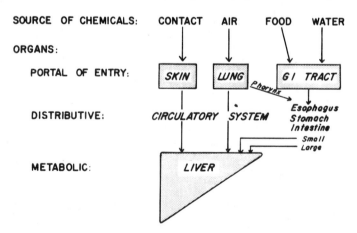

FIG. 1. Dynamics of exposure of the organism to environmental chemicals: portals of entry and initial distribution. Skin, lung, and gastrointestinal tract are the portal of entry organs for environmental chemicals. The entering chemicals are carried in the circulatory system to the liver, a major organ of metabolism.

of magnitude smaller than emulsion particles), with the polar portion of the bile acid facing the aqueous phase and the lipoidal region of the molecule to the center. Fatty acid and β-monoglyceride enter the micelle with the aliphatic hydrocarbon portion of the molecules oriented toward the lipoidal center and the polar portion of the molecule facing the aqueous phase.

Most environmental agents are ingested during feeding. Water-insoluble, lipophilic compounds such as DDT and polychlorinated biphenyls (PCBs) partition into the fat emulsion in the stomach and proximal small intestine and probably remain in the oil phase during the earlier stages of digestion. The behavior of ingested cholesterol and of fat-soluble vitamins is a model for the subsequent disposition of these substances. As the oil droplets are dissipated by digestion, cholesterol and fat-soluble vitamins pass from the oil phase into the micelles. These substances have relatively low solubility in micelles composed of bile acids alone. They dissolve well in bile acid-fatty acid-monoglyceride micelles formed after digestion of triglyceride, since they pack between the liquid hydrocarbon chains of the products of lipolysis. At a given bile acid concentration, solubility of such substances increases in proportion to concentration of products of lipolysis. These mixed micelles permit formation of relatively concentrated solutions of highly lipophilic substances, as well as provide the vehicle for transport from the oil phase to the cell membrane.

Micellar solubilization is essential for "normal" absorption of cholesterol and fat-soluble vitamins as well as for DDT and PCBs. Since these substances are virtually water-insoluble, their concentration in the aqueous phase is low, unless solubilized by micelles. In normal individuals, triglycerides constituting the oil phase are virtually completely digested. At this stage, water-insoluble substances dissolved in the oil phase precipitate, and their absorption is minimal. In the micelle, concentrations several times greater than that in the aqueous medium are achieved. The micelles permit delivery to the mucosa at high concentrations that greatly increase absorption rates. Dietary fat probably enhances absorption of DDT and PCBs as it does cholesterol. After entering the mucosal cell, these substances, like cholesterol, probably enter chylomicrons and dissolve in triglyceride synthesized by the enterocyte. Lipids are absorbed proximal to the ileum, and bile acids themselves are absorbed in the ileum.

Since normal individuals have a large reserve for digestion and absorption of fat, a high-fat diet promotes absorption of lipophilic substances such as DDT and PCBs. Conversely, patients with fat maldigestion should show impaired absorption. A defect in lipolysis (e.g., deficiency of pancreatic lipase) should produce a greater defect in DDT and PCB absorption than mucosal diseases causing malabsorption of fat after normal digestion (e.g., celiac sprue). If digestion is normal, mixed micelles form. This allows a higher concentration to be presented to the mucosa than in the state of fat maldigestion, where lipophilic substances remain in the emulsion and are carried in the fat to the colon. Although bacterial lipases hydrolyze much of the fat after it enters the colon, micelles do not form at this site, since adequate concentrations of bile acids are lacking. Hence, calcium soaps of fatty acids precipitate as the oil droplets are dissipated by digestion. Other water-insoluble lipophilic substances would also precipitate. Undigested fat excreted in the stool carries dissolved lipophilic compounds.

Luminal contents of the alimentary tract are a multicompartmental system with solid as well as the liquid components discussed above. The chief solid components remaining in the small intestine after digestion are those in fiber. The liquid phase of luminal contents is chiefly an aqueous electrolyte solution containing digestion products of food, chiefly carbohydrate and protein. Most components of the liquid phase are absorbed before the stool is excreted.

Physical Dimensions of the Luminal Milieu

Concentrations of environmental agents in luminal contents will be relatively low because of the large volumes of fluid entering the alimentary tract (Fig. 2) (51). In addition to water intake of 2 liters/day, salivary, gastric, biliary, and pancreatic secretions add 6 liters/day. To this 8-liter volume entering the proximal small intestine is added 6 liters/day of small intestinal secretions. When the luminal contents pass from distal small intestine across the ileocecal valve to enter the colon, this 14-liter volume is reduced to 1.5 liters/day. As the luminal contents traverse the large intestine, most of the water is absorbed in cecum and ascending colon, and at excretion in the stool, the volume of water is 0.1 to 0.2 liters/day. Thus, concentrations of unabsorbed and poorly absorbed agents in luminal contents increase in distal small intestine and attain their highest levels in the distal large intestine and rectum, where luminal volumes are lowest.

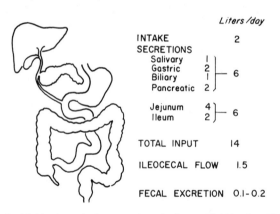

Liters/day

INTAKE		2
SECRETIONS		
Salivary	1	
Gastric	2	6
Biliary	1	
Pancreatic	2	
Jejunum	4	6
Ileum	2	
TOTAL INPUT		14
ILEOCECAL FLOW		1.5
FECAL EXCRETION		0.1-0.2

FIG. 2. Intraluminal fluid volume in the gastrointestinal tract. Fluid intake of 2 liters/day added to salivary, gastric, biliary, and pancreatic secretions totaling 6 liters/day introduces a total of 8 liters/day of fluid into the proximal jejunum. To this is added six liters/day of secretions by the small intestine. This total volume of input into proximal small intestine represents the potential volume containing environmental chemicals. This volume has been reduced to 1.5 liters/day at the time of exit from the small intestine at the ileocecal valve. The greatest increase in concentration of environmental chemicals that remains unabsorbed occurs in the colon where the intraluminal volume is reduced to 0.1 to 0.2 liters/day by the time the contents are excreted in stool. This volume-flow pattern is consistent with presentation of the highest concentration of unabsorbed chemicals to the colon.

Physiology and Biochemistry of the Luminal Milieu

Behavior of environmental agents after entering the alimentary tract is determined by anatomic, physiologic, and biochemical characteristics of the organ system. Anatomic factors are discussed below.

pH

The pH range of gastric contents is usually 1 to 3.5; most commonly 1 to 2.5. Gastric contents delivered into the duodenum increase in pH to 5 to 7 as the jejunum is traversed. Pancreatic, biliary, and intestinal secretions are alkaline, and the pH of intestinal contents gradually increases to 7 to 8 as they pass into the ileum. Colonic secretions are alkaline.

Acids and bases enter the membranes of cells lining the gastrointestinal tract only in their unionized form, where they have maximal lipid solubility. The low pH of gastric contents produced by hydrochloric acid secretion ensures that weak acids are essentially unionized and in their lipid-soluble form. Thus, weak acids, e.g., salicylic acid and aspirin, are best absorbed from the stomach. The lowest pK_a of an acid compatible with rapid absorption is about 3. Contrasting with the behavior of acids, environmental agents that are weak bases form salts with hydrochloric acid in the stomach, are ionized, and in this polar form are not absorbed. When these salts of basic compounds enter the small intestine, the increase in pH to 5 to 7 as the acid is neutralized forms the free base, which is lipid soluble. The lowest pK_a for a base that permits formation of free base at pH 5 to 7 is about 7.8. Strong bases retain the salt form, remain ionized, and are not absorbed from small or large intestine. Similarly, strong acids ($pK_a < 3$) do not combine with hydrogen ion in the stomach to form the neutral lipophilic molecule. Hence, they are not absorbed from the stomach and remain completely ionized and unabsorbed as they traverse the distal gut.

Motility

Effects of environmental agents may differ depending on whether the agent enters the stomach during fasting or with a meal. Gastric emptying is influenced by many factors. The fasting stomach empties rapidly, 30 min or less. After a high-fat meal, several hours may elapse before the stomach empties. Emptying rate is influenced by (a) the nature of the contents, including volume, viscosity, temperature, caloric density, buffering capacity, etc.; (b) individual factors, including age, state of health, emotion, activity, posture, etc.; and (c) extraneous factors including drugs, e.g., anticholinergics. Rate of transit through proximal small intestine is rapid, measured by minutes in the duodenum and by hours in the ileum. Transit through the colon requires 1 to 2 days. Differences in mucosal contact time determined by motility are critical in determining absorption and effects of environmental agents.

Digestion

Gastric secretions contain the proteolytic enzyme pepsin, which is active only at low pH. The main site of enzymatic activity is the small intestine. The most important intraluminal enzymes are the pancreatic proteases, carbohydrases, and lipases. Digestive enzymes in pancreatic secretions, such as glucuronidases and sulfatases, are of particular interest with respect to interactions with environmental factors. Compounds secreted into bile after conjugation with glucuronic or sulfuric acid are polar, anionic molecules that are poorly absorbed at the pH of the small intestinal contents. Deconjugation of these molecules permits their reabsorption. After absorption these compounds are carried in the portal circulation to the liver where they may be reconjugated, resecreted into bile, and where they reenter the intestine, thereby causing continuing exposure to their actions. The intestinal burden of glutethimide, griseofulvin, chloramphenicol, and indomethacin is amplified by enterohepatic recirculation, and toxicity is promoted. Indomethacin produces intestinal ulcerations by this amplification of dose (12). Studies of cumulative biliary excretion show that sensitivity to indomethacin-related lesions correlates with dose amplification by enterohepatic recirculation in a variety of animal species. The dose amplification in man is about 20-fold. Treatment is available to attenuate or prevent such dose amplification, e.g., by use of chemicals such as D-glucaro-1,4-lactone (37), an inhibitor of glucuronidase.

Intestinal mucosal digestive enzymes are integral components of the structure of the cell membrane and act at the cell surface, but small amounts of activity enter the lumen, e.g., with desquamated mucosal cells. Bile enters and mixes with duodenal contents and is essential for normal absorption of lipids. Because of their detergent properties, bile salts form mixed micelles with lipophilic molecules solubilizing them and facilitating their absorption. Deficiency of pancreatic lipase leads to malabsorption of fat. Steatorrhea promotes fecal excretion of environmental agents with lipophilic properties.

Nonabsorbed Agents

Luminal contents of the alimentary tract are considered to be outside the body, i.e., in the external, not the internal milieu. Many agents are relatively insoluble in contents of the alimentary tract. The fraction of agent remaining undissolved may be excreted from the alimentary tract in the feces in the same form it entered, without affecting the organism. Some substances suspended in the gut lumen exert significant effects. Although environmental agents are not taken in amounts sufficient to cause osmotic effects that change intraluminal fluid distribution, interactions occur between nonabsorbed agents and compounds in the lumen or at the limiting membrane of cells lining the alimentary tract. One example of a nonabsorbed endogenous agent is intestinal mucus. Mucus is a glycoprotein with affinity for a variety of substances, and its secretion is increased in diseases such as celiac sprue and colitis. Mucus binds the polymer polyvinylpyrrolidone and holds it in the intestinal lumen (55).

Experiments have demonstrated that nonabsorbed substances are important in influencing intraluminal concentrations and distribution of environmental agents and in altering their absorption. The ability of nonabsorbed agents to retain drugs and chemicals in the gut lumen is dramatically illustrated by activated charcoal, which adsorbs a variety of different compounds. Oral activated charcoal accelerates clearance of phenobarbital from the body (4) and is used for treatment of phenobarbital overdose (20). Charcoal also accelerates clearance of digoxin by the intestine (8) and has been used to treat digitoxin overdose (44). Cholestyramine, an ion-exchange resin, binds anions such as bile salts and glucuronide and sulfate conjugates excreted in bile. Cholestyramine treatment causes a small increase in fecal fat excretion and malabsorption of fat-soluble vitamins. Absorption of a wide variety of other substances is impaired by cholestyramine: inorganic and hemoglobin iron, vitamin B_{12}, phenylbutazone, warfarin, and thyroid hormones. Intraluminal cholestyramine protects against lethal digitalis intoxication in rat and guinea pig (9) and accelerates the excretion of chlordecone in workers exposed to this polychlorinated cyclic ketone (22). Cholestyramine and other anion exchange resins protect against toxic effects of cyclamate and amaranth (FD&C Red No. 2) (13). Intraluminal perfusion of the nonabsorbed hydrocarbons liquid paraffin and squalene increases the excretion of hexachlorobenzene into the gut lumen (49). These studies illustrate not only the ability of nonabsorbed luminal agents to retain environmental agents in the gut lumen, but also their potential for promoting removal of these agents from the body.

Bacteria

The colon is normally massively colonized with bacteria, and bacteria are also present in ileum. Both exogenous and endogenous substances may be metabolized by enzymes of the host's flora. This includes a wide range of substances from drugs (21) to carcinogens. In bacterial overgrowth syndrome (see below), this effect may be greatly amplified.

Fiber

The nature of the diet, particularly its fiber content, by providing additional unabsorbed luminal contents modifies distribution of both unabsorbed and absorbed substances. Fiber comprises indigestible plant components of the diet. The chemical composition of fiber is variable and includes celluloses, hemicelluloses, pectin, lignins, and other substances. Fiber itself is assumed to be virtually inert physiologically and to exert its effects through its physical and physiochemical properties.

Dietary fiber may play a role with respect to actions of environmental agents. Fiber may interact with ingested chemical agents and alter their entry into the body from the lumen (58). Hence, fiber may act on environmental agents intraluminally or at the brush border membrane-lumen interface. Fiber could be protective against effects of environmental pathogens by two mechanisms: (a) adsorption, thereby preventing their absorption; and (b) by effects on motility, increasing rate of passage through the alimentary tract, decreasing absorption, and changing distribution in the gut. Fiber adsorbs bile salts (32), depressing their normal reabsorption in distal ileum and increasing their fecal excretion. The modification by fiber of toxic dietary effects of carcinogens, toxic chemicals, infectious agents, and X-irradiation has been reviewed (33).

Fiber dilutes concentration of nonabsorbed and absorbed agents, particularly at distal sites, and may modify responses in large intestine, particularly the rectum and anus. Too low a level of dietary fiber has been linked with cancer of the colon and rectum and with diverticular disease of the colon. Presumably, the appropriate amount of fiber in diet would be preventive for these diseases. Excessive amounts of dietary fiber could be deleterious despite its inertness: fiber by its bulk would require that larger amounts of food be eaten to supply nutrients, particularly calories. Excessive amounts of fiber might also cause depletion of calcium, magnesium, trace metals (48), etc. Thus, fiber probably shows properties of nearly all environmental agents—damaging if present in too small or large an amount, with an optimal intermediate dose.

In addition to fiber, examples of other solid components remaining intraluminally after digestion include particulates such as asbestos fibers and fly-ash. They occur in small amounts and are of unknown significance. These substances may be ingested directly, as in drinking water, or inhaled and subsequently coughed up and swallowed. Human studies have shown that at least a small fraction of ingested asbestos fibers is absorbed: fibers originating in drinking water are excreted in urine (11). Penetration of asbestos fibers (introduced intragastrically) through the digestive tract and accumulation in tissues have been shown in the rat (46). Other particulates such as coal fly-ash are mutagenic (10), and there is evidence that membrane uptake of chemical carcinogens may be particle-mediated (35). In addition to the substances listed above, stool solids contain large numbers of dead bacteria and small amounts of many substances, including divalent cation salts of fatty acids.

Adsorption at the Gut Membrane-Lumen Interface and Storage in Mucosal Cells

Gut contents may be adsorbed on to the intestinal wall. For example, mineral oil can coat the alimentary tract, metabolic products of senna laxatives can be bound by the colonic mucosa *(melanosis coli)*, and bacteria, particularly pathogens, have the ability to attach to the gut wall. Some substances adsorbed to and taken up by cells lining gut wall may traverse the cell so slowly that a large proportion reenters the lumen as the mucosal cells age, die, and slough into the luminal contents. Iron taken up by duodenal mucosal cells is an example. Metals such as copper, zinc, and cadmium are bound by metallothionein in mucosal cells and lost in this way. The degree of binding by intestinal mucosa can differ, depending on physiologic state, e.g., more of an orally administered dose of radioactive cadmium is bound to mucosa of animals fed a low level of dietary calcium than those fed a normal level (62). The low-calcium diet increases mucosal calcium-binding protein, which causes enhanced binding of both calcium and cadmium.

ROLE OF THE GUT MUCOSA: TRANSPORT AND METABOLISM IN THE GUT WALL

General

The stomach and colon have reservoir function, and their epithelia are characterized as "tight." The small intestine is an absorbing-conducting structure with a "leaky" epithelium as regards electrolyte movements and transport of environmental agents. Surface area is also smaller in stomach and colon than in small intestine, where most of the absorption of the majority of environmental agents occur.

Cells lining the surface of the alimentary tract exercise barrier, transport, and metabolic functions. The structure of the surface of the small intestine, i.e., villi with intervening crypts, increases surface area. Highly specialized mucosal cells with their digestive-absorptive luminal surface, the brush border membrane, are the major surface structure of the villi. Many of the environmental agents in luminal contents are absorbed as they contact the surface of these cells. Hence, mucosal cells contain the highest concentrations of environmental agents. Mucus-secreting goblet cells are interspersed among the absorbing cells. Mucus acts as a barrier and mucous secretion changes in disease.

In contrast to the absorptive processes occurring in the villi, is the secretion taking place in the crypts. Crypts contain undifferentiated cells, the precursors of mucosal absorptive cells, Paneth, goblet, and endocrine cells: all are secretory. Damage to the undifferentiated cells, e.g., by radiation or by gliadin in patients with celiac sprue (see below) decreases the population of villous absorptive cells and leads to malabsorption of nutrients and environmental agents.

The colonic wall is folded with a smooth surface indented with crypts. Mucus-producing goblet cells are prominent in the colon and are depleted of mucus by inflammation. The colonic mucosal cells can provide appreciable absorptive capacity for environmental agents delivered to this distal site.

Membrane Properties: Transport

The membrane of mucosal cells is a protein-lipid bilayer that behaves as if it were discontinuous and penetrated at intervals by water-filled pores lined by fixed negative charges. Uncharged water-soluble substances of small molecular size, less than 4 Å in diameter, such as urea, are absorbed by simple diffusion through the water-filled channels. Most molecules, including environmental agents, are too large to be absorbed through pores and traverse the cell membrane itself. The protein-lipid bilayer serves as solvent for lipoidal molecules during passive transport. In this process the driving force is concentration gradient: the environmental agent moves from a higher concentration in the lumen, into the cell membrane, then into the cell.

Membranes of the alimentary tract behave as if they contain sites with special properties designated as carriers. These carrier sites enhance absorption of many molecules whose polar structure would otherwise greatly limit their entry rate. Carriers may act to enhance transport of an agent by facilitated diffusion or active transport. In facilitated diffusion the agent-substrate reacts with the carrier component of the membrane, and transfer between the two faces of the membrane is greatly facilitated without expenditure of cellular energy. The process is identical on both sides of the membrane.

Active transport is similar to facilitated diffusion except that the agent-substrate can be moved out of the lumen into the cell against its concentration gradient. This requires expenditure of energy and is largely unidirectional. Active transport can control rate of transport and thereby the internal environment or concentration of specific substances. Hydrolysis of adenosine triphosphate (ATP) provides the energy for most active transport processes.

One site of action of toxic chemicals should be the transport processes, since these are exposed on the surface of the cell. The concept of membrane lesions in toxicity of environmental chemicals has recently been reviewed (31) and has been the subject of a symposium (24,47). A strong case can be made for a membrane theory of toxicity with heavy metals and organochlorine compounds, notably DDT. DDT and PCBs inhibit $Na^+K^+ATPase$ and osmoregulatory sodium transport by intestinal and gill epithelia of teleosts adapted to seawater. A typical heavy metal, mercury, inhibits carrier-mediated influx of glucose across intestinal brush border vesicles of the flounder (quoted in ref. 47). Crude oil inhibits the mediated but not the nonmediated component of L-leucine uptake by intestine of herring gull chicks (38).

Most environmental agents are absorbed by passive diffusion whereas most nutrients, e.g., monosaccharides, amino acids, and vitamins such as thiamine, niacin, riboflavin, pyridoxine, are absorbed by carriers. Environmental agents that are acids or bases also enter the organism by diffusion, but their entry depends on pH in the lumen and at the interface as described above. In general, charged molecules do not enter and penetrate the membrane. Rates of intestinal transport of environmental chemicals might also differ greatly, simply on the basis of individuals factors, as discussed below.

Pinocytosis is cellular uptake by the process of engulfing particles or dissolved material through formation of a vesicle using the surface membranes of the cell. This is a type of active transport and requires energy. Intestinal cells of newborn mammals have a particular ability to absorb immunoglobulins by pinocytosis. This is the mechanism of transfer of maternal immunoglobulins in the milk to transmit passive immunity. Although present at birth, this capacity largely disappears within a short time, corresponding to several replacements of intestinal epithelium. This fetal and newborn mechanism persists into adulthood, at least to a minor extent, as shown by pinocytotic vesicles in adult rodents. Absorption of intact macromolecules by adult humans causes allergic phenomena. Such sensitization is probably caused by proteins absorbed by pinocytosis, but macromolecules may also enter through the desquamation zone at the tip of the villus. Immune responses to environmental antigens absorbed through the gastrointestinal tract have been reviewed (41). Particles such as asbestos fibers, which have been shown to penetrate through the digestive tract of rats (46), probably enter by this mechanism. A persorption mechanism for entry of macromolecules and solid particles has been described (60).

The discussion above has focused on the alimentary tract as a portal of entry for environmental agents. Less information is available regarding the gut as an excretory organ. Compounds excreted in bile are lost from the body if not deconjugated and reabsorbed. Anion binders can accelerate excretion of such compounds, as illustrated by use of cholestyramine to increase excretion of digoxin and chlordecone (9,22). The intestinal mucosa mediates exchange of a variety of compounds from blood to lumen. Thus, although biliary diversion causes the hepatic metabolite, chlordecone alcohol, to disappear from the stool, excretion of chlordecone itself continues in both man and rat (22). Hexachlorobenzene is not excreted in bile, although its main route of excretion is via the gut, and excretion is increased by feeding liquid paraffin (reviewed in ref. 49). The transport process is probably passive, since luminal concentrations attain those in plasma (49). Secretory intestinal transport mechanisms have been demonstrated for cardiac glycosides, quaternary ammonium salts, and organic acids (8,61). These compounds are transported more rapidly from blood to lumen than lumen to blood and are transported against a concentration gradient into the lumen.

Intracellular Processes

Intestinal mucosa is capable of metabolizing a wide variety of substrates (2,23). Metabolic processes occurring within the mucosal cell are critical in determining results of interactions between environmental agents and the alimentary tract. Absorption rates of such agents are also critical, since they determine delivery rates of agents into the cells, thereby influencing metabolism. Chemical agents present in the environment and ingested are analogous to drugs. Total body rates of metabolism of a given drug differ among individuals by factors of 3 to 40. These large variations between individuals disappear among genetically identical subjects (monozygotic twins) but persist in dizygotic twins. Since other factors were controlled, genetic factors appear to cause the variability observed (59). Individual variability in the metabolism of environmental factors by the alimentary tract has not been defined.

Metabolism of drugs and chemicals is also highly dependent on individual factors not genetically determined. Many drugs and chemicals induce hepatic microsomal enzymes. Such enzymes are also induced in the alimentary tract, particularly the small intestine (27,28). Environmental chemicals induce enzymes in the alimentary tract that alter their own absorption, metabolism, and distribution in the body, as well as that of other agents. Effects of natural foods differ from those of semisynthetic diets, and even the way in which food is prepared has an effect. Studies were performed in man and rat using phenacetin (42,43). An enzyme system present in mucosal cells metabolizes phenacetin to N-acetyl-p-aminophenol. Activity of this enzyme system is increased by treatment with environmental factors such as cigarette smoke, 3,4-benzpyrene, or 3-methylcholanthrene. This increased metabolism by the intestine probably decreases the amount of phenacetin absorbed unchanged in the bloodstream. Thus, cigarette smoking in man enhances metabolism and lowers plasma concentration of orally administered phenacetin without changing half-life in plasma. Composition of diet (natural foods vs semisynthetic diets) and differences in preparation of food (raw vs cooked vs charcoal-broiled ground beef) altered intestinal metabolism of phenacetin. These results suggest that normal diets of natural food or differences in the means for cooking food alter intestinal metabolism of environmental factors and thereby could decrease their absorption and effects on the organism.

Other nutritional factors also influence oxidative metabolism of antipyrene and theophylline (30). Increasing dietary carbohydrate prolongs drug half-lives, whereas protein supplements decrease drug half-lives. A high-cholesterol diet enhances mucosal activities of several enzymes, including aryl hydrocarbon hydroxylase; in contrast, PCBs decrease mucosal enzyme activities (25). Lipid diets decrease activities of drug hydroxylation and glucuronidation by duodenal mucosa (26).

PHYSIOLOGY OF DISTRIBUTION OF ENVIRONMENTAL CHEMICALS IN THE BODY

As shown in Fig. 3, ingested agents (after leaving the mouth, pharynx, and esophagus) progress to the stomach, then small intestine, and finally to the colon. Absorption of most environmental agents probably parallels that of nutrients and

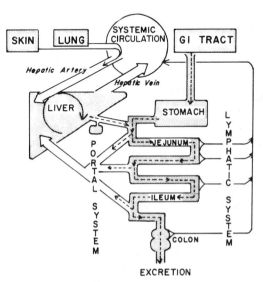

FIG. 3. Environmental chemicals: distribution, cycling, and gut excretion. Absorption of chemicals in food and water is chiefly from small intestine. The portal venous system carries nearly all absorbed substances to the liver except for fats and lipoidal compounds, which are carried in lymphatics to the systemic circulation. Here they join chemicals taken up by skin and lungs to be carried in the arterial circulation to the liver. In the liver chemicals are transformed, conjugated, and reexcreted into the alimentary tract. Within the lumen, conjugates are hydrolyzed and the deconjugated compounds are reabsorbed, completing an enterohepatic cycle that may be repeated many times.

occurs chiefly in the small intestine. The colon is the target organ for poorly absorbed or unabsorbed agents, or those secreted in bile into the small intestine and not reabsorbed. Most substances are absorbed before reaching the colon. Concentrations of environmental agents are relatively high in mucosal cells during absorption. As these agents move out of the cell into extracellular fluid down their concentration gradients, they are greatly diluted as they enter the blood and lymph to be distributed throughout the body. Rate of transfer out of the mucosa into the organism is determined by physiochemical properties of the agent and the concentration gradient. Concentration of absorbed environmental agents is maintained at a low level in blood and lymph by dilution, protein binding, metabolism, and excretion, e.g., back into the alimentary tract in the bile or by kidney, lung, or skin.

After traversing the intestinal mucosa, most substances enter the portal venous system and are carried to the liver, where oxidation, reduction, and conjugation are carried out. After absorption, highly lipophilic substances, particularly if taken with dietary fat, enter the lymphatics dissolved in the chylomicrons synthesized from glycerol and absorbed fatty acids in the mucosal cell. Concurrent ingestion of fat may accelerate the exit of lipophilic substances from the mucosa. As shown in Fig. 3, agents carried in the lymphatic system from the gut, as well as those taken up by the lungs and skin, enter the systemic circulation and are also carried to the liver. Entry into the liver is by way of the hepatic artery. Hence, regardless of entry route, environmental agents reach the liver and may appear in bile.

INDIVIDUAL FACTORS MODIFYING RESPONSE TO ENVIRONMENTAL AGENTS

General

The response to environmental agents must depend on many factors, including age, genetic constitution, sex, general health, nutritional state, usage of drugs (particularly those causing enzyme induction in liver or gut), ethanol, tobacco, occupational exposure to chemicals, diet, etc. For example, feeding a low-calcium diet increases susceptibility to lead (57) and cadmium (45,62) toxicity. Pregnancy and lactation change disposition of environmental agents: lead and cadmium absorption as well as calcium absorption increases. Lactation results in excretion of persistent organochlorine compounds in milk fat, thereby lowering body burden of these compounds. Disease states that alter hormonal status or function of gastrointestinal tract, liver, heart, or kidney will modify the effects of agents. Thus, physiologic disposition of environmental agents is altered in bowel disease (see below). We can only speculate about the role of many of these individual factors.

Age

All alimentary tract functions change with age. Gastric acid secretion in newborns approximates that in adults for the first 24 to 48 hr of life. After 48 hr, acidity declines steadily to a minimum level at 20 days. Gastric activity then increases until the third year of life, when adult levels are approached. In the adult, gastric acidity decreases with aging, and low gastric acidity is common in the elderly. Since gastric acidity enhances absorption of acids and depresses absorption of bases, their rate and site of absorption will vary with the age of the subject.

Nursing infants are unique in their exposure to pollutants in breast milk (50). The highly lipid soluble chlorinated hydrocarbons DDT and PCB concentrate in fat in breast milk. These persistent environmental agents resist physical and chemical degradation, are widely distributed in the environment, and excreted extremely slowly. Lactation is the only normal process by which large amounts of these residues can be excreted. Nursing infants can be regarded as at the top of the food chain in terms of exposure. No data are available regarding toxic effects of these agents on newborn babies. However, no specific illnesses have been associated with transmission of environmental chemicals in breast milk at the usual levels of contamination.

Infancy is the most vulnerable period for lead intoxication, particularly preweaning, as demonstrated by absorption studies in the rat (18) and balance studies in infants (63). Lactose feeding itself also enhances lead absorption (7).

Age alters the pharmacokinetics of drugs and of environmental agents. In the elderly these changes are secondary to decreased function of heart, liver, kidneys, and gastrointestinal tract. Since cardiac output declines by approximately 1% per year from age 19 to 86 years, the decrease in blood flow alters transport, metabolism, and excretion of environmental agents. Weight loss with concomitant increase in body fat (from 18%–36% of total body weight in men and from 33%–48% in women) that accompanies aging alters distribution of environmental agents. Age-related effects on the metabolizing capacity for environmental agents are unpredictable. The hepatic drug-metabolizing enzyme, cytochrome P-450, exists in multiple forms, differing in their regulation and specificity. Enzyme activity is usually low in the fetus, higher in the neonate, and peaks in the preadolescent. By middle age, values have declined to half the peak levels and decline further in the elderly. All of these factors will affect the impact of environmental agents on the organism.

Genetic Factors

Hereditary defects in membrane transport and membrane digestion usually lead to osmotic diarrhea and depressed absorption of nutrients and environmental agents. Membrane transport defects, such as glucose-galactose malabsorption and congenital chloridorrhea, are rare. Most membrane digestive defects, such as congenital lactase deficiency and sucrase-isomaltase deficiency, are also rare. In the newborn, during suckling, and in childhood, lactase activity of small intestinal mucosa is high. Most of the world's population develops some degree of lactase deficiency, i.e., acquired-adult lactase deficiency. Mucosal lactase levels decline before adolescence, and lactase deficiency is the norm for adults. Only northern Europeans, their emigrant populations to other parts of the world, and certain other ethnic groups with a dairying technology have levels of intestinal lactase in adults adequate for rapid digestion of dairy products such as milk and ice cream. Thus, most adults experience abdominal discomfort from increased motility due to osmotic diarrhea after lactose ingestion and tend to avoid milk products. Ingestion of lactose by these individuals increases the volume of the luminal milieu (Fig. 2) and alters its distribution. This probably also alters the handling of environmental agents. Osmotic diarrheal states increase fecal fat and nitrogen excretion (36), and increased excretion of environmental agents is also to be expected.

Bacterial Overgrowth Syndrome

Bacteria are absent or present in very low concentrations in the stomach and proximal small intestine. Appreciable concentrations of bacteria are present in the ileum, and the colon is normally massively colonized with bacteria. Abnormalities in the flow of luminal contents through the alimentary tract alter the normal distribution of bacterial flora in the gut. The proximal small intestine becomes colonized with bacteria (16). Bacterial overgrowth causes a secretory diarrhea if the organisms are capable of deconjugating bile salts or hydroxylating unsaturated fatty acids. This water and electrolyte diarrhea alters fluid distribution in the gut and intraluminal distribution of environmental agents. Bacterial overgrowth syndromes of this type can result from motility disorders or altered anatomy of the alimentary tract. Disturbances of gut motility may result from intrinsic disease of the organ system or its innervation, or from systemic disease. These diseases include primary visceral myopathy (15,56); diabetes, which produces visceral autonomic neuropathy involving the stomach most prominently; primary systemic sclerosis and amyloidosis involving smooth muscle of the gastrointestinal tract; and vagotomy with delayed gastric emptying and hypochlorhydria. Anatomic factors causing bacterial overgrowth include stasis of luminal contents in blind loops, in diverticula, or proximal to strictures. Toxicity of environmental agents is modified in bacterial overgrowth syndromes. Methyl mercury is much more toxic than ingested elemental mercury, which passes through the gastrointestinal tract largely unchanged. Methyl-mercury formation is increased by an order of magnitude in rats with experimental blind loops of the small intestine as compared with controls (1) and produces symptoms of mercury poisoning in blind loop animals.

INTESTINAL DISEASES CAUSED BY ENVIRONMENTAL AGENTS

General

In this section, diseases in which an environmental agent may be involved are considered. The list is arbitrary and limited. For some diseases, e.g., celiac and tropical sprue, the etiologic role of environmental factors is well established. For others, such as cancer of the colon, it is highly probable that environmental factors play a significant role. In certain other instances—e.g., Crohn's disease and ulcerative colitis, two diseases of unknown etiology—only a possible association can be postulated. Diseases of the small and large intestine caused by environmental agents are of particular interest: the disease itself, by altering function of the main portal of entry, alters response to environmental agents. These diseases will ordinarily produce malabsorption of nutrients and chemicals and decrease exposure. When diseases cause extensive inflammation, e.g., in Crohn's disease, permeability of the gut wall increases, and macromolecules not otherwise absorbed or secreted readily pass the mucosa. Also included are selected examples of drug-induced diseases or syndromes, e.g., antibiotic-associated colitis and phosphorus-depletion syndrome. These are included to illustrate mechanisms whereby environmental agents may act to produce disease and to provide a frame of reference for thinking about how environmental diseases may occur.

Small Intestine

Celiac Sprue

The disease nontropical (celiac) sprue is caused by damage to proximal small intestinal mucosa by peptides in the gliadin fraction of wheat gluten. Despite the increased rate of mucosal cell division in response to cell damage, villous atrophy occurs, and malabsorption of virtually all nutrients results. These patients also have nutritional deficiencies affecting nearly all organ systems. Damage to the mucosa increases permeability, and large polar molecules that otherwise are not absorbed penetrate the mucosa. For example, sucrose is absorbed intact and excreted in the urine. Permeability of the mucosa of the alimentary tract to ^{51}Cr ethylenediaminetetraacetic acid (EDTA) is increased in patients with celiac sprue in relapse, and the increased permeability persists even in patients in remission (3). Thus, these patients may have malabsorption of most environmental agents, but others ordinarily not absorbed may penetrate the mucosa. This is probably also true of most diseases with mucosal damage, including inflammatory bowel diseases.

Tropical Sprue

Tropical sprue is a chronic disease prevalent throughout the world in underdeveloped countries. It occurs in natives of developed countries after living in endemic areas and remits on return to developed country. It causes impairment of absorption of nearly all nutrients, and inefficient utilization of nutrients in the diet causes generalized nutritional deficiency. Inhabitants of underdeveloped countries eat a marginal diet, and any interference with absorption magnifies the effect of marginal intake. The disease has a multifactorial etiology, sometimes occurring in epidemics in a form different from the endemic form. It is a self-perpetuating disease, since the poor nutrition caused by the disease itself causes the malabsorption to worsen by damaging structure and altering function of the alimentary tract.

Crohn's Disease

Crohn's disease can involve any part of the alimentary tract (e.g., esophagus, stomach, duodenum), but distal small intestine (regional ileitis) and colon (Crohn's colitis) are most often affected. Although this pattern of distribution may be consistent with response to an environmental agent, the cause of Crohn's disease is unknown; indeed, it is not even known if it is a disease complex of multiple etiologies. The incidence of Crohn's disease appears to be increasing (5,6,14,29, 34,39,40), but it is not known whether the increase is real or the result of greater awareness. Although the incidence of Crohn's disease is greater in industrialized societies than in developing countries, it is not clear if this is simply a difference in recognition. Because Crohn's disease has been recognized only recently and appears to have the highest incidence in industrialized societies, and since its incidence appears to be increasing, Crohn's disease may be triggered by or be the result of some factor in the environment. Clearly, constitutional factors in Crohn's disease are also important: Whites develop the disease two to five times more frequently than nonwhites; the disease occurs two to three times more frequently in Jews than in non-Jews; incidence of inflammatory bowel disease (both ulcerative colitis and Crohn's disease) is greatly increased in relatives of patients. Thus, evidence is not available to determine the possible role of environmental agents in this disease complex.

Phosphorus Depletion Syndrome

Patients taking high doses (240–360 ml) of aluminum-containing antacids develop hypophosphatemia and hypophosphaturia. Increased intestinal absorption of calcium and hypercalciuria develop, probably secondary to increased 1,25-dihydroxyvitamin D production caused by hypophosphatemia. Weakness, anorexia, central nervous system dysfunction and debility represent a few of the complications of severe hypophosphatemia (17). 2,3-Diphosphoglyceric acid deficiency in erythrocytes cause a shift in the oxygen-dissociation curve of hemoglobin, resulting in decreased tissue oxygenation.

Neomycin-Induced Malabsorption

A wide variety of reversible defects in intestinal absorption of the following are produced by neomycin: fat, cholesterol, carotene, vitamin K, nitrogen, disaccharide, monosaccharide, vitamin B_{12}, iron. Two mechanisms are involved: (a) neomycin has a direct toxic effect on the mucosa; (b) neomycin is a cationic molecule and combines with anions such as fatty acid and bile salts. The latter effect disrupts micelles and leads to malabsorption of fat, fat-soluble vitamins, and cholesterol.

Large Intestine

Ulcerative Colitis

Ulcerative colitis was first distinguished from other diarrheal diseases in 1875, long before Crohn's disease was identified in 1932. Yet both are relatively new diseases and could be associated with environmental factors from industrialization.

Ulcerative colitis is being recognized with increasing frequency. Its geographic distribution was originally thought to be Europe and North America. The disease is now being diagnosed in South America and Central America, Japan, Thailand, India, and other far eastern countries. The extent to which this is the result of improved diagnostic facilities and of increased awareness rather than with the spread of industrial agents is unknown. Clearly, constitutional factors predispose to ulcerative colitis as discussed above for Crohn's disease. Ulcerative colitis is rare in unrelated members of the same household, ruling out the sole operation of an environmental factor. The most favored current hypothesis of genetic or immunologic etiology for ulcerative colitis does not even consider the role of environmental agents.

Antibiotic-Associated Colitis

Diarrhea is frequently associated with antibiotic treatment. When a pseudomembrane is identified by proctoscopy in the affected patient, the disease is an antibiotic-associated colitis. Although any antibiotic may produce the disease, the incidence is unusually high with lincomycin and clindamycin (19). Antibiotic treatment is clearly the initiating event, although many other factors, including the change in bacterial flora and superinfection by a pathogen, may supervene. Direct toxic action of the antibiotic may be a minor factor.

Cancer

A large number of epidemiological studies have demonstrated that environmental factors play a key role in determining incidence and site of cancer. These factors may be part of the "natural" environment or the result of the introduction of chemicals and drugs. Mutagens and carcinogens, both natural and introduced, are part of the daily diet. The most important cancer of the alimentary tract is cancer of the colon and rectum, and a large body of information has been accumulated regarding colon and rectal cancer as an environmental disease (54).

CONCLUSION

Environmental diseases of the gastrointestinal tract are matters of concern to all of us. Research needs in this area have been identified (52), and more questions are arising almost daily.

REFERENCES

1. Abdullah, M., Arnesjö, B., and Ihse, I. (1973): Methylation of mercury in intestinal diseases. *Scand. J. Gastroenterol.*, 8:565–567.
2. Bachur, N. R. (1976): Cytoplasmic aldo-keto reductases: a class of drug metabolizing enzymes. *Science*, 193:595–597.
3. Bajarnasen, I., Veale, N., and Peters, T. J. (1983): A simple clinical method for detecting alterations of intestinal permeability: demonstration of a persistent defect in celiac disease. *Clin. Sci.*, 64:74P.
4. Berg, M. J., Berlinger, W. G., Goldberg, M. J., Spector, R., and Johnson, G. F. (1982): Accel-

eration of the body clearance of phenobarbital by oral activated charcoal. *N. Engl. J. Med.*, 307:642–644.

5. Bergman, L., and Krause, U. (1975): The incidence of Crohn's disease in Central Sweden. *Scand. J. Gastroenterol.*, 10:725–729.

6. Brahme, F., Lindstrom, C., and Wenkert, A. (1975): Crohn's disease in a defined population. *Gastroenterology*, 69:342–351.

7. Bushnell, P. J., and DeLuca, H. F. (1981): Lactose facilitates the intestinal absorption of lead in weanling rats. *Science*, 211:61–63.

8. Caldwell, J. H., Caldwell, P. B., Murphy, J. W., and Beachler, C. W. (1980): Intestinal secretion of digoxin in the rat. Augmentation by feeding activated charcoal. *Nauyn Schmiedebergs Arch. Pharmacol.*, 312:271–275.

9. Caldwell, J. H., and Greenberger, N. J. (1971): Interruption of the enterohepatic circulation of digitoxin by cholestyramine. 1. Protection against lethal digitoxin intoxication. *J. Clin. Invest.*, 50:2626–2637.

10. Chrisp, C. E., Fisher, G. L., and Lammert, J. E. (1978): Mutagenicity of filtrates from respirable coal fly ash. *Science*, 199:73–75.

11. Cook, P. M., and Olson, G. F. (1979): Ingested mineral fibers: elimination in human urine.*Science*, 204:195–198.

12. Duggan, D. E., Hooke, K. F., Noll, R. M., and Chiu Kwan, K. (1975): Enterohepatic circulation of indomethacin and its role in intestinal irritation. *Biochem. Pharmacol.*, 24:1749–1754.

13. Ershoff, B. H. (1976): Protective effects of cholestyramine in rats fed low fiber diets containing toxic doses of sodium cyclamate and amaranth. *Proc. Soc. Exp. Biol. Med.*, 152:253–256.

14. Evans, J. G., and Acheson, E. D. (1965): An epidemiological study of ulcerative colitis and regional enteritis in the Oxford area. *Gut*, 6:311–324.

15. Faulk, D. L., Anuras, S., Gardner, G. D., Mitros, F. A., Summers, R. W., and Christensen, J. (1978): A familial visceral myopathy. *Ann. Intern. Med.*, 89:600–606.

16. Finegold, S. M. (1977): *Anaerobic Bacteria in Human Disease*, pp. 578–589. Academic Press, New York.

17. Fitzgerald, F. (1978): Clinical hypophosphatemia. *Annu. Rev. Med.*, 19:177–189.

18. Forbes, G. B., and Reina, J. C. (1972): Effect of age on gastrointestinal absorption (Fe, Sr, Pb) in the rat. *J. Nutr.*, 102:647–652.

19. Gibson, G. E., Rowland, R., and Hecker, R. (1975): Diarrhoea and colitis associated with antibiotic treatment. *Aust. N. Z. J. Med.*, 5:340–347.

20. Goldberg, M. J., and Berlinger, W. G. (1982): Treatment of phenobarbital overdose with activated charcoal. *JAMA*, 247:2400–2401.

21. Goldman, P., Peppercorn, M. A., and Goldin, B. R. (1974): Metabolism of drugs by microorganisms in the intestine. *Am. J. Clin. Nutr.*, 27:1348–1355.

22. Guzelian, P. S. (1982): Chlordecone poisoning: A case study in approaches for detoxification of humans exposed to environmental chemicals. *Drug Metab. Rev.*, 13:663–679.

23. Hartiala, K. (1973): Metabolism of hormones, drugs, and other substances by the gut. *Physiol. Rev.*, 53:496–534.

24. Hayes, A. W. (1979): Transport processes as sites of action of toxic chemicals. *Fed. Proc.*, 38:2218–2219.

25. Hietanen, E., Laitinen, M., Lang, M., and Vainio, H. (1975): Inducibility of mucosal drug-metabolizing enzymes of rats fed on a cholesterol-rich diet by polychlorinated biphenyl, 3-methylcholanthrene and phenobarbitone. *Pharmacology*, 13:287–296.

26. Hietanen, E., Laitinen, M., Vaino, H., and Hänninen, O. (1975): Dietary fats and properties of endoplasmic reticulum: II. Dietary lipid induced changes in activities of drug metabolizing enzymes in liver and duodenum of rat. *Lipids*, 10:467–472.

27. Hoensch, H., Woo, C. H., Raffin, S. B., and Schmid, R. (1976): Oxidative metabolism of foreign compounds in rat small intestine: Cellular localization and dependence of dietary iron. *Gastroenterology*, 70:1063–1070.

28. Hoensch, H. P., Hutt, R., and Hartmann, F. (1979): Biotransformation of xenobiotics in human intestinal mucosa. *Environ. Health Perspect.*, 33:71–78.

29. Hoj, L., Jensen, P., Bounerie, O., and Riis, P. (1973): An epidemiological study of regional enteritis and acute ileitis in Copenhagen county. *Scand. J. Gastroenterol.*, 8:381–384.

30. Kappas, A., Anderson, K. E., Conney, A. H., and Alvares, A. P. (1976): Influence of dietary

protein and carbohydrate on antipyrine and theophylline metabolism in man. *Clin. Pharm. Therap.*, 20:643–653.

31. Kinter, W. B., and Pritchard, J. B. (1977): Altered permeability of cell membranes. In: *Handbook of Physiology, Section 9: Reactions to Environmental Agents*, pp. 563–576. American Physiological Society, Washington, D.C.

32. Kritchevsky, D., and Story, J. A. (1974): Binding of bile salts by non-nutritive fiber. *J. Nutr.*, 104:458–462.

33. Kritchevsky, D. (1977): Modification by fiber of toxic dietary effects. *Fed. Proc.*, 36:1692–1695.

34. Kyle, J. (1971): An epidemiological study of Crohn's disease in northeast Scotland. *Gastroenterology*, 61:826–833.

35. Lakowicz, J. R., McNamara, M., and Steenson, L. (1978): Particle-mediated membrane uptake of chemical carcinogens studied by fluorescence spectroscopy. *Science*, 199:305–307.

36. Leichter, J., and Tolensky, A. F. (1975): Effect of dietary lactose on the absorption of protein, fat and calcium in the post-weaning rat. *Am. J. Clin. Nutr.*, 28:238–241.

37. Marselos, M., Dutton, G., and Hanninen, O. (1975): Evidence that D-glucaro-1,4-lactone shortens the pharmacological action of drugs being disposed via the bile as glucuronides. *Biochem. Pharmacol.*, 24:1855–1858.

38. Miller, D. S., Peakall, D. B., and Kinter, W. B. (1978): Ingestion of crude oil: Sublethal effects in herring gull chicks. *Science*, 199:315–317.

39. Monk, M., Mendeloff, A., Siegel, C., and Lilienfeld, A. (1967): An epidemiological study of ulcerative colitis and regional enteritis among adults in Baltimore. I. Hospital incidence and prevalence, 1960 to 1963. *Gastroenterology*, 53:198–210.

40. Monk, M., Mendeloff, A., Siegel, C., and Lilienfeld, A. (1969): An epidemiological study of ulcerative colitis and regional enteritis among adults in Baltimore. II. Social and demographic factors. *Gastroenterology*, 56:847–857.

41. Parker, C. W. (1977): Immune responses to environmental antigens absorbed through the gastrointestinal tract. *Fed. Proc.*, 36:1732–1735.

42. Pantuck, E. J., Hsiao, K. C., Kuntzman, R., and Conney, A. H. (1975): Intestinal metabolism of phenacetin in the rat: Effect of charcoal-broiled beef and rat chow. *Science*, 187:744–746.

43. Pantuck, E. J., Hsiao, K. C., Conney, A. H., Garland, W. A., Kappas, A., Anderson, K. E., and Alvares, A. P. (1976): Effect of charcoal-broiled beef on phenacetin metabolism in man. *Science*, 194:1055–1057.

44. Pond, S., Jacobs, M., Marks, J., Garner, J., Goldschlager, N., Hansen, D. (1981): Treatment of digitoxin overdose with oral activated charcoal. *Lancet*, 2:1177–1178.

45. Pond, W. G., and Walker, E. F. (1975): Effect of dietary Ca and Cd level of pregnant rats on reproduction and on dam and progeny tissue mineral concentrations. *Proc. Soc. Exp. Biol. Med.*, 148:665–668.

46. Pontefract, R. D., and Cunningham, H. M. (1973): Penetration of asbestos through the digestive tract of rats. *Nature*, 243:352–353.

47. Pritchard, J. B. (1979): Toxic substances and cell membrane function. *Fed. Proc.*, 38:2220–2225.

48. Reinhold, J. B., Faradji, B., and Adabi, P. (1976): Decreased absorption of calcium, magnesium, zinc, and phosphorus by humans due to increased fiber and phosphorus consumption as wheat bread. *J. Nutr.*, 106:493–503.

49. Richter, E., and Schäfer, S. G. (1981): Intestinal excretion of hexachlorobenzene. *Arch. Toxicol.*, 47:233–239.

50. Rogan, W. J., Bagriewska, A., and Damstra, T. (1980): Pollutants in breast milk. *N. Engl. J. Med.*, 302:1450–1453.

51. Schedl, H. P. (1974): Water and electrolyte transport: Clinical aspects. *Med. Clin. North Am.*, 58:1429–1448.

52. Schedl, H. P. (1977): Gastrointestinal tract. In: *Human Health and the Environment—Some Research Needs: Report of the Second Task Force for Research Planning in Environmental Health Science*, pp. 373–377. U.S. Department of Health, Education, and Welfare, National Institute of Environmental Health Sciences, DHEW Publication No. NIH 77-1277.

53. Schedl, H. P. (1977): Environmental factors and the development of disease and injury in the alimentary tract. *Environ. Health Perspect.*, 20:39–54.

54. Schedl, H. P. (1979): Intestinal disease in the urban environment. *Environ. Health Perspect.*, 33:115–126.

55. Schedl, H. P., and Clifton, J. A. (1962): Polyvinylpyrrolidone-I[131] as an indicator of net intestinal water flux: Its binding by intestinal mucus. *Proc. Soc. Exp. Biol. Med.*, 110:381–384.
56. Schuffler, M. D., Lowe, M. C., and Bill, A. H. (1977): Studies of idiopathic intestinal pseudoobstruction. I. Hereditary hollow visceral myopathy: clinical and pathological studies. *Gastroenterology*, 73:327–338.
57. Six, K. M., and Goyer, R. A. (1970): Experimental enforcement of lead toxicity by low dietary calcium. *J. Lab. Clin. Med.*, 76:933–942.
58. Trowell, H. (1976): Definition of dietary fiber and hypotheses that it is a protective factor in certain diseases. *Am. J. Clin. Nutr.*, 29:417–427.
59. Vesell, E. S. (1975): Pharmacogenetics—the individual factor in drug response. *Triangle*, 14:125–130.
60. Volkheimer, G., and Schulz, F. H. (1968): The phenomenon of persorption. *Digestion*, 1:213–218.
61. Von Lauterbach, F. (1975): Resorption und sekretion von arzneistoffen durch die mukosaepithelien des gastroinestinaltraktes. *Arzneimittelforsch.*, 25:479–488.
62. Washko, P. W., and Cousins, R. J. (1977): Role of dietary calcium and calcium binding protein in cadmium toxicity in rats. *J. Nutr.*, 107:920–928.
63. Ziegler, E. E., Edwards, B. B., Jensen, R. L., Mahaffey, K. R., and Fomon, S. J. (1978): Absorption and retention of lead by infants. *Pediatr. Res.*, 12:29–34.

Intestinal Toxicology, edited by C. M. Schiller.
Raven Press, New York © 1984.

Summary and Conclusions

Carol M. Schiller

*Laboratory of Pharmacology, National Institute of Environmental Health Sciences,
Research Triangle Park, North Carolina 27709*

Considerable progress has been made in relating to the intestines as a primary organ. This primacy reflects concern for the intestines as an essential metabolic organ for the homeostasis of the entire organism. Both development and differentiation of the intestines have been a growing focus for researchers with interests in nutrition, transport, immunology, and metabolism. More than ever, studies indicate the importance of the intestines as a port of entry for nutrients and other dietary essentials as well as a significant target for possible deleterious effects of natural and man-made toxins that are present in our food chain and water supplies.

Absorption of nutrients and pharmaceuticals by the intestines has been the traditional focus of gastrointestinal studies. Now, various animal model systems and *in vitro* techniques are being used to examine other aspects of intestinal function/dysfunction. Although the rapid differentiation and turnover of the intestinal epithelium may provide a challenge to the gastroenterologists in terms of experimental design and limitation, these processes also allow for a fertile basis of study unlike any other mammalian cell. This uniqueness of the intestinal epithelium is intertwined with the relatively limited understanding of many basic intestinal processes and of how many intestinal toxins act. The tissue specificity (independent of route of administration) of some toxins, e.g., 1,2-dimethylhydrazine, provides an unending challenge for the determined investigator.

The future offers an opportunity to examine the emerging role of the intestines as a key target organ. The potential interactions between ingested chemicals (natural and man-made) and the intestinal microflora within the unique milieu of the intestinal mucosal surface are staggering. As the recognition of intestinal disease as a major medical concern increases, there will be an even greater demand for basic information about the intestines and about the unique responses of the intestines to toxic insults.

Subject Index

Subject Index

233